AF757354

Guided Internet-Based Treatments in Psychiatry

Nils Lindefors • Gerhard Andersson
Editors

Guided Internet-Based Treatments in Psychiatry

Springer

Editors
Nils Lindefors
Stockholm
Sweden

Gerhard Andersson
Linköping
Sweden

ISBN 978-3-319-06082-8 ISBN 978-3-319-06083-5 (eBook)
DOI 10.1007/978-3-319-06083-5

Library of Congress Control Number: 2015960761

Springer Cham Heidelberg New York Dordrecht London
© Springer International Publishing Switzerland 2016
This work is subject to copyright. All rights are reserved by the Publisher, whether the whole or part of the material is concerned, specifically the rights of translation, reprinting, reuse of illustrations, recitation, broadcasting, reproduction on microfilms or in any other physical way, and transmission or information storage and retrieval, electronic adaptation, computer software, or by similar or dissimilar methodology now known or hereafter developed.
The use of general descriptive names, registered names, trademarks, service marks, etc. in this publication does not imply, even in the absence of a specific statement, that such names are exempt from the relevant protective laws and regulations and therefore free for general use.
The publisher, the authors and the editors are safe to assume that the advice and information in this book are believed to be true and accurate at the date of publication. Neither the publisher nor the authors or the editors give a warranty, express or implied, with respect to the material contained herein or for any errors or omissions that may have been made.

Printed on acid-free paper

Springer International Publishing AG Switzerland is part of Springer Science+Business Media (www.springer.com)

Preface

Many psychiatric disorders entail symptoms and problems treatable with cognitive behaviour therapy (CBT). Research in this field is extensive and expanding and evidence for significant reduction of burden of disease following CBT is ample. Treatment guidelines in many countries recommend CBT as a first-line treatment for, for example, major depression and anxiety disorders. However, most if not all countries suffer from a worldwide troublesome shortage in the number of trained CBT therapists. Although we know from extensive evidence that CBT is cost-effective and well received in clinical psychiatry, patients are often recommended other means of treatment when asking for CBT due to this problematic shortage in therapists. To assist the development of disseminated CBT with quality-assured means, this book present methods and discuss related issues for Internet-based CBT (ICBT). The focus is on therapist-guided ICBT.

ICBT is a novel contribution to modern health care in the domain of eHealth. According to the World Health Organization (WHO), eHealth is the use of information and communication technologies (ICT) for health. Possible domains for eHealth development suggested by WHO include treating patients, conducting research, educating the health workforce, tracking diseases and monitoring public health. In line with this, we conclude that ICBT provides an important promising relatively new contribution to global eHealth and ICBT should be tested further in large-scale international trials.

ICBT may provide a direct safe electronic supply chain for information and communication between therapist and patient. ICBT is less resource demanding than conventional face-to-face interventions, without compromising treatment effectiveness. Furthermore, ICBT add a sustainable treatment option as it reduces the patients' need for transport to health centres or clinics for therapist interaction. This will most probably reduce the carbon dioxide emission accompanying the treatment

We suggest that the global burden of disease due to psychiatric disorders treatable with CBT imply such a movement. In addition and to support dissemination, cost-effectiveness data are urgent to release funding for large-scale development for IT platforms needed for further methods development and an opportunity for widespread dissemination of ICBT.

Published scientific findings and extensive clinical experiences presented and discussed in this book suggest that ICBT provides means for flexible dissemination of CBT, where each therapist may guide more individuals through treatment compared to in clinical live CBT. In addition, new hand-held devices and the development of other means and gadgets that may assist the individual through the ICBT will most probably further reduce dependence of professional therapists and to allow real-life monitoring and thus enable the limited number of therapists to focus on those not eligible for ICBT.

The health-care sector consists of a significant part of the gross national products (GNP) in most countries, and due to the development of new and often expensive methods and materials, the cost of health care is increasing fast. The demand for clinically effective, cost-effective and value-based methods in general is thus urgent. Methods to systematically collect measures of patient outcome and other important markers for delivered patient value by treatments are largely missing in clinical practice. In psychiatry, this demand is displayed by lack of well-defined and standardised diagnostic procedures, value-based outcome measures and shortage of reliable tools to monitor side effects and safety issues in disorders treatments.

This book is compiled of chapters with world-leading ICBT researchers and clinicians selected for their specific expertise. The scope to provide extensive evidence-based ICBT programmes for psychiatry cannot be fulfilled completely due to limited evidence, but due to the relative novelty of ICBT, we think that the evidence for effectiveness of this treatment format in clinical psychiatry is very promising and demands further development.

We thank Springer for giving us the opportunity to edit this book and to our families for their support during the process. Finally, we thank our co-workers in the field of ICBT and the many patients who have contributed to the research.

Stockholm, Sweden Nils Lindefors
September 2015 Gerhard Andersson

Contents

History and Current Status of ICBT

1

Gerhard Andersson, Per Carlbring, and Nils Lindefors

Abstract

We begin this chapter with a discussion of the history of ICBT and its roots in bibliotherapy and computerised CBT. We then provide a brief description of one way of administering guided ICBT, including the role of the therapist and data security issues. This description is followed by examples of conditions that are not covered later in the book, such as specific phobias and addictions. We end this chapter with a discussion of technical developments, cost-effectiveness and implementation.

Cognitive Behaviour Therapy (CBT)

In order to uncover the origin of Internet-based cognitive behaviour therapy (ICBT), it is important to acknowledge the different strands in the literature. One source of differentiation is choice of treatment format. There are two treatment formats of particular importance. The first is cognitive behaviour therapy (CBT), which is the most well researched form of psychotherapy. CBT is also increasingly used in

G. Andersson, PhD (✉)
Department of Behavioural Sciences and Learning, Linköping University, Linköping SE 581 83, Sweden

Department of Clinical Neuroscience, Karolinska Institutet, Stockholm, Sweden
e-mail: Gerhard.andersson@liu.se

P. Carlbring, PhD
Department of Psychology, Stockholm University, Stockholm, Sweden
e-mail: per.carlbring@psychology.su.se

N. Lindefors, MD, PhD
Division of Psychiatry, Department of Clinical Neuroscience, Karolinska Institutet, Stockholm, Sweden
e-mail: nils.lindefors@ki.se

© Springer International Publishing Switzerland 2016

N. Lindefors, G. Andersson (eds.), *Guided Internet-Based Treatments in Psychiatry*, DOI 10.1007/978-3-319-06083-5_1

health care, particularly for the treatment of mild to moderate psychiatric conditions (Andersson et al. 2005a). Arguably the most evidence-based psychological treatment, CBT is now disseminated on a wide scale in countries like the United Kingdom (Layard and Clark 2014). It is beyond the scope of this book to discuss CBT in detail, but we can outline a few of its key characteristics. The first step in CBT is a case conceptualisation, which can be more or less behavioural in its orientation. The next step is typically to present a treatment rationale to the patient. The subsequent treatment steps may vary depending on the agreed-upon treatment goals, but behaviour problems (too much or too little) and irrational beliefs are common targets, so specific treatment techniques have been developed to address them (Westbrook et al. 2011). These specific treatment techniques include behavioural activation in the treatment of depression and exposure when treating anxiety and avoidance. These techniques are framed using a rationale based on a cognitive and/or a behavioural conceptualisation. CBT is often focused on problems "here and now", and recipients of CBT are instructed to practise techniques both during sessions and between sessions in the form of homework. The duration of the treatments may vary, but time constraints typically limit treatment to 10–20 weeks. However, there are examples of shorter treatments (like one-session treatments of specific phobia) and longer treatments (like dialectical behaviour therapy for borderline personality disorder, in which the first phase alone can last a year). Finally, relapse prevention and follow-up sessions may be included as well by the end of the treatment. While that concludes our overview of the execution of CBT, there are many more CBT techniques and procedures that we did not discuss, such as relaxation techniques, mindfulness, response prevention and specific cognitive techniques like Socratic questioning (this is sometimes, but not always regarded as a CBT technique). The key to CBT's success is likely the fact that treatments are adjusted according to the problem at hand (Barlow 2004). Thus, CBT for chronic pain will differ from CBT for something else, such as post-traumatic stress disorder (PTSD), even if there is some overlap. Another factor that uniquely characterises CBT is the way it is delivered. Whereas standard psychotherapy is typically done in the form of individual face-to-face treatment, CBT has been conducted in many different forms, such as group, family and couple therapy. CBT has even been done in a large lecture format. However, most noteworthy to us is the vast literature on CBT as self-help (Watkins 2008).

CBT as Guided Self-Help

CBT has been the topic of self-help research for a long time, which is often referred to as bibliotherapy (not to be confused with self-help groups led by patients themselves that are unrelated to CBT). Particularly, guided self-help using text material (mostly books) has been studied in controlled trials, with results showing moderate to large effects for a range of psychiatric and somatic conditions (Watkins and Clum 2008). Although ICBT was not developed until later, ICBT programmes are influenced by or even identical to the information presented in these evidence-based self-help books. There is a confusion in the literature because early bibliotherapy studies are sometimes collapsed with ICBT studies in reviews (Cuijpers et al. 2010). It is possible that guided bibliotherapy and guided ICBT are about as equally effective when therapist guidance is involved. For example, while two of the authors of the present chapter were treating social anxiety disorder (SAD), they found no difference between the two formats when the same text was used as either a book or as part of an online programme (Furmark et al. 2009). However, ICBT and bibliotherapy are not identical because while undergoing ICBT, a patient will be required to complete at least some tasks using the online programme and/or while interacting with a therapist using modern information technology (Marks et al. 2007).

Computerised Treatments

Another important field with a close affiliation to the ICBT community is the field of computerised psychological treatments and programmes (Marks et al. 1998). Many of these treatments and programmes were developed before the Internet. *Beating the blues*, a programme for mild to moderate depression (Proudfoot et al. 2004), was recommended by the National Institute for Health and Clinical Excellence (NICE) in 2006 after several controlled trials (Marks et al. 2007). Just like bibliotherapy and ICBT, computerised CBT (sometimes referred to as CCBT often delivered on a CD-ROM) and ICBT share many similarities. The main differences are the platform needed to deliver the programme (any computer vs. a computer with Internet connection) and the way support is provided (by phone vs. by Internet/e-mail). Apart from these differences, computerised CBT and ICBT programmes can appear identical. However, literature on computerised assessments points to another slight difference between computerized CBT and ICBT (Epstein and Klinkenberg 2001): ICBT assessments are often online (such as online questionnaires), whereas, computerized CBT assessments are given offline.

There are two additional promising roles for computers in CBT. The first is through virtual reality treatment, which research has shown to be effective in exposure therapy (Côté and Bouchard 2008). Virtual reality treatment could also be integrated with ICBT, which would reduce equipment costs. This is a rapidly changing field with ongoing research on augmented reality (Baus and Bouchard 2014), and applications for conditions other than phobias and serious gaming are in the process of development (Mohr et al. 2013). The second use for computers in CBT is cognitive bias modification, which is a treatment format based on laboratory research done on various forms of selective information processing. This treatment is markedly different from regular CBT and ICBT. For example, instead of reading text and doing homework assignments to learn to avoid getting fixated on negative faces, one could do regular exercises in front of the computer (Amir et al. 2009). In most studies, these interventions were delivered in the laboratory, but in a series of studies with largely negative findings, attention training was delivered through the Internet (Carlbring et al. 2012). This is a scattered field with mixed findings, and a recent meta-analysis indicates that the effect sizes are small (Cristea et al. 2015). Some research shows that patients may benefit from attention training alone (Kuckertz et al. 2014) or as an adjunct to ICBT (Williams et al. 2013), but there are also findings that suggest there are no significant benefits of attention training (Boettcher et al. 2014a). These conflicting findings indicate that this is a field in need of more research (Boettcher et al. 2013).

In sum, computers have been used in various ways to deliver psychological treatments. According to Marks et al. (2007), computer-aided psychotherapy "refers to any computing system that aids talking treatments by using patient input to make at least some computations and treatment decisions" (Marks et al. 2007, p. 6). ICBT partly fits this description, although the focus is more on the mode of delivery than the actual use of automated decisions. In this book, we focus on ICBT, but we are aware of the blurred distinctions between ICBT and other fields. Therefore, we acknowledge the existence and contributions of related fields such as virtual reality treatment and face-to-face treatment using web cameras (Storch et al. 2011).

ICBT Begins

This leads us to the topic of this book – ICBT. The terminology is far from consistent, and various names are used and have previously been used both interchangeably to describe the same online treatments and as separate terms to describe differing treatments (Barak 2013). For example, not even the term "Internet" is used consistently to refer to Internet-based interventions. A few alternative terms are "web based", "online therapy", "computerized psychotherapy", "digital interventions", "e-therapy", "telepsychiatry", "cybertherapy", "robot-based psychotherapy", "Internet interventions" and "CCBT". This is of course problematic when reviewing the literature, and the often very short descriptions of the interventions do not help to clarify. Here we will use the term ICBT, by which we mean an intervention that is mainly delivered using the Internet and modern information technology (e.g. accessed via different platforms) and that is based on cognitive behaviour therapy. Most of the studies and applications covered in the book will be therapist guided, but automated ICBT is mentioned.

The question of how it all began depends on who tells the story. Our presentation here is inevitably coloured by our own history, and the fact that as researchers, we based our findings on peer-reviewed publications. We acknowledge that it is possible that some clinicians have been using the treatment practices discussed in the research, but have not published any documentation (as is the case with clinicians using telecommunication software such as Skype in therapy). In research, there is also often a long lag between starting a project and finally getting the research published, which can take years. Because we know that early on multiple CBT researchers began to comment on the potential uses of the Internet (Riley and Veale 1999), it is likely that several research groups had more or less the same idea at about the same time. Researchers in Australia were early, with MoodGYM's research on depressive symptoms (Christensen and Griffiths 2002) and the late Jeff Richards' research on anxiety disorders (Klein and Richards 2001). Other early research took place in the Netherlands, such as research on Interapy treatment (Lange et al. 2000). These researchers began their work in the mid- to late 1990s, as did researchers in the United States such as Lee Ritterband et al. (2003). In Sweden, we were fairly early as well, with the first project starting in 1998, which subsequently lead to the first controlled trial on the treatment of headaches using the Internet (Ström et al. 2000). This was followed by a long line of research projects, but it is worth mentioning here the early work on tinnitus (ringing in the ears) that was rapidly implemented in regular health care at the audiology department in Uppsala, Sweden, by the turn of the century. This was followed by a controlled trial (Andersson et al. 2002), and the effectiveness data was published soon after (Kaldo-Sandström et al. 2004). This is probably one of the earliest implementations of ICBT in regular health care, and the treatment is still being used as a standard healthcare practice (Kaldo et al. 2013).

Early work in Sweden was also done on psychiatric conditions, beginning with panic disorder (Carlbring et al. 2001) and depression (Andersson et al. 2005b). This leads to a collaboration between clinical psychiatry and academic psychology (hence the three of us writing this chapter together), which subsequently resulted in a clinical implementation at the Stockholm health care services in Sweden known as the Internet Psychiatry Unit (internetpsychiatry.se). This work began as projects during 2002, and subsequently in 2007, the unit was opened for public use in regular health care in the Stockholm county region. There were several other implementations at about the same time in other countries around the world, but the implementation varied according to the country's healthcare system. There are distinct differences among tax-funded healthcare systems in countries like the Netherlands, centralised units in Australia and general practices in the United Kingdom like IAPT (increasing access to psychological therapies). In general practice systems such as that of the United Kingdom, the implementation of ICBT lagged behind the research activities.

On the subject of research activities, it is remarkable that so many controlled trials have been conducted over a fairly short period of about 15 years (Andersson 2014). The number of controlled trials on ICBT for a range of conditions has greatly surpassed many other related fields, such as virtual reality, possibly bibliotherapy and some forms of psychotherapy that have been around for much longer. We suggest three reasons why ICBT has been possible to study in more than 100 controlled trials (Hedman et al. 2012). First, many time-consuming routine tasks in research, such as entering data from questionnaires, are not needed in ICBT research. Second, recruitment is publicised through advertisements (in both social media and regular newspapers). Interested participants then enter the screening phase and then are finally interviewed by a clinician. Third, in contrast to many high-quality CBT trials, a vast majority of ICBT trials in Sweden have been done using psychologist student therapists with little training apart from their basic CBT training. Interestingly, and to our initial surprise, as feedback from the guided ICBT trials, ICBT appears to benefit participants as much as face-to-face CBT.

ISRII and ESRII

One of us, along with help from the other two authors and a PhD student, initiated the formation of an organisation devoted to ICBT. Andersson and Lindefors invited researchers for an initial informal meeting on "Internet and CBT" in 2004 at the Karolinska University Hospital in Stockholm. During the meeting, a decision was made to form an association named the *International Society for Research on Internet Interventions* (ISRII) (see www.isrii.org). The next meeting was held in 2006 at a somewhat less fashionable hospital setting, but more people attended compared to the first meeting and it became clear that this new field was advancing rapidly, with many new trials completed just 2 years after the first meeting (Ritterband et al. 2006). Following Per Carlbring who handled a mailing list, Lee Ritterband assumed the role of managing the second mailing list and first website. The third meeting of ISRII was later held at the University of Virginia in Charlottesville, Virginia, USA, in 2007. By that time, the organisation was very active with increasing number of people on the mailing list. The fourth ISRII meeting was in Amsterdam, Netherlands, and was combined with a national meeting, but many ISRII members attended and presented separately for the ISRII community. The Amsterdam meetings were hosted by the Netherlands Institute of Mental Health and Addiction Trimbos instituut, the Vrije Universiteit of Amsterdam and the University of, in 2009. The following meeting was in Sydney, Australia, in 2011, hosted by the Australian National University. More people, over 160, attended the meetings during those warm days in Australia. It was then time to return to the United States, where the sixth meeting was held in Chicago in 2013 with more than 260 people in attendance. The most recent meeting was in 2014 in Europe, this time in Valencia, Spain, and almost 300 delegates came. The steadily increasing number of ISRII members corresponds nicely to organisation's goal of bringing together researchers in the field of Internet interventions and other interested parties. There are now national associations for Internet intervention research and development. Additionally, there is the *European Society for Research on Internet Interventions* (ESRII; www.esrii.org), which has had three meetings already, beginning with one in Lüneburg, Germany, in 2012, followed by another meeting in Linköping, Sweden, in 2013, and the most recent meeting in Warsaw, Poland, in 2015.

The ISRII and the ESRII developed a scientific journal called *Internet Interventions*. Andersson is the editor-in-chief and Carlbring, Helen Riper and Nick Titov are the associate editors. The journal was launched in 2014 and is now in its second year of publication. The journal has already and will continue to publish high-quality and innovative new studies including consensus statements.

In sum, ICBT is a steadily advancing field that already includes two international associations and one scientific journal. Additionally, studies on ICBT are frequently presented at conferences in psychiatry and clinical psychology, and most major journals in those fields publish ICBT studies as well. The materialisation of implementation from innovation likely would have been longer without the ISRII and the ESRII and the scientific publications.

How ICBT Can Be Done

In each of the following chapters, different conditions, programmes and outcome studies will be presented. We will not assume that all readers are familiar with ICBT, so we will now present a brief overview on how clinician-guided ICBT can be conducted. Several texts are available for a more detailed description (Andersson 2014), but the basic parts will be outlined here.

The first thing needed for ICBT is a stable and secure electronic treatment platform. The treatment platform is where the treatment is presented online using an Internet-connected device, where direct communication between a patient and the clinician takes place, and often as well as where assessments are given. Even if there are different technical solutions and regulations regarding data security issues (Bennett et al. 2010), most contemporary systems will require a secure login and often resemble Internet bank systems, e.g. used to pay online bills. In other words, systems are encrypted and often use a double authentication procedure at login. For example, a patient may need to first use a password to log in, and then a separate number via a card reader or a text message sent to their personal mobile phone (2015). For the future, we would expect that safer and more reliable systems will increase information integrity and improve user friendliness with smart individual authentication in the individual's personal Internet device.

Most ICBT systems have questionnaire data capacities embedded in the systems. This is a separate but related topic and there are numerous studies on the psychometric properties of online administered questionnaires. Here it suffices to say that online data collection is often both efficient and reliable, but that it may be best to use the same format consistently rather than switching between online and paper-and-pencil administration (Carlbring et al. 2007).

The second necessary component of ICBT is a proper treatment programme. In almost all programmes, the main format of delivery has been text, usually in the form of book-length text materials (Andersson et al. 2008). Programmes tend to be based on face-to-face manuals and self-help books, but streamed videos and audio files are increasingly included. With high-speed Internet access, it has also been easier to use interactive programmes and even virtual reality components. Modern smartphone applications (apps) are also increasingly integrated into ICBT. The duration of the treatments mirror face-to-face CBT. For example, 10 weeks is the treatment time required for panic disorder both in face-to-face CBT and ICBT (Carlbring et al. 2006). However, ICBT programmes are sometimes shorter in research, and there are examples of programmes that have been extended in time when implemented into regular health care (El Alaoui et al. 2015). In the remaining chapters of this book, more information will be provided on the actual components included for the particular mental illness (e.g. major depression), but here we can note that clinician-guided ICBT includes homework assignments, followed by feedback and encouragement on the assignments delivered through the securely closed platform. In addition to feedback, the clinician can answer questions on the programme, but most correspondence usually takes the form of support and advice on how to complete the assignments and progress through the treatment (Andersson 2014).

There are conflicting results on the third aspect of guided ICBT, clinician guidance. Several systematic reviews have found that guidance reduces dropout and probably increase the effects (Baumeister et al. 2014), but it is possible that the need for a therapist differs depending on the conditions. It may also be true that access to a clinician when the patient asks for it and automated reminders are enough for some patients (Titov et al. 2013). However, some studies clearly support the superiority of clinician guidance (Kleiboer et al. 2015). Additionally, although it is not trivial how the correspondence with the patient is handled, it is probably the case that for a vast majority of patients it does not really matter who the person is giving them guidance (Almlöv et al. 2011; Almlöv et al. 2009). Moreover, the support can be mainly technical and practical in nature and does not need to be psychotherapeutically oriented (Titov et al. 2010). On the other hand, there may be therapist behaviours that are especially helpful for some patient groups, like a forgiving attitude towards non-completion of homework in the treatment of generalised anxiety disorder (Paxling et al. 2013).

A Few Words on Ethics and Negative Outcomes

As with any treatment for psychiatric disorders and in health care in general, ICBT raises questions regarding ethics and possible side effects. Although there are general aspects to consider such as human rights and the principle of doing no harm, there are also some considerations that are unique to ICBT. For example, whether it is acceptable to provide psychological treatment from a distance using the Internet may differ between countries like Sweden and Norway. In the United States, regulations may vary depending on which state the practitioner resides in. There is an emerging albeit small literature on the ethical aspects of ICBT (Dever Fitzgerald et al. 2010). The current consensus is that ICBT should be subject to the same ethical regulations as face-to-face therapy, but there are some additional aspects to consider in ICBT such as data protection/security, clinician responsibility, the possibility of anonymous treatment, etc.

One important aspect of ICBT is the possibility that adverse events will follow the intervention and that there is a clear link between those events/symptoms and the treatment. The literature on this topic is growing and recommendations to report negative outcomes in trials have been published (Rozental et al. 2014). There are also empirical studies on the topic. Data from four large clinical trials (total $N = 558$) revealed that 9.3 % of patients reported some type of negative effects (Rozental et al. 2015a). Another study from the same group reported that 14 % experienced negative effects in a trial on social anxiety disorder (SAD). These "negative effects" were defined as unwanted negative events that the patients related to the treatment (Boettcher et al. 2014b). Even though severely negative outcomes following ICBT are fairly uncommon, they should be reported, which has been the case in recent studies.

Conditions Not Covered in this Book

In this book most, but not all, psychiatric conditions for which ICBT has been developed are included. Here we will discuss some of the conditions that have been researched using controlled studies, as well as comment on the large literature on somatic conditions and studies on subclinical problems like perfectionism.

There are a few studies that have focused on guided ICBT for the treatment of specific phobias (Andersson 2014) and some studies that do not focus on, but include, patients with specific phobias, such as research done on the Internet version of the programme FearFighter (Schneider et al. 2005). Another example is a fairly large (N=212) recent trial done in the Netherlands. There was a high rate of attrition, and the results of the trial showed a small effect (I am not 100 % sure this is what you mean by "small effects"), which is noteworthy because these results differ from those of many other trials in the field (Kok et al. 2014). This study did not only include specific phobia patients; other patients were included as well. To our knowledge, only two controlled trials exclusively done on adults with specific phobias exist. These two small studies from Sweden compared live one-session exposure to guided ICBT (Andersson et al. 2009, 2013). In the first trial, 30 participants with spider phobias were included, and the results showed that both the one-session treatment and the ICBT condition were effective, but the one-session live treatment condition participants did better on a behavioural approach test (BAT). Following treatment, evaluation revealed that 46.2 % of the ICBT group and 85.7 % of the live-exposure group achieved clinically significant improvement. In the second trial (Andersson et al. 2013), 30 participants with snake phobias were included. Results were similar with no difference in self-reported outcomes, but again there was a difference in BAT scores. The post-treatment evaluation revealed that 61.5 % of the ICBT group and 84.6 % of the one-session group achieved a clinically significant improvement. In a Cochrane review on guided ICBT for anxiety disorder, only one trial could be included (Olthuis et al. 2015), and the 2009 trial from Sweden was selected. One uncontrolled trial on guided ICBT for children with specific phobias has also been published (Vigerland et al. 2013) and will be covered in a separate chapter in this book. Thus, there are only a few small studies on guided ICBT for the treatment of specific phobias, so there is a need for larger replications of the Swedish findings. It is possible that online versions of virtual reality treatments or augmented reality using smartphones will be the next step, rather than the self-guided exposure treatment that has been the focus of the previous ICBT trials on specific phobias.

In this book, we did not include chapters specifically on drug/alcohol addictions or pathological gambling, which are both potential fields for ICBT. There has only been one controlled trial done on ICBT for pathological gambling. This study tested the effects of an 8-week treatment (Carlbring and Smit 2008). The study included 66 pathological gamblers who did not suffer from severe co-morbid depression. Results showed favourable outcomes in pathological gambling, anxiety, depression and quality of life, with a large average between-group effect size when compared to the waiting list control group (Cohen's $d=0.83$). Importantly, follow-up results at 6, 18 and 36 months post-treatment showed that the results were stable. However, it is important to note that this group demanded a lot of attention and guidance. A larger open study on this programme has also been published (Carlbring et al. 2011). This way of treating gamblers has later been implemented in Finland (Castren et al. 2013). There is a fairly large body of literature on Internet treatment for drug addictions, but there has only been a small amount of research done on using guided ICBT to treat addiction issues such as problematic alcohol and cannabis use (Tait et al. 2013; Riper et al. 2011). In a recent meta-analysis on studies using guided treatments, only 4 out of 16 trials involved therapist guidance and there was no difference in effect (overall small effects). Only two studies provided direct comparisons between guided and unguided interventions, and in these two studies, there was a small difference in favour of guided interventions (Blankers et al. 2011; Doumas and Hannah 2008). We believe there is room for improvement and that more trials on guided ICBT, perhaps considering treatment of co-morbid psychiatric conditions (i.e. tailored treatment)) could be feasible.

Guided ICBT interventions have been developed and tested for a range of somatic conditions that are commonly co-morbid with anxiety and depression, such as chronic pain, headache, tinnitus, irritable bowel syndrome, diabetes, cancer, erectile dysfunction, multiple sclerosis and a growing number of other health problems beyond the scope of this chapter and book. However, insomnia is covered in a chapter of this book. There is also evidence in favour of evidence favouring guided ICBT for several other health-related problems, including stress (Andersson 2014). Researchers are increasingly focusing on specific target groups, such as people with diabetes and depressive symptoms (van Bastelaar et al. 2011) and teachers with depressive symptoms (Ebert et al. 2014).

Another fairly recent notion is the idea of developing programmes for non-clinical conditions. There are already studies on perfectionism (Arpin-Cribbie et al. 2012), infertility distress (Haemmerli et al. 2010) and procrastination (Rozental et al. 2015b), and the number of target problems being studied is continually increasing. For example, at Linköping University, Sweden, a project focuses on Internet treatment of interpersonal violence.

Discussion and Future Directions

In this chapter, we focused on our view of the history of ICBT. There are several future challenges and some additional aspects that we want to comment on. The first has to do with technology. ICBT is now not only delivered via computers, but also through modern mobile phones (smartphones), which are used either as stand-alone treatments or as complements to other platforms. Indeed, the platforms from which a patient can access a treatment are increasingly more varied, not only in appearance but also in terms of functionality. For example, smartphones can be used to collect other forms of data relevant to the study, such as heart rate. Additionally, smartphones can be used to track treatment progress and monitor activity completion. As previously mentioned, virtual reality and augmented reality may become more common as costs now are reduced and the techniques are more mobile. While the focus and expertise of this book are not on serious games (Mohr et al. 2013), we would like to comment that programmes like Sparx (Merry et al. 2012), if delivered online, could be a more modern and potentially more interesting way to present ICBT to young people.

In the following chapters, the issue of the cost-effectiveness of the interventions will be raised. This is important because it was assumed early on that ICBT should be cost-effective because it involves less therapist time (Ström et al. 2000). But from a societal perspective that might not be true even if it is likely if guided ICBT is as effective as face-to-face CBT. To investigate the question, costs pertaining not only to intervention costs but also to the costs of sick leave and other indirect costs needs to be considered (Drummond et al. 2005). Indeed, in a recent systematic review of cost-effectiveness studies on ICBT, the authors found that 9/16 papers endorsed a societal perspective (Donker et al. 2015). The authors found that for several conditions (e.g. anxiety and depression), guided ICBT was likely to be cost-effective when compared against control conditions. It appeared to be the case that unguided ICBT was less cost-effective than guided ICBT (in the case of cost-utility analyses), but the authors were careful to mention that there is a need for more high-quality cost-effectiveness studies. Here we conclude that in the history of ICBT, cost-effectiveness has always been regarded as important.

The third topic to discuss is the dissemination of ICBT into regular clinical settings. We mention effectiveness studies (a term for studies that are more representative of ordinary clinical conditions) in several chapters of this book. While there are many more efficacy studies (studies less representative of clinical settings that recruit participants through advertisements), effectiveness studies are essential in establishing a treatment as both effective and possible for clinicians in the general population to administer. There are important distinctions between specialist clinics (Andersson et al. 2010) and general practice settings because the conditions for service delivery may differ markedly between the two. The research to date clearly suggests that guided ICBT can be as effective in effectiveness studies as in efficacy studies (Andersson and Hedman 2013), but we need more studies and a large series of patients to confirm this. However, dissemination is more than just a discussion of research trials. Attitudes of both clinicians and patients towards the treatment, means of funding services, regulations and clinical guidelines may all impact how possible it is to introduce ICBT.

ICBT in routine health care has been implemented in Stockholm health care services since 2007 at the Internet Psychiatry Unit (internetpsychiatry.se). The unit undertakes development and clinical trials in association with the Karolinska Institutet. ICBT for major depression, panic disorder and social anxiety disorders is available in routine mental health care. Continuous evaluation shows that satisfactory effects for these disorders are maintained in routine health care as compared with previous clinical trials (El Alaoui et al. 2015; Hedman et al. 2013, 2014). Trials for various other disorders, such as insomnia, obsessive-compulsive disorder, health anxiety and irritable bowel disorder are also conducted at the Internet Psychiatry Unit.

In conclusion, in a short time, ICBT has been established as a treatment option for a range of psychiatric and somatic problems. It has also generated a research field, including a scientific journal and a number of academic organisations. While technology is evolving rapidly, we believe that (at least for the next few years) the approach presented in this book will be disseminated more broadly as a viable treatment alternative, as well as a supplement to other psychiatric services.

References

Almlöv J, Carlbring P, Berger T, Cuijpers P, Andersson G (2009) Therapist factors in internet-delivered CBT for major depressive disorder. Cogn Behav Ther 38:247–254. doi:10.1080/16506070903116935

Almlöv J, Carlbring P, Källqvist K, Paxling B, Cuijpers P, Andersson G (2011) Therapist effects in guided internet-delivered CBT for anxiety disorders. Behav Cogn Psychother 39:311–322. doi:10.1017/S135246581000069X

Amir N, Beard C, Taylor CT, Klumpp H, Elias J, Burns M et al (2009) Attention training in individuals with generalized social phobia: a randomized controlled trial. J Consult Clin Psychol 77:961–973. doi:10.1037/a0016685

Andersson G (2014) The internet and CBT: a clinical guide. CRC Press, Boca Raton

Andersson G, Hedman E (2013) Effectiveness of guided internet-delivered cognitive behaviour therapy in regular clinical settings. Verhaltenstherapie 23:140–148. doi:10.1159/000354779

Andersson G, Strömgren T, Ström L, Lyttkens L (2002) Randomised controlled trial of internet based cognitive behavior therapy for distress associated with tinnitus. Psychosom Med 64:810–816

Andersson G, Asmundson GJG, Carlbring P, Ghaderi A, Hofmann SG, Stewart SH (2005a) Is CBT already the dominant paradigm in psychotherapy research and practice? Cogn Behav Ther 34:1–2. doi:10.1080/16506070510008489

Andersson G, Bergström J, Holländare F, Carlbring P, Kaldo V, Ekselius L (2005b) Internet-based self-help for depression: a randomised controlled trial. Br J Psychiatry 187:456–461. doi:10.1192/bjp.187.5.456

Andersson G, Bergström J, Buhrman M, Carlbring P, Holländare F, Kaldo V et al (2008) Development of a new approach to guided self-help via the Internet. The Swedish experience. J Technol Human Serv 26:161–181. doi:10.1080/15228830802094627

Andersson G, Waara J, Jonsson U, Malmaeus F, Carlbring P, Öst L-G (2009) Internet-based self-help vs. one-session exposure in the treatment of spider phobia: a randomized controlled trial. Cogn Behav Ther 38:114–120. doi:10.1080/16506070902931326

Andersson G, Carlbring P, Kaldo V, Cuijpers P (2010) Challenges and potential solutions in integrating internet-based CBT into specialist services. In: Bennett-Levy J, Christensen H, Farrand P, Griffiths K, Kavanagh D, Klein B et al (eds) Oxford guide to low intensity CBT interventions. Oxford University Press, Oxford, pp 495–501

Andersson G, Waara J, Jonsson U, Malmaeus F, Carlbring P, Öst L-G (2013) Internet-based vs. one-session exposure treatment of snake phobia: a randomized controlled trial. Cogn Behav Ther 42:284–291. doi:10.1080/16506073.2013.844202

Arpin-Cribbie C, Irvine J, Ritvo P (2012) Web-based cognitive-behavioral therapy for perfectionism: a randomized controlled trial. Psychother Res 22(2):194–207. doi:10.1080/10503307.2011.637242

Barak A (2013) Concepts, definitions, and applications: the terminology chaos of Internet-supported psychotherapeutic interventions. In: Paper presented at the The International Society for Research on Internet Interventions 6th Chicago Meeting

Barlow DH (2004) Psychological treatments. Am Psychol 59:869–878
Baumeister H, Reichler L, Munzinger M, Lin J (2014) The impact of guidance on internet-based mental health interventions – a systematic review. Intern Intervent 1(4):205–215. doi:10.1016/j.invent.2014.08.003
Baus O, Bouchard S (2014) Moving from virtual reality exposure-based therapy to augmented reality exposure-based therapy: a review. Front Hum Neurosci 8:112. doi:10.3389/fnhum.2014.00112
Bennett K, Bennett AJ, Griffiths KM (2010) Security considerations for e-mental health interventions. J Med Internet Res 12(5):e61. doi:10.2196/jmir.1468
Blankers M, Koeter MW, Schippers GM (2011) Internet therapy versus internet self-help versus no treatment for problematic alcohol use: a randomized controlled trial. J Consult Clin Psychol 79(3):330–341. doi:10.1037/a0023498
Boettcher J, Leek L, Matson L, Holmes EA, Browning M, MacLeod C et al (2013) Internet-based attention modification for social anxiety: a randomised controlled comparison of training towards negative and training towards positive cues. PLoS One 8:e71760. doi:10.1371/journal.pone.0071760
Boettcher J, Hasselrot J, Sund E, Andersson G, Carlbring P (2014a) Combining attention training with internet-based cognitive-behavioural self-help for social anxiety: a randomized controlled trial. Cogn Behav Ther 43:34–48. doi:10.1080/16506073.2013.809141
Boettcher J, Rozental A, Andersson G, Carlbring P (2014b) Side effects in internet-based interventions for social anxiety disorder. Intern Intervent 1:3–11. doi:10.1016/j.invent.2014.02.002
Carlbring P, Smit F (2008) Randomized trial of internet-delivered self-help with telephone support for pathological gamblers. J Consult Clin Psychol 76:1090–1094. doi:10.1037/a0013603
Carlbring P, Westling BE, Ljungstrand P, Ekselius L, Andersson G (2001) Treatment of panic disorder via the internet- a randomized trial of a self-help program. Behav Ther 32:751–764. doi:10.1016/S0005-7894(01)80019-8
Carlbring P, Bohman S, Brunt S, Buhrman M, Westling BE, Ekselius L et al (2006) Remote treatment of panic disorder: a randomized trial of internet-based cognitive behavioral therapy supplemented with telephone calls. Am J Psychiatry 163:2119–2125. doi:10.1176/appi.ajp.163.12.2119
Carlbring P, Brunt S, Bohman S, Austin D, Richards JC, Öst L-G et al (2007) Internet vs. paper and pencil administration of questionnaires commonly used in panic/agoraphobia research. Comput Hum Behav 23:1421–1434. doi:10.1016/j.chb.2005.05.002
Carlbring P, Degerman N, Jonsson J, Andersson G (2011) Internet-based treatment of pathological gambling with a three-year follow-up. Cogn Behav Ther 40:321–334. doi:10.1080/16506073.2012.689323
Carlbring P, Apelstrand M, Sehlin H, Amir N, Rousseau A, Hofmann S et al (2012) Internet-delivered attention training in individuals with social anxiety disorder – a double blind randomized controlled trial. BMC Psychiatry 12:66
Castren S, Pankakoski M, Tamminen M, Lipsanen J, Ladouceur R, Lahti T (2013) Internet-based CBT intervention for gamblers in Finland: experiences from the field. Scand J Psychol 54:230–235. doi:10.1111/sjop.12034
Christensen H, Griffiths KM (2002) The prevention of depression using the internet. Med J Australia 177:S122–S125
Côté S, Bouchard S (2008) Virtual reality exposure for phobias: a critical review. J CyberTher Rehabilitation 1:75–91
Cristea IA, Kok RN, Cuijpers P (2015) Efficacy of cognitive bias modification interventions in anxiety and depression: meta-analysis. Br J Psychiatry 206:7–16. doi:10.1192/bjp.bp.114.146761
Cuijpers P, Donker T, van Straten A, Andersson G (2010) Is guided self-help as effective as face-to-face psychotherapy for depression and anxiety disorders? A meta-analysis of comparative outcome studies. Psychol Med 40:1943–1957. doi:10.1017/S0033291710000772
Dever Fitzgerald T, Hunter PV, Hadjistavropoulos T, Koocher GP (2010) Ethical and legal considerations for internet-based psychotherapy. Cogn Behav Ther 39:173–187. doi:10.1080/16506071003636046

Donker, T., Blankers, M., Hedman, E., Ljótsson, B., Petrie, K., & Christensen, H. (2015). Economic evaluations of Internet interventions for mental health: a systematic review. *Psychological Medicine*, 45:3357–3376. doi:10.1017/s0033291715001427

Doumas DM, Hannah E (2008) Preventing high-risk drinking in youth in the workplace: a web-based normative feedback program. J Subst Abuse Treat 34:263–271. doi:10.1016/j.jsat.2007.04.006

Drummond MF, Sculpher MJ, Torrance GW, O'Brien BJ, Stoddart GL (2005) Methods for the economic evaluation of health care programmes, 3rd edn. Oxford University Press, Oxford

Ebert D, Lehr F, Boß L, Riper H, Cuijpers P, Andersson G et al (2014) Efficacy of an internet-based problem-solving training for teachers: results of a randomized controlled trial. Scand J Work Environ Health 40:582–596. doi:10.5271/sjweh.3449

El Alaoui S, Hedman E, Kaldo V, Hesser H, Kraepelien M, Andersson E et al (2015) Effectiveness of internet-based cognitive behavior therapy for social anxiety disorder in clinical psychiatry. J Consult Clin Psychol 83:902–914

Epstein J, Klinkenberg WD (2001) From Eliza to internet: a brief history of computerized assessment. Comp Hum Behav 17:295–314

Furmark T, Carlbring P, Hedman E, Sonnenstein A, Clevberger P, Bohman B et al (2009) Guided and unguided self-help for social anxiety disorder: randomised controlled trial. Br J Psychiatry 195:440–447. doi:10.1192/bjp.bp.108.060996

Haemmerli K, Znoj H, Berger T (2010) Internet-based support for infertile patients: a randomized controlled study. J Behav Med 33:135–146. doi:10.1007/s10865-009-9243-2

Hedman E, Ljótsson B, Lindefors N (2012) Cognitive behavior therapy via the internet: a systematic review of applications, clinical efficacy and cost-effectiveness. Expert Rev Pharmacoecon Outcomes Res 12:745–764. doi:10.1586/erp.12.67

Hedman E, Ljótsson B, Rück C, Bergström J, Andersson G, Kaldo V et al (2013) Effectiveness of internet-based cognitive behaviour therapy for panic disorder in routine psychiatric care. Acta Psychiatr Scand 128:457–467. doi:10.1111/acps.12079

Hedman E, Ljótsson B, Kaldo V, Hesser H, El Alaoui S, Kraepelin M et al (2014) Effectiveness of internet-based cognitive behaviour therapy for depression in routine psychiatric care. J Affect Disord 155:49–58. doi:10.1016/j.jad.2013.10.023

Kaldo V, Haak T, Buhrman M, Alfonsson S, Larsen H-C, Andersson G (2013) Internet-based cognitive behaviour therapy for tinnitus patients delivered in a regular clinical setting – outcome and analysis of treatment drop-out. Cogn Behav Ther 42:146–158

Kaldo-Sandström V, Larsen HC, Andersson G (2004) Internet-based cognitive-behavioral self-help treatment of tinnitus: clinical effectiveness and predictors of outcome. Am J Audiol 13:185–192. doi:10.1044/1059-0889(2004/023)

Kleiboer A, Donker T, Seekles W, van Straten A, Riper H, Cuijpers P (2015) A randomized controlled trial on the role of support in internet-based problem solving therapy for depression and anxiety. Behav Res Ther 72:63–71. doi:10.1016/j.brat.2015.06.013

Klein B, Richards JC (2001) A brief internet-based treatment for panic disorder. Behav Cogn Psychother 29:113–117

Kok RN, van Straten A, Beekman AT, Cuijpers P (2014) Short-term effectiveness of web-based guided self-help for phobic outpatients: randomized controlled trial. J Med Internet Res 16, e226. doi:10.2196/jmir.3429

Kuckertz JM, Gildebrant E, Liliequist B, Karlström P, Väppling C, Bodlund O et al (2014) Moderation and mediation of the effect of attention training in social anxiety disorder. Behav Res Ther 53:30–40

Lange A, Schrieken B, van den Ven J-P, Bredweg B, Emmelkamp PMG, van der Kolk J et al (2000) "Interapy": the effects of a short protocolled treatment of posttraumatic stress and pathological grief through the internet. Behav Cogn Psychother 28:175–192

Layard R, Clark DM (2014) Thrive. The power of evidence-based psychological therapies. Allen Lane, London

Marks IM, Shaw S, Parkin R (1998) Computer-assisted treatments of mental health problems. Clin Psychol 5:51–170. doi:10.1111/j.1468-2850.1998.tb00141.x
Marks IM, Cavanagh K, Gega L (2007) Hands-on help. Computer-aided psychotherapy (Maudsley monograph no. 49). Psychology Press, Hove
Merry SN, Stasiak K, Shepherd M, Frampton C, Fleming T, Lucassen MF (2012) The effectiveness of SPARX, a computerised self help intervention for adolescents seeking help for depression: randomised controlled non-inferiority trial. Br Med J 344:e2598. doi:10.1136/bmj.e2598
Mohr DC, Burns MN, Schueller SM, Clarke G, Klinkman M (2013) Behavioral intervention technologies: evidence review and recommendations for future research in mental health. Gen Hosp Psychiatry 35:332–338. doi:10.1016/j.genhosppsych.2013.03.008
Olthuis JV, Watt MC, Bailey K, Hayden JA, Stewart SH (2015) Therapist-supported Internet cognitive behavioural therapy for anxiety disorders in adults. Cochrane Database Syst Rev (3):CD011565. doi:10.1002/14651858.cd011565
Paxling B, Lundgren S, Norman A, Almlöv J, Carlbring P, Cuijpers P et al (2013) Therapist behaviours in internet-delivered cognitive behaviour therapy: analyses of e-mail correspondence in the treatment of generalized anxiety disorder. Behav Cogn Psychother 41:280–289
Proudfoot J, Ryden C, Everitt B, Shapiro DA, Goldberg D, Mann A et al (2004) Clinical efficacy of computerised cognitive-behavioural therapy for anxiety and depression in primary care: randomised controlled trial. Br J Psychiatry 185:46–54. doi:10.1192/bjp.185.1.46
Riley S, Veale D (1999) The internet and its relevance to cognitive behavioural psychotherapists. Behav Cogn Psychother 27:37–46
Riper H, Spek V, Boon B, Conijn B, Kramer J, Martin-Abello K et al (2011) Effectiveness of E-self-help interventions for curbing adult problem drinking: a meta-analysis. J Med Internet Res 13(2):e42. doi:10.2196/jmir.1691
Ritterband LM, Gonder-Frederick LA, Cox DJ, Clifton AD, West RW, Borowitz SM (2003) Internet interventions: in review, in use, and into the future. Professional Psychol Res Pract 34:527–534
Ritterband LM, Andersson G, Christensen HM, Carlbring P, Cuijpers P (2006) Directions for the International Society for Research on Internet Interventions (ISRII). J Med Internet Res 8:e23. doi:10.2196/jmir.8.3.e23
Rozental A, Andersson G, Boettcher J, Ebert D, Cuijpers P, Knaevelsrud C et al (2014) Consensus statement on defining and measuring negative effects of internet interventions. Internet Interventions 1:12–19. doi:10.1016/j.invent.2014.02.001
Rozental A, Boettcher J, Andersson G, Schmidt B, Carlbring P (2015a) Negative effects of internet interventions: a qualitative content analysis of patients' experiences with treatments delivered online. Cogn Behav Ther 44:223–236. doi:10.1080/16506073.2015.1008033
Rozental A, Forsell E, Svensson A, Andersson G, Carlbring P (2015b) Internet-based cognitive behavior therapy for procrastination: a randomized controlled trial. J Consult Clin Psychol 83:808–824. doi:10.1037/ccp0000023
Schneider AJ, Mataix-Cols D, Marks IM, Bachofen M (2005) Internet-guided self-help with or without exposure therapy for phobic and panic disorders. Psychother Psychosom 74:154–164
Storch EA, Caporino NE, Morgan JR, Lewin AB, Rojas A, Brauer L et al (2011) Preliminary investigation of web-camera delivered cognitive-behavioral therapy for youth with obsessive-compulsive disorder. Psychiatry Res 189:407–412. doi:10.1016/j.psychres.2011.05.047
Ström L, Pettersson R, Andersson G (2000) A controlled trial of self-help treatment of recurrent headache conducted via the internet. J Consult Clin Psychol 68:722–727. doi:10.1037/0022-006X.68.4.722
Tait RJ, Spijkerman R, Riper H (2013) Internet and computer based interventions for cannabis use: a meta-analysis. Drug Alcohol Depend 133:295–304. doi:10.1016/j.drugalcdep.2013.05.012
Titov N, Andrews G, Davies M, McIntyre K, Robinson E, Solley K (2010) Internet treatment for depression: a randomized controlled trial comparing clinician vs technician assistance. PLoS One 5:e10939. doi:10.1371/journal.pone.0010939

Titov N, Dear BF, Johnston L, Lorian C, Zou J, Wootton B et al (2013) Improving adherence and clinical outcomes in self-guided internet treatment for anxiety and depression: randomised controlled trial. PLoS One 8:e62873. doi:10.1371/journal.pone.0062873

van Bastelaar KM, Pouwer F, Cuijpers P, Riper H, Snoek FJ (2011) Web-based depression treatment for type 1 and type 2 diabetic patients: a randomized, controlled trial. Diabetes Care 34:320–325. doi:10.2337/dc10-1248

Vigerland S, Thulin U, Svirsky L, Öst L-G, Ljótsson B, Lindefors N et al (2013) Internet-delivered CBT for children with specific phobia: a pilot study. Cogn Behav Ther 42:303–314. doi:10.1080/16506073.2013.844201

Vlaescu G, Carlbring P, Lunner T, Andersson G (2015) An e-platform for rehabilitation of persons with hearing problems. Am J 24:271–275. doi:10.1044/2015_AJA-14-0083

Watkins PL (2008) Self-help therapies: past and present. In: Watkins PL, Clum GA (eds) Handbook of self-help therapies. Routledge, New York, pp 1–24

Watkins PL, Clum GA (eds) (2008) Handbook of self-help therapies. Routledge, New York

Westbrook D, Kennerly H, Kirk J (2011) Cognitive behaviour therapy. Skills and applications, 2nd edn. Sage, Los Angeles

Williams AD, Blackwell SE, Mackenzie A, Holmes EA, Andrews G (2013) Combining imagination and reason in the treatment of depression: a randomized controlled trial of internet-based cognitive-bias modification and internet-CBT for depression. J Consult Clin Psychol 81: 793–799. doi:10.1037/a0033247

ICBT for Depression

2

Gerhard Andersson, Birgit Wagner, and Pim Cuijpers

Abstract

Major depression and depressive symptoms are widely prevalent and there is a need for cost-effective and easily available psychological treatments. There is a large and growing literature on guided Internet-based CBT (ICBT) for depression and depressive symptoms. In this chapter, we give examples of programs and review the evidence. When compared against waiting list controls, guided ICBT has large effects, and studies also suggest that guided ICBT is probably as effective as face-to-face CBT. There are studies on long-term effects and effectiveness data showing that effects can endure and that ICBT can be effective in clinically representative settings. There are yet few studies on the cost-effectiveness of guided ICBT for depression, and more studies are needed in which Internet and face-to-face CBT are blended. Moreover, most studies have been on adults and studies are needed with adolescents and older adults as target groups.

G. Andersson, PhD (✉)
Department of Behavioural Sciences and Learning, Linköping University,
Linköping SE 581 83, Sweden
e-mail: Gerhard.andersson@liu.se

B. Wagner, PhD
MSB Medical School Berlin, Hochschule für Gesundheit und Medizin,
Villa Siemens, Calandrellistraße 1-9, Berlin 12247, Germany
e-mail: birgit.wagner@medicalschool-berlin.de

P. Cuijpers, PhD
Department of Clinical, Neuro and Developmental Psychology, Vrije Universiteit
Amsterdam, Van der Boechorststraat 1, Amsterdam BT 1081, The Netherlands
e-mail: p.cuijpers@psy.vu.nl

© Springer International Publishing Switzerland 2016

N. Lindefors, G. Andersson (eds.), *Guided Internet-Based Treatments in Psychiatry*, DOI 10.1007/978-3-319-06083-5_2

Background

Depression is a common condition across the world (Ebmeier et al. 2006). Even if the way depression is manifested may differ markedly, a diagnosis of major depression requires that the person has a depressed mood most of the day and nearly every day during a 2-week period or has a markedly diminished interest or pleasure in all, or almost all, activities most of the day, nearly every day. In addition to the two key symptoms, the diagnosis involves other symptoms during at least a 2-week period such as significant weight loss, insomnia or hypersomnia, psychomotor agitation or retardation, fatigue or loss of energy, feelings of worthlessness or excessive or inappropriate guilt, diminished ability to think or concentrate or indecisiveness, or recurrent thoughts of death (American Psychiatric Association 2013). It is required that at least five of these symptoms are present. Dysthymic disorder is a special kind of depression in which a person has a depressed mood for most of the days, for more days than not, for at least 2 years. In addition, at least two of the other symptoms of major depression have to be present. Unfortunately, relapse is a common problem in depression. The first episode can last between 3 and 12 months (Spijker et al. 2002), but then it is likely that the person has a second episode (around a third), and for each new episode, it becomes more likely for another episode to occur. Thus, a challenge for clinicians is not only to treat depression when it occurs but also to prevent relapse. In addition, minor depression can also be treated and this can be a cost-effective way to prevent the onset of a full depressive episode (van Zoonen et al. 2014). In this chapter, we will review guided internet-based CBT treatments for depression, but first, we will comment on the different types of psychological treatments that are common.

Treatment

There are numerous ways to treat depression including different forms of pharmacotherapy and several psychological treatments. The most common is antidepressant medication which can be effective and add to psychological treatments (Cuijpers et al. 2012). However, as a stand-alone treatment antidepressant medication may not be as effective as CBT in the long run (Cuijpers et al. 2013). This chapter focuses on Internet-delivered CBT (ICBT), but is worth mentioning that other psychological treatments such as psychodynamic internet treatment (Johansson et al. 2012a) and physical exercise (Ström et al. 2013) have been found to be effective as well in the treatment of depression. Even interpersonal psychotherapy has been tested as an unguided Internet intervention for depressive symptoms (Donker et al. 2013).

An important question when it comes to ICBT for depression is how it is conducted. This was included in the history chapter, but is worth commenting on briefly here as well. We restrict the discussion to guided ICBT as there is evidence to suggest that fully automated treatments tend to be less effective when it comes to depression (Johansson and Andersson 2012).

ICBT Programs for Depression

As the literature on ICBT for depression is growing rapidly, and given the fact that many treatment programs never are tested in research, it will not be possible to present even a majority of the existing ICBT programs in any detail (Johansson and Andersson 2012). However, the ones that have been developed and tested are often based on CBT. Thus, it is common that they include a rationale, behavioral activation, cognitive restructuring, and relapse prevention. There are, however, several other aspects that may differ between programs. *First*, early programs were largely text based and had few if any interactive features. This could be referred to as "net bibliotherapy" (Marks et al. 2007). Then gradually programs became more interactive and automated. Thus, pictures, streamed videos, animations, audio files, and even online lessons are now fairly common, and there is even a program for subclinical depression based on a manga format, which is a Japanese cartoon style (Imamura et al. 2014). However, it is still the case that many ICBT programs for depression mainly rely on text and downloadable text files. *Second*, the level of client-therapist interaction differs widely. A common approach is to provide "minimal" guidance in the form of e-mail correspondence (Titov 2010) within a secure web platform. This "minimal contact" often takes the form of encouragement and feedback on homework assignments and usually does not take more time than 10 min per client per week in a regular ICBT program (see history chapter for more information). Analyses have revealed a significant correlation between the amount of therapist time in minutes per participant and the between-group effect sizes of Internet-based interventions (Palmqvist et al. 2007). Andersson and colleagues have suggested that it can be sufficient for the therapist to spend about 100 min per patient over a 10-week program giving comments on patients' homework and providing feedback (Andersson et al. 2009). Studies indicate that increasing therapist contact time beyond a certain threshold may not facilitate further treatment gains (Vernmark et al. 2010). Interestingly, it may be that this form of process feedback does not require specialist clinicians but may be handled by lay persons under supervision (Titov et al. 2010). A way to reduce the contact time even further is to provide automated e-mails (Titov et al. 2013). A different approach is to provide more clinician contact. For example, real-time contact with scheduled chat sessions has been tested but requires more time and is less flexible than mainly self-guided ICBT (Kessler et al. 2009). There is also a program called Interapy with much text-based interaction between the clinician and the client (Ruwaard et al. 2009). *Third*, it may be the case that differences between how programs are delivered (e.g., process of delivery and presentation) are more important than the actual contents of the programs. When it comes to depression, there are reasons to believe that different forms of ICBT are about as effective, but the way ICBT is delivered could be important. Referral patterns (self-referral or being referred from a clinic), diagnostic procedures, therapist support during the intervention, a clear deadline for completion of the treatment, treatment duration, and many other "structural" factors could be of importance.

Different approaches within CBT are reflected in the ICBT programs. Basically, most programs rely on both behavioral and cognitive therapy techniques, but there is also a form of ICBT based on problem solving (Warmerdam et al. 2008) that has been adapted for Internet delivery. There are transdiagnostic treatments as well with one form being derived from what is common across different disorders (e.g., anxiety and mood disorders) (Titov et al. 2011) and the other approach being tailored ICBT in which the treatment is tailored according to the different problems the patient presents (Johansson et al. 2012b). Not only do programs differ in terms of what they emphasize but also the target group for which the intervention is aimed. For example, there are programs for children/adolescents (Van Voorhees et al. 2007), adults (Andersson et al. 2005), older adults (Dear et al. 2013), and one program aimed for persons with residual depressive symptoms (Holländare et al. 2011). A few examples of the contents of programs are presented in Table 2.1.

Empirical Studies

There is now a fairly large number of trials on guided ICBT for depression that have been summarized in systematic reviews and meta-analyses. Many reviews do not distinguish between computerized treatments in general and Internet-delivered treatments, but increasingly studies on ICBT dominate reviews as few new studies on computerized treatments appear (e.g., delivered via CD-ROM in a clinic, like the Beating the Blues program). First, we will comment on the overall effects as presented in meta-analytic reviews. Then we will cover long-term effects of ICBT for depression and after that comparisons against face-to-face CBT. Finally, effectiveness data will be mentioned.

One early meta-analytic review by two of us included both computerized interventions and ICBT, but there were only two studies out of 12 that did not involve the Internet (Andersson and Cuijpers 2009). We found an average effect size vs. control groups at posttest of $d=0.41$, but it was also clear that this estimate was moderated by a significant difference between guided ($d=0.61$) and unguided ($d=0.25$) treatments. Subsequent reviews have included more studies but have largely found the same results (Richards and Richardson 2012; Johansson and Andersson 2012), with a linear association between support and outcome. Even the effect size of $d=0.61$ might be higher when considering subsequent studies. Johansson and Andersson (2012) found that totally unguided treatments had a between-group effect $d=0.21$, whereas studies with contact before treatment only had an effect of $d=0.44$. When there was contact with a person/staff contact during treatment, the effect was $d=0.58$, and finally when there was contact both before and during the intervention, the effect was $d=0.76$. This latter effect size is in line with what is found for face-to-face psychotherapies in general (Cuijpers et al. 2011). A more recent update showed that only in the period between January 2013 to September 2014, as many as 11 controlled trials on Internet treatment for depression have been published only on guided treatments (Andersson et al. 2014a).

The literature in this area is expanding rapidly. From the early controlled trials on, e.g., unguided (Clarke et al. 2002; Christensen et al. 2004) and guided ICBT (Andersson et al. 2005), a considerable number of controlled trials have followed.

Table 2.1 Examples of contents of different guided ICBT programs for depression

Program and *country of origin*	Duration and number of modules/lessons	Main contents	Mode of presentation	Reference example supporting use
Relapse prevention program (ISIDOR) *Sweden*	10 weeks 9 basic modules and 7 optional advanced modules with more specific information	Psychoeducation Adding positively reinforced activities Handling negatively reinforced activities Cognitive restructuring Improving sleep Mindfulness Reducing anxiety Physical activity Long-term goals	Downloadable pdf files and text on screen Secure contact handling system for homework and guidance via that system	Holländare et al. (2011)
Tailored Internet intervention for depression (Taylor) *Sweden*	Up to 10 weeks but flexible 25 modules that are prescribed according to symptom profile 4 modules are fixed: psychoeducation, cognitive restructuring, and relapse prevention	Modules on depression, panic, social anxiety, worry, trauma, stress management, concentration problems, problem solving, mindfulness, and relaxation	As above	Johansson et al. (2012a)
Sadness program *Australia*	8 weeks 6 online lessons	Behavioral activation Cognitive restructuring Problem solving Assertiveness skills	Lessons online with illustrated case stories, printable summary, additional resource documents (text files on sleep, panic, and other comorbid problems) Therapist support via e-mail, automated reminders	Perini et al. (2009)

(continued)

Table 2.1 (continued)

Program and *country of origin*	Duration and number of modules/ lessons	Main contents	Mode of presentation	Reference example supporting use
Interapy depression *Netherlands*	11 weeks 8 treatment phases	Divided into phases with written instructions 1. Inducing awareness: writing 2. Inducing awareness: monitoring 3. Structuring activities 4. Challenging negative thoughts 5. Behavioral experiments 6. Positive self-verbalization 7. Social skills 8. Relapse prevention	A personal interactive workbook is used by participants and a manual with templates for therapists Communication via e-mail (within the system) Homework assignments are included	Ruwaard et al. (2009)

For example, guided ICBT for depression has been found to work in controlled trials from Australia (Perini et al. 2009), Switzerland (Berger et al. 2011), Germany (Wagner et al. 2014), the Netherlands (Warmerdam et al. 2008; Ruwaard et al. 2009), and the United States (Mohr et al. 2013). Several formats of ICBT have been tested as well such as e-mail therapy (Vernmark et al. 2010), acceptance-oriented CBT (Carlbring et al. 2013), but also trials on smartphone-delivered CBT together with Internet support (Ly et al. 2014). Another example is a study from Japan in which an intervention incorporating manga pictures for mild depression was tested (Imamura et al. 2014). As mentioned earlier, there are also studies on different subgroups, for example, persons with diabetes and depression (van Bastelaar et al. 2011) and postpartum depression (O'Mahen et al. 2014), adolescents (Saulsberry et al. 2013), and older adults (Titov et al. 2015a), and programs have been translated and adapted to for other non-Western languages such as Chinese (Choi et al. 2012). While most studies have focused on mild to moderate depression, with an increasing number using validated instruments to diagnose depression, there is at least one example of a relapse prevention program from Sweden showing promising results (Holländare et al. 2011), also at a 2-year follow-up (Holländare et al. 2013).

Earlier in this chapter, transdiagnostic and tailored ICBT were mentioned. One advantage with transdiagnostic and tailored approaches is the possibility to target comorbid problems that are known to exist alongside depression, anxiety being one example (Andersson and Titov 2014). In one controlled trial, tailored ICBT was found to be more effective for the more severe clients in the trial when compared against standard ICBT (Johansson et al. 2012b). More research is needed to confirm this observation as different depression treatments usually tend to lead to equivalent outcomes. For example, the previously mentioned psychodynamic Internet treatment yielded large treatment effects in one trial (Johansson et al. 2012a). An interesting way to study differences between treatments is to allow clients to choose treatment form, which was done in one trial showing largely equivalent findings but a preference for ICBT over the psychodynamic Internet treatment (Johansson et al. 2013).

Some studies in the ICBT field have included longer-term follow-ups, often included in the original publication. For example, in one controlled trial where ICBT was compared against face-to-face group treatment, data from a 3-year follow-up were included suggesting sustained treatment effects and no differences between the two formats (Andersson et al. 2013b). In another study, 3.5-year follow-up data were presented showing maintained effects (Andersson et al. 2013a), and other studies showing long-term effects up to 3 years posttreatment have been published (Ruwaard et al. 2009). A limitation of these studies however is that they have not documented the course of depression during the follow-up period.

With regard to the contrast between ICBT and face-to-face CBT, there are few direct comparisons, possibly because such trials are more costly and time consuming. In a recent review, Andersson and coworkers compiled the studies that had directly compared face to face and ICBT within the same trial (four trials) (Andersson et al. 2014a). The overall random effects effect size was a nonsignificant Hedges' $g = 0.12$ (95 % CI: −0.08 ~ 0.32) favoring guided ICBT over face-to-face therapy and with no signs of heterogeneity ($I2 = 00$ %). This finding is in line with other reviews suggesting the guided self-help in general (Cuijpers et al. 2010), and ICBT (Andersson et al. 2014b) appears to be as effective as face-to-face therapy when directly compared in controlled trials.

It is probably the case that patients recruited via advertisement to research settings differ from patients seen in regular care, which calls for separate studies in these two settings. This is referred to as the difference between efficacy and effectiveness, with the latter being studies conducted in clinically representative settings with regular patients and clinicians (Hunsley and Lee 2007). An increasing number of studies on ICBT delivered in regular clinic have been published (Andersson and Hedman 2013), some of which are on depression. For example, effectiveness data have been published on the Dutch Interapy program (Ruwaard et al. 2012), the Swedish Internet psychiatry unit treatment (Hedman et al. 2014), and the Australian Sadness program (Williams and Andrews 2013). Data on the effectiveness of unguided treatments for depression have also been published (Leykin et al. 2014). In general, these studies indicate that the effects of ICBT interventions found in trials are comparable to those found in regular care.

In sum, the research to date clearly supports that guided ICBT is effective for depression and that the effects may be durable. It is possible that guided ICBT is as effective as face-to-face CBT, but it is important to remember that most studies have been on mild to moderate depression and not more severe forms. In addition, research suggests that guided ICBT is effective for different target groups, but most research has been on adults.

Case Description

Inger had been depressed once in her 20s but is now a 45-year-old middle manager at a large company and has a family with two kids and a husband. She could never expect that she would be depressed again. During winter holiday, the family went skiing and she managed to fall and break her leg. In addition to staying away from work a few weeks, she did not get an expected promotion and finally her oldest son (16 years old) had problems at school and spent much time in front of the computer. All this eventually lead to her feeling depressed and increasingly more passive. For example, she ceased doing her regular exercise and avoided her friends. She only managed to focus on work and on her family and felt easily distracted and annoyed when things went against her. Family had noted her changed mood and the fact that she had problems with sleep. When she eventually went to the GP, she was recommended that she should seek help at the Internet psychiatry unit in Stockholm, Sweden. She lived in another city close by. To her surprise, she was offered a consultation with a psychiatrist within 2 weeks and then an interview with a clinical psychologist who described how guided ICBT would work if she decided to start treatment now. As she was not too severely depressed and had a university degree, she thought that this would be a good alternative for her as she did not need to take time off from work. She started with the treatment that lasted for 10 weeks with guidance from a psychologist at the unit (Erik) who supported her and gave feedback on homework assignments. Scheduling of activities was fairly easy for her but the most appreciated part of the treatment was to work with cognitive therapy techniques as she had always had tendencies toward negative thinking and found the registrations and homework assignments helpful. In addition, the advice given for sleep management was beneficial even if she fairly rapidly started to sleep better once she had control over her days and started to engage in rewarding activities (like getting back to exercise and seeing her friends). The last thing she did in the treatment was to do a relapse prevention plan. She was interviewed after the treatment and received feedback from the therapist. During the treatment, symptoms were monitored and she noted already after a few weeks that things were getting better. Afterward, she felt she had done a good job and that her therapist had supported her.

Cost-Effectiveness

There is not much research on the cost-effectiveness of guided ICBT for depression, but there are some studies on unguided ICBT (de Graaf et al. 2008). However, Warmerdam and colleagues showed that both guided ICBT and problem solving therapy were cost-effective (Warmerdam et al. 2010), and results from a trial on real-time ICBT conducted in the United Kingdom showed similar findings (Hollinghurst et al. 2010). Moreover, cost data were reported in a trial on ICBT for older adults (Titov et al. 2015a). In a trial on depressive symptoms among employees, the intervention was partly cost-effective, but not for the employers (Geraedts et al. 2015). The literature is yet uncertain when it comes to the cost-effectiveness of guided ICBT for depression (Arnberg et al. 2014), and more studies are needed.

Clinical Implementation and Dissemination

As mentioned previously in the chapter, effectiveness data are increasingly published and there are also reports from clinics like the MindSpot clinic in Australia with large series of patients (Titov et al. 2015b). It is hard to give an overview of how well guided ICBT for depression has been disseminated, in particular as not all who provide treatment publish research. Moreover, unguided programs like MoodGYM can be delivered by clinicians as an adjunct, and thus the treatment is blended with face-to-face services (Høifødt et al. 2013). In Sweden, guided ICBT for depression is offered in a few places (like the internet psychiatry unit at Karolinska University Hospital), but a national treatment platform has been developed which most likely will increase access to ICBT in Sweden. Moreover, in many places in the world, health care is insurance based, and programs from private companies like Deprexis in Germany are gradually being introduced as a treatment option (Meyer et al. 2015), and in the Netherlands, several programs are disseminated (e.g., Interapy). In the United Kingdom, Norway, and Sweden, tax-funded health care has been part of the implementation process. To conclude, the field of dissemination is highly dependent on legal and ethical considerations, but increasingly ICBT for depression is being incorporated into clinical guidelines.

Discussion and Future Challenges

Here we will comment on the role of the therapist, patient experiences, new venues for research, and limitations. First, as attested by many studies, ICBT for depression benefits from having a person guiding the patient through the treatment (Andersson 2014). The question is then if it matters who that person is? Titov and coworkers have, as previously mentioned, found that support can probably be provided from mainly a technical perspective (Titov et al. 2010), and there appear to be small differences in effectiveness between different therapists (Almlöv et al. 2009). It is also possible that therapeutic support is conveyed directly in the program/text material (Richardson et al. 2010), and thus the role of the therapist is mainly to encourage the patient. On the other hand, ratings of therapeutic alliance tend to be high in ICBT studies (Andersson et al. 2012; Preschl et al. 2011), and our clinical experience is that patients develop a bond with their online therapist. This is an important area for future research, as it is a different form of alliance than in face-to-face therapy as the patients do not see their therapist in person. Second, there is an increasing number of qualitative studies on how patients experience Internet treatments, and in one study on depression, it was observed that some patients tended to go through their program as "readers," thus not changing anything in their lives in spite of taking part of the treatment material (Bendelin et al. 2011). This can occur in face-to-face treatments as well, but is a clinical observation that should be considered as adherence in general does not seem to be worse than in face-to-face treatments (van Ballegooijen et al. 2014).

Although these preliminary findings provide some evidence that ICBT might be as effective as face-to-face interventions, it remains unclear whether the factors that are responsible for symptom reduction in face-to-face therapy operate in the same way in ICBT settings. Therapeutic factors such as decreased social presence and missing face-to-face contact were originally seen as disadvantages of Internet-based interventions. However, it might be exactly these factors that offer an advantage in comparison to face-to-face interventions (Wagner et al. 2014). Online participants might be more focused on the structured treatment manual as they are responsible for continuation of the intervention. Less personal guidance puts a stronger focus on self-responsibility to conduct the treatment modules and homework assignments than the face-to-face intervention. This might lead to a greater treatment manual adherence than in face-to-face therapy. DeRubeis and Feeley (1990) differentiated between two types of adherence to cognitive behavioral therapies, concrete and abstract adherence. Concrete adherence involves methods to support use by the patients of cognitive behavioral tools such as cognitive restructuring worksheets, homework assignments, and behavioral techniques. In contrast to this, abstract adherence to CBT involves broader discussions of therapy-relevant issues with focus put upon understanding the patients' situation and beliefs and conversations about the patients' well-being and therapy progress. In ICBT, there is a clear focus on concrete adherence through use of homework assignments, psychoeducation, and behavioral observation techniques. Usually, only a small part of the therapeutic contact involves abstract adherence, such as conversations about the patient's current personal situation. Face-to-face CBT still gives the patients more opportunities to discuss problematic current situations, alongside pure adherence to the treatment modules (Wagner et al. 2014).

Future challenges in this field are plentiful. There is a lack of studies on bipolar disorder using guided ICBT as an adjunct to medication (there is at least one trial on online psychoeducation) and only initial work on suicidal ideation in association with depression (van Spijker et al. 2014), even if such symptoms may decrease overall following internet interventions (Watts et al. 2012). While studies are being published on smartphone applications as adjuncts to face-to-face treatments for depression (Ly et al. 2015), there are still few studies in which regular face-to-face and ICBT are truly blended. This is a promising area for research as clinicians may be more positive toward blending services than replacing face to face with Internet treatment (van der Vaart et al. 2014). Another research challenge relates to moderators and mediators of treatment outcome. Here, we see a role for patient-level meta-analyses which can be useful for finding moderators as large data sets can be collected (Bower et al. 2013). When it comes to mediators, there are also possibilities as weekly measures often are embedded in ICBT programs (Hedman et al. 2014). With the use of modern mobile phone applications (apps), new ways of collecting data become easily available, with, for example, sensor data being one example (Cuijpers et al. 2015). Another area of research concerns cognitive-bias modification (CBM) and possibilities to boost the effects of ICBT (Williams et al. 2013).

As with the possibilities, there are also several limitations. First, as is often the case with psychotherapy research in general, many patients in the controlled trials have been well educated, and it is not clear how much ICBT needs to be adapted for patients with minor educational background or if ICBT would work if the treatment was delivered via sound or movies (audiobook and streamed video lectures). Second, antidepressant medication is very common and may boost the effects of psychotherapy for depression, in particular when the depression is more severe (Cuijpers et al. 2011). In many trials on ICBT, patients have been on medication (stabilized), but it is not yet clear how much ICBT and antidepressants interact. Third, attitudes toward ICBT may differ between different settings, countries, and stakeholders. For example, it may be that patients are more positive than clinicians overall (Gun et al. 2011), but may also be that for many face-to-face therapy it is the preferred option (Mohr et al. 2010) rendering blended treatments a possible way to integrate ICBT in order to be able to help more patients at a lower cost. In conclusion, there are several challenges in research, but the research to date clearly suggests that ICBT for depression is a viable treatment option.

References

Almlöv J, Carlbring P, Berger T, Cuijpers P, Andersson G (2009) Therapist factors in Internet-delivered CBT for major depressive disorder. Cogn Behav Ther 38:247–254. doi:10.1080/16506070903116935

American Psychiatric Association (2013) Desk reference to the diagnostic criteria from DSM-5. American Psychiatric Press, Washington

Andersson G (2014) The internet and CBT: a clinical guide. CRC Press, Boca Raton

Andersson G, Cuijpers P (2009) Internet-based and other computerized psychological treatments for adult depression: a meta-analysis. Cogn Behav Ther 38:196–205. doi:10.1080/16506070903318960

Andersson G, Hedman E (2013) Effectiveness of guided Internet-delivered cognitive behaviour therapy in regular clinical settings. Verhaltenstherapie 23:140–148. doi:10.1159/000354779

Andersson G, Titov N (2014) Advantages and limitations of Internet-based interventions for common mental disorders. World Psychiatry 13:4–11. doi:10.1002/wps.20083

Andersson G, Bergström J, Holländare F, Carlbring P, Kaldo V, Ekselius L (2005) Internet-based self-help for depression: a randomised controlled trial. Br J Psychiatry 187:456–461. doi:10.1192/bjp.187.5.456

Andersson G, Carlbring P, Berger T, Almlöv J, Cuijpers P (2009) What makes Internet therapy work? Cogn Behav Ther 38(S1):55–60. doi:10.1080/16506070902916400

Andersson G, Paxling B, Wiwe M, Vernmark K, Bertholds Felix C, Lundborg L et al (2012) Therapeutic alliance in guided Internet-delivered cognitive behavioral treatment of depression, generalized anxiety disorder and social anxiety disorder. Behav Res Ther 50:544–550. doi:10.1016/j.brat.2012.05.003

Andersson G, Hesser H, Hummerdal D, Bergman-Nordgren L, Carlbring P (2013a) A 3.5-year follow-up of Internet-delivered cognitive behaviour therapy for major depression. J Ment Health 22:155–164

Andersson G, Hesser H, Veilord A, Svedling L, Andersson F, Sleman O et al (2013b) Randomized controlled non-inferiority trial with 3-year follow-up of internet-delivered versus face-to-face group cognitive behavioural therapy for depression. J Affect Disord 151:986–994. doi:10.1016/j.jad.2013.08.022

Andersson G, Bergman Nordgren L, Buhrman M, Carlbring P (2014a) Psychological treatments for depression delivered via the Internet and supported by a clinician: an update. Span J Clin Psychol 19:217–225. doi:10.5944/rppc.vol.19.num.3.2014.13903

Andersson G, Cuijpers P, Carlbring P, Riper H, Hedman E (2014b) Internet-based vs. face-to-face cognitive behaviour therapy for psychiatric and somatic disorders: a systematic review and meta-analysis. World Psychiatry 13:288–295. doi:10.1002/wps.20151

Arnberg FK, Linton SJ, Hultcrantz M, Heintz E, Jonsson U (2014) Internet-delivered psychological treatments for mood and anxiety disorders: a systematic review of their efficacy, safety, and cost-effectiveness. PLoS One 9:e98118. doi:10.1371/journal.pone.0098118

Bendelin N, Hesser H, Dahl J, Carlbring P, Zetterqvist Nelson K, Andersson G (2011) Experiences of guided Internet-based cognitive-behavioural treatment for depression: A qualitative study. BMC Psychiatry 11:107. doi:10.1186/1471-244X-11-107

Berger T, Hämmerli K, Gubser N, Andersson G, Caspar F (2011) Internet-based treatment of depression: a randomized controlled trial comparing guided with unguided self-help. Cogn Behav Ther 40:251–266. doi:10.1080/16506073.2011.616531

Bower P, Kontopantelis E, Sutton AP, Kendrick T, Richards D, Gilbody S et al (2013) Influence of initial severity of depression on effectiveness of low intensity interventions: meta-analysis of individual patient data. Br Med J 346:f540. doi:10.1136/bmj.f540

Carlbring P, Hägglund M, Luthström A, Dahlin M, Kadowaki Å, Vernmark K et al (2013) Internet-based behavioral activation and acceptance-based treatment for depression: a randomized controlled trial. J Affect Disord 148:331–337. doi:10.1016/j.jad.2012.12.020

Choi I, Zou J, Titov N, Dear BF, Li S, Johnston L et al (2012) Culturally attuned Internet treatment for depression amongst Chinese Australians: a randomised controlled trial. J Affect Disord 136:459–468. doi:10.1016/j.jad.2011.11.003

Christensen H, Griffiths KM, Jorm A (2004) Delivering interventions for depression by using the internet: randomised controlled trial. Br Med J 328:265–268. doi:10.1136/bmj.37945.566632.EE

Clarke G, Reid E, Eubanks D, O'Connor E, DeBar LL, Kelleher C et al (2002) Overcoming depression on the Internet (ODIN): a randomized controlled trial of an Internet depression skills intervention program. JMIR 4:e14. doi:10.2196/jmir.4.3.e14

Cuijpers P, Donker T, van Straten A, Andersson G (2010) Is guided self-help as effective as face-to-face psychotherapy for depression and anxiety disorders? A meta-analysis of comparative outcome studies. Psychol Med 40:1943–1957. doi:10.1017/S0033291710000772

Cuijpers P, Andersson G, Donker T, van Straten A (2011) Psychological treatment of depression: results of a series of meta-analyses. Nord J Psychiatry 65:354–364. doi:10.3109/08039488.2011.596570

Cuijpers P, Reynolds CF II, Donker T, Juan L, Andersson G, Beekman A (2012) Personalized treatment of adult depression: medication, psychotherapy or both? A systematic review. Depress Anxiety 29:855–864. doi:10.1002/da.21985

Cuijpers P, Hollon S, Van Straten A, Bockting C, Berking M, Andersson G (2013) Does cognitive behaviour therapy have an enduring effect that is superior to keeping patients on continuation pharmacotherapy? A meta-analysis. BMJ Open 3:e002542. doi:10.1136/bmjopen-2012-002542

Cuijpers P, Riper H, Andersson G (2015) Internet-based treatment of depression. Curr Opin Psychol 4:131–135. doi:10.1016/j.copsyc.2014.12.026

de Graaf LE, Gerhards SA, Evers SM, Arntz A, Riper H, Severens JL et al (2008) Clinical and cost-effectiveness of computerised cognitive behavioural therapy for depression in primary care: design of a randomised trial. BMC Public Health 8:224. doi:10.1186/1471-2458-8-224

Dear BF, Zou J, Titov N, Lorian C, Johnston L, Spence J et al (2013) Internet-delivered cognitive behavioural therapy for depression: a feasibility open trial for older adults. Aust N Z J Psychiatry 47:169–176. doi:10.1177/0004867412466154

Donker T, Bennett K, Bennett A, Mackinnon A, van Straten A, Cuijpers P et al (2013) Internet-delivered interpersonal psychotherapy versus internet-delivered cognitive behavioral therapy for adults with depressive symptoms: randomized controlled noninferiority trial. JMIR 15:e82. doi:10.2196/jmir.2307, v15i5e82 [pii]

Ebmeier KP, Donaghey C, Steele JD (2006) Recent developments and current controversies in depression. Lancet 367:153–167. doi:10.1016/S0140-6736(06)67964-6

Geraedts AS, van Dongen JM, Kleiboer AM, Wiezer NM, van Mechelen W, Cuijpers P et al (2015) Economic evaluation of a web-based guided self-help intervention for employees with depressive symptoms: results of a randomized controlled trial. J Occup Environ Med 57:666–675. doi:10.1097/jom.0000000000000423

Gun SY, Titov N, Andrews G (2011) Acceptability of Internet treatment of anxiety and depression. Australas Psychiatry 19:259–264. doi:10.3109/10398562.2011.562295

Hedman E, Ljótsson B, Kaldo V, Hesser H, El Alaoui S, Kraepelin M et al (2014) Effectiveness of Internet-based cognitive behaviour therapy for depression in routine psychiatric care. J Affect Disord 155:49–58. doi:10.1016/j.jad.2013.10.023

Høifødt RS, Lillevoll KR, Griffiths KM, Wilsgaard T, Eisemann M, Waterloo K et al (2013) The clinical effectiveness of web-based cognitive behavioral therapy with face-to-face therapist support for depressed primary care patients: randomized controlled trial. J Med Internet Res 15:e153. doi:10.2196/jmir.2714

Holländare F, Johnsson S, Randestad M, Tillfors M, Carlbring P, Andersson G et al (2011) Randomized trial of internet-based relapse prevention for partially remitted depression. Acta Psychiatr Scand 124:285–294. doi:10.1111/j.1600-0447.2011.01698.x

Holländare F, Johnsson S, Randestad M, Tillfors M, Carlbring P, Andersson G et al (2013) Two-year outcome for Internet-based relapse prevention for partially remitted depression. Behav Res Ther 51:719–722. doi:10.1016/j.brat.2013.08.002

Hollinghurst S, Peters TJ, Kaur S, Wiles N, Lewis G, Kessler D (2010) Cost-effectiveness of therapist-delivered online cognitive-behavioural therapy for depression: randomised controlled trial. Br J Psychiatry 197:297–304. doi:10.1192/bjp.bp.109.073080

Hunsley J, Lee CM (2007) Research-informed benchmarks for psychological treatments: efficacy studies, effectiveness studies, and beyond. Prof Psychol Res Pract 38:21–33. doi:10.1037/0735-7028.38.1.21

Imamura K, Kawakami N, Furukawa TA, Matsuyama Y, Shimazu A, Umanodan R et al (2014) Effects of an Internet-based cognitive behavioral therapy (ICBT) program in Manga format on improving subthreshold depressive symptoms among healthy workers: a randomized controlled trial. PLoS One 9(5):e97167. doi:10.1371/journal.pone.0097167

Johansson R, Andersson G (2012) Internet-based psychological treatments for depression. Expert Rev Neurother 12:861–870. doi:10.1586/ern.12.63

Johansson R, Ekbladh S, Hebert A, Lindström M, Möller S, Petitt E et al (2012a) Psychodynamic guided self-help for adult depression through the Internet: a randomised controlled trial. PLoS One 7(5):e38021. doi:10.1371/journal.pone.0038021

Johansson R, Sjöberg E, Sjögren M, Johnsson E, Carlbring P, Andersson T et al (2012b) Tailored vs. standardized Internet-based cognitive behavior therapy for depression and comorbid symptoms: a randomized controlled trial. PLoS One 7(5):e36905. doi:10.1371/journal.pone.0036905

Johansson R, Nyblom A, Carlbring P, Cuijpers P, Andersson G (2013) Choosing between Internet-based psychodynamic versus cognitive behavioral therapy for depression: a pilot preference study. BMC Psychiatry 13:268. doi:10.1186/10.1186/1471-244X-13-268

Kessler D, Lewis G, Kaur S, Wiles N, King M, Weich S et al (2009) Therapist-delivered internet psychotherapy for depression in primary care: a randomised controlled trial. Lancet 374: 628–634. doi:10.1016/S0140-6736(09)61257-5

Leykin Y, Muñoz RF, Contreras O, Latham MD (2014) Results from a trial of an unsupported internet intervention for depressive symptoms. Internet Interv 1:175–181. doi:10.1016/j.invent.2014.09.002

Ly KH, Trüschel A, Jarl L, Magnusson S, Windahl T, Johansson R et al (2014) Behavioral activation vs Mindfulness-based guided self-help treatment administered through a smartphone application: a randomized controlled trial. BMJ Open 4:e003440. doi:10.1136/bmjopen-2013-003440

Ly KH, Topooco N, Cederlund H, Wallin A, Bergström J, Molander O et al (2015) Smartphone-supported versus full behavioural activation for depression: a randomised controlled trial. PLoS One 10:e0126559. doi:10.1371/journal.pone.0126559

Marks IM, Cavanagh K, Gega L (2007) Hands-on help. Computer-aided psychotherapy (Maudsley monograph no. 49). Psychology Press, Hove

Meyer B, Bierbrodt J, Schröder J, Berger T, Beeverse CG, Weissa M et al (2015) Effects of an internet intervention (Deprexis) on severe depression symptoms: randomized controlled trial. Internet Intervent 2:48–59. doi:10.1016/j.invent.2014.12.003

Mohr DC, Siddique J, Ho J, Duffecy J, Jin L, Fokuo JK (2010) Interest in behavioral and psychological treatments delivered face-to-face, by telephone, and by internet. Ann Behav Med 40:89–98. doi:10.1007/s12160-010-9203-7

Mohr DC, Duffecy J, Ho J, Kwasny M, Cai X, Burns MN et al (2013) A randomized controlled trial evaluating a manualized TeleCoaching protocol for improving adherence to a web-based intervention for the treatment of depression. PLoS One 8(8):e70086. doi:10.1371/journal.pone.0070086

O'Mahen HA, Richards DA, Woodford J, Wilkinson E, McGinley J, Taylor RS et al (2014) Netmums: a phase II randomized controlled trial of a guided Internet behavioural activation treatment for postpartum depression. Psychol Med 44:1675–1689. doi:10.1017/s0033291713002092

Palmqvist B, Carlbring P, Andersson G (2007) Internet-delivered treatments with or without therapist input: does the therapist factor have implications for efficacy and cost? Expert Rev Pharmacoecon Outcomes Res 7:291–297. doi:10.1586/14737167.7.3.291

Perini S, Titov N, Andrews G (2009) Clinician-assisted Internet-based treatment is effective for depression: randomized controlled trial. Aust N Z J Psychiatry 43:571–578. doi:10.1080/00048670902873722

Preschl B, Maercker A, Wagner B (2011) The working alliance in a randomized controlled trial comparing online with face-to-face cognitive-behavioral therapy for depression. BMC Psychiatry 11:189. doi:10.1186/1471-244X-11-189

Richards D, Richardson T (2012) Computer-based psychological treatments for depression: a systematic review and meta-analysis. Clin Psychol Rev 32:329–342. doi:10.1016/j.cpr.2012.02.004

Richardson R, Richards DA, Barkham M (2010) Self-help books for people with depression: the role of the therapeutic relationship. Behav Cogn Psychother 38:67–81

Ruwaard J, Schrieken B, Schrijver M, Broeksteeg J, Dekker J, Vermeulen H et al (2009) Standardized web-based CBT of mild to moderate depression: a randomized controlled trial with a long-term follow-up. Cogn Behav Ther 38:206–221

Ruwaard J, Lange A, Schrieken B, Dolan CV, Emmelkamp P (2012) The effectiveness of online cognitive behavioral treatment in routine clinical practice. PLoS One 7(7):e40089. doi:10.1371/journal.pone.0040089

Saulsberry A, Marko-Holguin M, Blomeke K, Hinkle C, Fogel J, Gladstone T et al (2013) Randomized clinical trial of a primary care internet-based intervention to prevent adolescent depression: one-year outcomes. J Can Acad Child Adolesc Psychiatry 22:106–117

Spijker J, de Graaf R, Bijl RV, Beekman AT, Ormel J, Nolen WA (2002) Duration of major depressive episodes in the general population: results from The Netherlands Mental Health Survey and Incidence Study (NEMESIS). Br J Psychiatry 181:208–213. doi:10.1192/bjp.181.3.208

Ström M, Uckelstam C-J, Andersson G, Hassmén P, Umefjord G, Carlbring P (2013) Internet-delivered therapist-guided physical activity for mild to moderate depression: a randomized controlled trial. PeerJ 1:e178. doi:10.7717/peerj.178

Titov N (2010) Email in low intensity CBT interventions. In: Bennett-Levy J, Christensen H, Farrand P, Griffiths K, Kavanagh D, Klein B et al (eds) Oxford Guide to low intensity CBT interventions. Oxford University Press, Oxford, pp 287–293

Titov N, Andrews G, Davies M, McIntyre K, Robinson E, Solley K (2010) Internet treatment for depression: a randomized controlled trial comparing clinician vs technician assistance. PLoS One 5:e10939. doi:10.1371/journal.pone.0010939

Titov N, Dear BF, Schwencke G, Andrews G, Johnston L, Craske MG et al (2011) Transdiagnostic internet treatment for anxiety and depression: a randomised controlled trial. Behav Res Ther 49:441–452. doi:10.1016/j.brat.2011.03.007

Titov N, Dear BF, Johnston L, Lorian C, Zou J, Wootton B et al (2013) Improving adherence and clinical outcomes in self-guided internet treatment for anxiety and depression: randomised controlled trial. PLoS One 8:e62873. doi:10.1371/journal.pone.0062873

Titov N, Dear BF, Ali S, Zou JB, Lorian CN, Johnston L et al (2015a) Clinical and cost-effectiveness of therapist-guided internet-delivered cognitive behavior therapy for older adults with symptoms of depression: a randomized controlled trial. Behav Ther 46:193–205. doi:10.1016/j.beth.2014.09.008

Titov N, Dear BF, Staples L, Bennett-Levy J, Klein B, Rapee RM et al (2015b) MindSpot Clinic: an accessible, efficient and effective online treatment service for anxiety and depression. Psychiatr Serv 66(10):1043–1050

van Ballegooijen W, Cuijpers P, van Straten A, Karyotaki E, Andersson G, Smit JH et al (2014) Adherence to Internet-based and face-to-face cognitive behavioural therapy for depression: a meta-analysis. PLoS One 9:e100674. doi:10.1371/journal.pone.0100674

van Bastelaar KM, Pouwer F, Cuijpers P, Riper H, Snoek FJ (2011) Web-based depression treatment for type 1 and type 2 diabetic patients: a randomized, controlled trial. Diabetes Care 34:320–325. doi:10.2337/dc10-1248

van der Vaart R, Witting M, Riper H, Kooistra L, Bohlmeijer ET, van Gemert-Pijnen LJ (2014) Blending online therapy into regular face-to-face therapy for depression: content, ratio and preconditions according to patients and therapists using a Delphi study. BMC Psychiatry 14:355. doi:10.1186/s12888-014-0355-z

van Spijker BA, van Straten A, Kerkhof AJ (2014) Effectiveness of online self-help for suicidal thoughts: results of a randomised controlled trial. PLoS One 9:e90118. doi:10.1371/journal.pone.0090118

Van Voorhees BW, Ellis JM, Gollan JK, Bell CC, Stuart SS, Fogel J et al (2007) Development and process evaluation of a primary care Internet-based intervention to prevent depression in emerging adults. Prim Care Companion J Clin Psychiatry 9(5):346–355

van Zoonen K, Buntrock C, Ebert DD, Smit F, Reynolds CF 3rd, Beekman AT et al (2014) Preventing the onset of major depressive disorder: a meta-analytic review of psychological interventions. Int J Epidemiol 43(2):318–329. doi:10.1093/ije/dyt175

Vernmark K, Lenndin J, Bjärehed J, Carlsson M, Karlsson J, Öberg J et al (2010) Internet administered guided self-help versus individualized e-mail therapy: a randomized trial of two versions of CBT for major depression. Behav Res Ther 48:368–376. doi:10.1016/j.brat.2010.01.005

Wagner B, Horn AB, Maercker A (2014) Internet-based versus face-to-face cognitive-behavioral intervention for depression: a randomized controlled non-inferiority trial. J Affect Disord 152–154:113–121. doi:10.1016/j.jad.2013.06.032

Warmerdam L, van Straten A, Twisk J, Riper H, Cuijpers P (2008) Internet-based treatment for adults with depressive symptoms: randomized controlled trial. JMIR 10:e44. doi:10.2196/jmir.1094

Warmerdam L, Smit F, van Straten A, Riper H, Cuijpers P (2010) Cost-utility and cost-effectiveness of internet-based treatment for adults with depressive symptoms: randomized trial. JMIR 12(5):e53. doi:10.2196/jmir.1436

Watts S, Newby JM, Mewton L, Andrews G (2012) A clinical audit of changes in suicide ideas with internet treatment for depression. BMJ Open 2:e001558. doi:10.1136/bmjopen-2012-001558

Williams AD, Andrews G (2013) The effectiveness of Internet cognitive behavioural therapy (ICBT) for depression in primary care: a quality assurance study. PLoS One 8:e57447. doi:10.1371/journal.pone.0057447

Williams AD, Blackwell SE, Mackenzie A, Holmes EA, Andrews G (2013) Combining imagination and reason in the treatment of depression: a randomized controlled trial of internet-based cognitive-bias modification and internet-CBT for depression. J Consult Clin Psychol 81: 793–799. doi:10.1037/a0033247

ICBT for Panic Disorder and Agoraphobia: From the Computer at Home to Real-Life 'In Vivo' Exposure

3

Wouter van Ballegooijen, Britt Klein, and Nils Lindefors

Abstract

Panic disorder with or without agoraphobia (PD/A) is a disabling disorder that involves physical anxiety symptoms, maladaptive cognitions and avoidance behaviour. Internet-based cognitive behavioural therapy (ICBT) can provide accessible mental health care to those who suffer from PD/A, which may increase the uptake of psychological treatment. The literature on ICBT for PD/A shows largely positive results, especially for therapist-guided ICBT among the general population. Unguided ICBT for PD/A is less studied. It has also demonstrated positive results, but is commonly associated with higher attrition than guided ICBT. There is also some evidence that guided ICBT for PD/A is effective for inpatients. Cost-effectiveness of ICBT for PD/A has only been minimally studied, but some evidence indicates it can be cost saving compared with face-to-face CBT. This chapter further describes the existing ICBT programmes for PD/A, a case study and implementation examples from Sweden and Australia. Finally, this chapter discusses the feasibility of minimally guided ICBT and current innovations in ICBT for PD/A, such as the use of mobile technology and virtual reality, and provides future directions for research and development.

W. van Ballegooijen (✉)
Department of Clinical Psychology and Psychiatry, Vrije Universiteit Amsterdam/GGZ inGeest, Amsterdam, The Netherlands
e-mail: w.van.ballegooijen@vu.nl

B. Klein
Department of Psychology, Federation University, Mount Helen, VIC, Australia
e-mail: brittklein@netspace.net.au

N. Lindefors
Department of Clinical Neuroscience, Karolinska Institutet, Solna, Sweden
e-mail: nils.lindefors@ki.se

© Springer International Publishing Switzerland 2016

N. Lindefors, G. Andersson (eds.), *Guided Internet-Based Treatments in Psychiatry*, DOI 10.1007/978-3-319-06083-5_3

Panic Disorder and Agoraphobia

Panic disorder and agoraphobia are common and disabling anxiety disorders with considerable impact on the individual and on society as a whole (Buist-Bouwman et al. 2006; De Graaf et al. 2010; Smit et al. 2006). Panic disorder is characterised by panic attacks that involve physical symptoms, such as breathing difficulties and palpitations, problematic cognitions (e.g. probability over estimations) and constant fear of having a panic attack (World Health Organisation 2014; American Psychiatric Association 2013). Agoraphobia commonly co-occurs with panic disorder and involves avoidance of situations and places where escape would be difficult or embarrassing in case a panic attack happens. Agoraphobia can also occur without panic attacks and can be diagnosed as a separate disorder. Panic disorder with or without agoraphobia is abbreviated as PD/A in this chapter. Lifetime prevalence rates of PD/A or agoraphobia without panic are 3.8 % and 0.9 %, respectively (De Graaf et al. 2010). Twelve-month prevalence rates are 1.2 % and 0.4 %, respectively, in the Netherlands (De Graaf et al. 2010). The 12-month prevalence rate is 2.6 % in Australia (Australian Bureau of Statistics 2007).

Common situations that are avoided by people with PD/A or agoraphobia include driving a car, going to the supermarket and travelling by public transportation. Therefore, ICBT, which can be accessed flexibly such as from one's home, has the potential of high acceptability for this group and may increase the uptake of psychological treatment. In this chapter, we give an overview of the literature about ICBT for PD/A and agoraphobia. Challenges, innovations and future directions will also be discussed.

Existing ICBT Programmes for Panic Disorder and Agoraphobia

Several studies describe Internet interventions for PD/A and agoraphobia. These interventions are based on cognitive behavioural therapy (CBT) and guided by a therapist or coach.

Panic Online

Panic Online was developed at Federation University Australia by Klein and colleagues in the late 1990s. It has been trialled vigorously on multiple occasions (e.g. Kiropoulos et al. 2008; Klein et al. 2006, 2008, 2009; Klein and Richards 2001; Pier et al. 2008; Richards et al. 2006; Shandley et al. 2008) with all studies attesting to its efficacy. The Panic Online programme consists of six core panic modules that are drawn from CBT treatment principles of panic disorder. These include psychoeducation, self-monitoring panic and anxiety, controlled breathing, progressive muscle relaxation, negative cognitions (probability over estimations and catastrophising), exposure to panic sensations and situations as well as relapse prevention. The programme makes use of interactivity on the Internet through the use of audio relaxation recordings, flash interactives, pictorial exposure exercises, provision of PDFs, online self-monitoring forms and use of email communications (for the therapist-assisted versions). Module length varies, but on average, each module is about eight web pages in length.

Panic Stop!

Panic Stop! was developed by Klein and colleagues in 2009 at Swinburne University, Australia, as part of a Federal Government grant to build a virtual psychological clinic (initially called Anxiety Online, now called Mental Health Online). Mental Health Online offers free self-guided CBT treatment for the anxiety disorders following automated psychological assessment via e-PASS internationally. e-PASS is an online self-report diagnostic assessment tool that assesses for 21 DSM-IV-TR (APA 2000) disorders and serves as the gateway into the self-help and therapist-assisted online programmes. e-PASS is automated and consists of over 540 items directly using the criteria specified in the DSM-IV-TR (APA 2000). In addition to addressing 21 DSM-IV-TR (APA 2000) disorders, it also screens for suicidal ideation and distorted thinking and checks for whether substance affects or medical conditions may better account for reported symptoms. e-PASS was designed to help consumers identify whether they are experiencing difficulties within a range of psychological symptoms and disorders and to ensure they were offered an appropriate online treatment programme based on their reported symptoms (see Klein et al. 2011 for a more detailed account). Panic Stop! is a longer, extended version of Panic Online consisting of 12 modules (as per Panic Online but typically two modules for each one from Panic Online). Panic Stop! includes numerous interactives, dynamic self-monitoring of panic and mood, numerous audio instructions (e.g. breathing control, PMR, mindfulness) and video-based exposure exercises (e.g. going over a bridge, entering a store, using public transport), homework instructions and email reminders. Module length varies, but on average, each module is 20 web pages in length. The evidence to date also suggests that Panic Stop! (self-guided version) is effective for panic (Klein et al. 2011) as well as co-morbid depression (AL-Asadi et al. 2014).

Internet Psychiatry Clinic

The Internet Psychiatry Clinic in Stockholm provides guided ICBT treatments in Swedish for depression, social anxiety disorder and PD/A. The PD/A treatment consists of ten modules and is supposed to extend over three months divided into ten separate and succeeding treatment modules. During treatment, communication between therapist and patient is executed using a web-based platform also containing treatment module information, facilities for self-assessments and various other means for support of the process (Hedman et al. 2013). The treatment consists of the following parts: (1) psychoeducation on anxiety, panic disorder and cognitive behaviour therapy; (2) identifying negative automatic thoughts, the vicious circle of thoughts, emotions and internal focus; (3) cognitive restructuring; (4–5) interoceptive exposure; (6–8) agoraphobic exposure; (9) recapitulating of all previous modules; and (10) relapse prevention. As soon as a treatment module is evaluated by the patient and therapist, the therapist releases the next module. Outcome is monitored and measured by pre- to post-measures during clinic visits and by a web-based 6-month follow-up. In addition, weekly self-assessments are collected via the treatment platform including PDSS-SR and MADRS-S (Montgomery Åsberg Depression rating Scale-Self-report; Svanborg and Åsberg 1994).

The Uppsala Model

The ICBT intervention described by Carlbring et al. (2006) consists of ten modules (modules 1–2, psychoeducation and socialisation; module 3, breathing retraining and hyperventilation test; modules 4–5, cognitive restructuring; modules 6–7, interoceptive exposure; modules 8–9, exposure in vivo; and finally, module 10, relapse prevention and assertiveness training). Each module consists of approximately 25 pages, includes information and exercises and ends with three to eight essay questions. Also included in each module is an interactive multiple-choice quiz, which has to be answered correctly in order to proceed. Otherwise, the participants receive immediate automatic feedback and the correct answer with an extensive explanation.

Open Unguided CBT Programme

This ICBT intervention (Farvolden et al. 2005) is an unguided version. The essential components include orientation to the cognitive behavioural model of panic disorder and agoraphobia, goal setting, exposure work exercises, cognitive restructuring, interoceptive exposure work, relaxation training and information about lifestyle change and stress management. Participants are assigned homework to complete each week, and at the beginning of each module, they are asked to respond to a number of questions about their symptoms, homework and progress to date (weekly review). These results as well as the results from the dynamic exercises completed during each module are stored in the user's Session Diary and can be viewed by the user at any time.

The Panic Programme

The Panic programme (Wims et al. 2010) consists of four components: six online modules, homework assignments, participation in an online discussion forum and regular email contact with a mental health clinician. The six online modules represent best practice principles used in CBT programmes for PD/A. Part of the content of each module is presented in the form of an illustrated story about a woman with panic and agoraphobia, who, with the help of a therapist, learns how to gain mastery over her symptoms. Principles and techniques of CBT described in the Panic programme include psychoeducation, graded exposure, cognitive restructuring, physiological de-arousal and relapse prevention. Each module includes a printable summary of the module and homework assignment. Participants can post messages and homework assignments on a secure and confidential online discussion forum, using an alias. This forum is moderated by a clinician. After completing each module, participants are also emailed by the therapist.

Interapy

The Panic programme of Interapy (Ruwaard et al. 2010) is also based on CBT. Compared with other interventions for PD/A, Interapy was designed to be more similar to face-to-face CBT. The treatment comprises homework assignments and scheduled therapeutic sessions, in which assignments are explained and tailored to the needs of the client. The homework assignments are based on a personal interactive workbook. At specific occasions indicated in the manual, therapists post feedback and further instructions on the basis of the contents of this workbook. Therapists take about 20–40 min to read a client's assignment and to prepare feedback. The manual includes 14 of these feedback sessions, so that a full treatment requires between 5 and 9 h of therapist time. Treatment integrity is high given the use of a computerised manual stipulating each step during treatment, including the order, the nature, and the contents of the assignments, and the timing of therapist feedback. Furthermore, the manual provides feedback templates, which the therapists adapt to the needs of their clients. These templates include suggested course of action given various scenarios, such as problems in completing a given assignment. The approximate duration of treatment is 11 weeks, in which clients work through seven treatment modules. During these 11 weeks, participants keep a panic diary and receive psychoeducation, awareness training, applied relaxation, cognitive restructuring and (interoceptive) exposure techniques. The programme includes several written assignments, such as writing a letter of advice to a hypothetical friend coping with similar fears and panic attacks.

Tailored ICBT for PD/A

In the study of Silfvernagel et al. (2012), a tailored ICBT intervention is described that can be tailored to the symptoms of the participant and contains content of various previous ICBT interventions for anxiety disorders and depression. The first module (introduction) and the last module (relapse prevention) are fixed, and the following 17 are optional for the therapists to prescribe: cognitive restructuring (2 modules), panic disorder (2 modules), agoraphobia (1 module), generalised anxiety (3 modules), social anxiety (2 modules), behavioural activation (2 modules), applied relaxation (1 module), stress (1 module), mindfulness (1 module), problem solving (1 module) and insomnia (1 module). The modules are all based on established and evidence-based CBT components. The panic modules consist of psychoeducation and interoceptive exposure. All modules include psychoeducation; most contain exposure exercises, and some contain behavioural experiments depending on the content. All modules include homework assignments, which consist of questions on the psychoeducational sections and tasks for the participant to complete, such as exposure exercises. The authors aimed to prescribe 6 to 8 modules within an 8-week time frame for each participant. A typical prescription for a participant could be an introduction, cognitive restructuring 1 and 2, panic disorder 1 and 2, agoraphobia, applied relaxation and relapse prevention.

Don't Panic Online

Don't Panic Online (DPO) is a Dutch, guided ICBT course (Van Ballegooijen et al. 2011, 2013). It was developed by the Trimbos Institute, which is the Netherlands Institute for Mental Health and Addiction, in collaboration with GGNet, a Dutch mental healthcare institute. The course's format was based on Colour Your Life, an evidence-based Internet intervention for depressive symptoms (Warmerdam et al. 2008; Spek et al. 2008), while the content was based on a face-to-face group treatment called Don't Panic (Meulenbeek et al. 2005, 2010). DPO consists of six modules, in which the participants learn to control their panic symptoms by applying various cognitive and behavioural techniques and skills. Each module consists of text, voice-over, animated diagrams and video. The pace of the voice-over and animation parts is set. A typical module takes about 30 min to walk through and contains an introduction, a discussion of the previous module's homework, new theory and homework for the following week. The course is designed to be followed on a weekly basis until module five, while the sixth module can be followed 4 weeks after the fifth. The course can be completed in 8 weeks, but participants were allowed to take 3 months. Besides the modules, the participants had several online resources available to them: a homework station, a panic attack log, a library for extra information, reading tips and a discussion board.

Participants in DPO start with information about panic attacks, anxiety, hyperventilation, sources of stress and the influence of lifestyle. This information is based on CBT, so it is explained that anxious thoughts, feelings and behaviour can create a vicious cycle. The participants keep track of their panic attacks in the panic attack log. The course further includes relaxation exercises and cognitive restructuring. Participants learn to challenge thoughts that enable feelings of panic, to replace these thoughts by more realistic, constructive thoughts that reduce anxiety and are instructed to practise this. There are also interoceptive exposure exercises, where participants actively induce panic symptoms, for example, by making themselves dizzy or holding their breath, to get used to these physical panic-like sensations. In the final stage, participants perform exposure in vivo by ranking activities from manageable to difficult and carrying them out in order of difficulty. The final module is followed 4 weeks after the fifth and addresses relapse prevention.

Effects in Research and Clinic

Overview of the Literature

Internet interventions for PD/A have been studied extensively. Overall effect sizes of guided ICBT interventions are favourable when compared with a control group (Hedge's $g=0.84$; Andrews et al. 2010). provides an overview of randomised controlled trials of guided ICBT for PD/A. Other studies have shown that guided ICBT for PD/A could be just as efficacious as gold standard face-to-face CBT (Kiropoulos et al. 2008), that the frequency of therapist contact by email does not make a difference in efficacy (Klein et al. 2009) and that email support from a psychologist can be equally efficacious as face-to-face support from a general practitioner (Shandley et al. 2009; Pier et al. 2008). ICBT has been compared with group-administered CBT in a randomised controlled trial being equally effective (Bergström et al. 2010). Adding a stress management component to ICBT for PD/A could result in better clinical outcomes immediately post-treatment, compared with ICBT alone (Richards et al. 2006), although this study found no difference at longer-term follow-up. Other studies have investigated transdiagnostic-guided ICBT for several anxiety disorders, sometimes also including depression. These interventions can consist of a fixed order of modules with generic content (e.g. Titov et al. 2011) or consist of optional modules where the participants follow the applicable ones (Carlbring et al. 2011). Transdiagnostic ICBT seems a useful development, considering anxiety disorders often coincide with each other and with depression (Kessler et al. 2005). These studies show favourable outcomes (Carlbring et al. 2011; Titov et al. 2011), also for PD/A specifically.

Unguided (or self-help) ICBT for PD/A has also been investigated, but less so than therapist assisted. Unguided ICBT has been studied in both naturalistic fully automated open-access studies and uncontrolled quasi-experimental studies (Farvolden et al. 2005; Klein et al. 2008, 2011; AL-Asadi et al. 2014). Naturalistic, fully automated open access studies (Farvolden et al. 2005; Klein et al. 2011; AL-Asadi et al. 2014) do not involve any involvement (i.e. screening, assessment, therapy) between the researchers and participants. The programme involves sophisticated programming so that the participant is guided through the entire programme via automated mechanisms. The results from these fully automated studies indicate that participants display a reduction in their panic symptoms at post-assessment (Farvolden et al. 2005; Klein et al. 2011; AL-Asadi et al. 2014) and reductions in psychological distress, panic and depression clinical severity and increases in self-confidence in managing their mental health care (Klein et al. 2011; AL-Asadi et al. 2014). Despite large intake numbers in all three studies, only a small percentage completed the post-treatment questionnaires.

When it comes to the use of ICBT for PD/A in clinical practice, two studies have investigated the feasibility and effectiveness of guided ICBT in this setting (Bergström et al. 2010; Hedman et al. 2013). Hedman et al. (2013) concluded that ICBT for PD/A could be as effective when delivered in a routine care context as in the previously published randomised controlled trials. Bergström et al. (2010) conducted a randomised controlled trial among inpatients in a psychiatry clinic and demonstrated that there was very little difference in efficacy between ICBT and an active gold standard control treatment with group-administered CBT.

Overall, these studies show promising results for guided and unguided ICBT for PD/A and also show some evidence that these interventions could be effective in clinical practice. The open-access fully automated nature of the unguided ICBT programmes could offer considerable cost benefits, but treatment acceptability and attrition are typically more of an issue than guided versions.

Don't Panic Online

Although most of the published randomised controlled trials show significant effects for guided ICBT for PD/A (Table 3.1), the effect sizes of these studies vary from each other to a large degree. One study shows a between-groups effect that is not significant (Van Ballegooijen et al. 2013), i.e. participants in the intervention did not improve significantly more than the participants on a waiting list. Completers-only analysis however did show that the outcome results were comparable to the other studies in Table 1 (Cohen's $d=0.60–0.94$), but due to the large number of dropouts, whose post-treatment scores were conservatively estimated by multiple imputation, the intention-to-treat analysis showed a non-significant effect. There are many factors that could affect the rate of treatment adherence, such as the content of the intervention, the technical aspects of the intervention, the type of guidance, the study procedures and the characteristics of the recruited sample. By taking a detailed look at this study (Van Ballegooijen et al. 2011; 2013), it might be possible to form a hypothesis about the low treatment adherence.

The intervention Don't Panic Online (DPO) has been described above. The participants in the intervention group were coached by Master's-level Clinical Psychology students who had received brief training and were supervised by one of the investigators. It should be noted that in the Netherlands, Master's-level Clinical Psychology students have very little practical experience. Every week, the participants received an email from their coach, asking how they were doing and whether they were experiencing any difficulty in following the programme. The coaches responded to questions about the course and the associated exercises. They were instructed to reply only briefly to questions about the participant's mental health. Participants were supported for a maximum of 3 months. The total weekly time spent on each participant differed considerably per participant and per week, but on average, it took between 5 and 10 min.

Participants in the randomised controlled trial were recruited from the general population, mostly from websites. Inclusion criteria were being aged 18 and above, mild to moderate panic symptoms (a score of 5–15 on the Panic Disorder Severity Scale-Self Report; PDSS-SR) and no or low suicide risk. No restrictions were imposed on diagnosis or the use of pharmacotherapy or psychotherapy. Of 368 applicants, 126 met these criteria and were randomly allocated to the intervention

Table 3.1 Randomised controlled trials of guided ICBT for panic disorder with or without agoraphobia

Author (year)	*N*	*n*	Conditions	Effect size (Cohen's *d*) between groups posttreatment	Drop-out *n* (%)
Carlbring (2001)	31	±15	ICBT	ICBT > Control, $d = \pm 1.44$ (BSQ)	4 (27 %)
		±15	WL		
Carlbring (2006)	60	30	ICBT	ICBT > Control, $d = 1.97$ (BSQ)	1 (3 %)
		30	WL		
Klein (2001)	23	11	ICBT	ICBT > Control	1 (9 %)
		12	Self-monitoring		
Klein (2006)	37	19	ICBT	ICBT > Control, $d = 2.52$ (PDSS)	1 (5 %)
		18	Information		
Richards (2006)	21	12	ICBT	ICBT > Control, $d = 1.36$ (PDSS)	2 (17 %)
		9	Information		
Ruwaard (2010)	58	27	ICBT	ICBT>Control, $d = 0.55$ (PDSS-SR)	3 (11 %)
		31	WL		
Silfvernagel (2012)	57	29	ICBT (tailored)	ICBT > Control, $d = 1.39$ (PDSS)	12 (41 %) <50 % sessions
		28	WL		
Van Ballegooijen (2013)	126	63	ICBT	ICBT = Control, $d = 0.30^{NS}$ (PDSS-SR)	46 (73 %) <67 % sessions
		63	WL		
Wims (2010)	59	29	ICBT	ICBT > Control, $d = 0.59$ (PDSS)	6 (21 %)
		25	WL		
Point estimate of pooled effect sizes				$d = 1.21$	

BSQ body sensations questionnaire, *ICBT* internet-based cognitive behavioural therapy, *NS* not significant, *PDSS* panic disorder severity scale, *PDSS-SR* panic disorder severity scale-self report, *WL* waiting list

($n = 63$) or to the control group ($n = 63$). Participants in the control group received access to DPO after completing the post-treatment measurement (3 months after baseline), although they did not receive guidance. While waiting, they had access to a website that contained information about the symptoms of panic and agoraphobia. This website included advice to contact a general practitioner, in case the participant had further questions about panic symptoms and its treatment. All of the participants in the control group and the intervention group were free to seek any (additional) help they might require. In the intervention group, 34 of 63 participants (54 %) completed the post-treatment questionnaires. Slightly more participants in the control group completed the post-treatment questionnaires (39 of 63 or 62 %).

As mentioned above, the intention-to-treat analyses did not yield a significant effect, while the completers-only analyses did. Completers were not actually full completers, but had completed the first four modules (or more) of the course ($n = 17$). Sixteen of these 17 participants also filled in post-treatment questionnaires. A track-and-trace system kept a record of the dates on which participants completed a module. Figure 3.1 shows the adherence of the intervention (guided) group and the waiting-control (unguided) group. Four participants in the intervention group (6 %) completed all six modules within 3 months. There were 30 participants in the intervention group who did respond to the post-treatment measurement but did not complete all six modules. These participants were asked why they had not finished. The most frequently reported reasons involved time constraints ($n = 13$), life events ($n = 5$) and symptoms so severe that the individual was unable to follow the programme (or parts thereof) or carry out the homework assignments ($n = 5$).

The treatment adherence was lower in the study on DPO than in previous studies of guided Internet interventions for PD/A (Table 3.1). There are a number of possible explanations (see Van Ballegooijen et al. 2013), where the type of guidance could be a main factor that explains the low adherence. When viewing Fig. 3.1, there is only a small difference between the adherence of participants in the guided intervention group and the participants in the unguided group that started once they completed their 3-month wait. This indicates that the guidance had little impact on the adherence. The adherence rate of both groups more closely resembles the figures of unguided Internet interventions for PD/A (Farvolden et al. 2005; Klein et al. 2011) than the adherence rates of previous studies of guided ICBT for PD/A. A completion rate of 1 % or 10 % is reported in the studies on unguided ICBT (Farvolden et al. 2005; Klein et al. 2011). As described above, the guidance to DPO was supposed to be minimal and focussed on retaining participants' motivation. Questions about the participant's mental health were only briefly addressed. Possibly, such minimal coaching is not sufficient to support participants in ICBT for PD/A and interaction with a therapist is needed. This is further discussed in the Discussion section of this chapter.

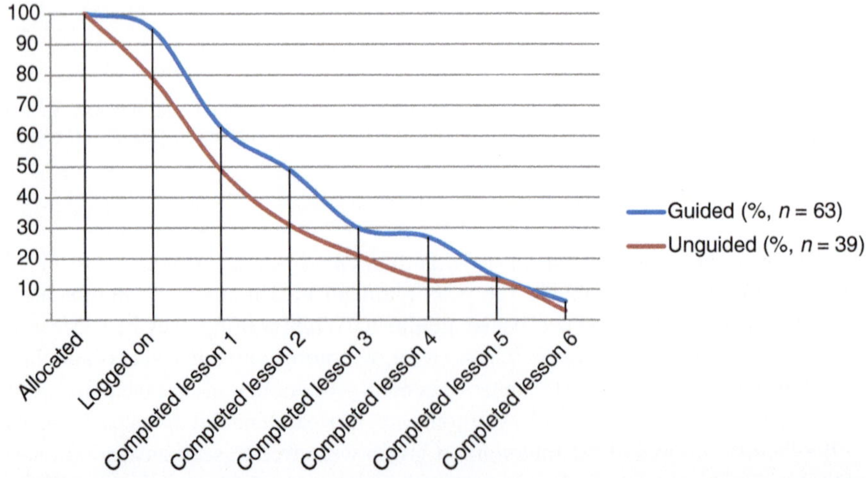

Fig. 3.1 Adherence to Don't Panic Online of the intervention group (guided) and the control group (unguided) in percentages

Panic Online Case Description

Below we will feature a case study on one participant's treatment experience (Lisa – not her real name) while undertaking the Panic Online therapist-assisted ICBT programme.

General Comments Around ICBT Programme Design and Content

The online therapist is an important factor, apart from how an ICBT programme is designed (e.g. navigation style, use and mixture of multimedia), module delivery (e.g. full access to all modules from the start, or sequentially released on a weekly basis), how the content is ordered (e.g. following a traditional CBT format for panic – physiological, cognition and behaviour or some other variant) and the tone of the content (e.g. whether it promotes feelings of self-efficacy, or motivation to persevere when things become more difficult). It is imperative the online therapist builds rapport from the first day and also consistently encourages and motivates participants, especially when working through the more confronting aspects of treatment. Participant concerns, anxieties and fears need to be monitored vigilantly via the participant self-monitoring forms, 'forensically' examining participant responses (and non-responses) within participant emails, as well as asking participants directly through therapist emails.

Modules 1 and 2

The first two modules of Panic Online provide panic and anxiety psychoeducation, treatment rationale building, building self-efficacy as well as introducing self-monitoring. Like many people with panic, Lisa talked about feeling overwhelmed by the prospect of starting the programme because this meant that she had to '*face her fears*'. On the other hand, Lisa admitted that she felt comforted by the online nature of the treatment. In the back of her mind, she knew that she could always close the programme '*if it got too rough or scary*'.

During the first 2 weeks of ICBT treatment, rapport was established quickly via email communications. Lisa also reported back how she went with the offline panic and mood-monitoring activities. A summary of these activities was also available to the therapist after participants submitted their self-monitoring forms via the system. At the end of the second week, Lisa reported that she felt better able to see her panic attack sequence profile and how her mood affected the frequency and severity of her panic attacks. Lisa reported feeling '*more in control*' as she could now identify the conditions where her panic attacks were more likely to occur and what the specific triggers were.

Module 3

Module 3 focuses on the physiological component – namely, relaxation. This relaxation consists of learning how to be calm and relaxed by teaching breathing control exercises and progressive muscle relaxation (PMR) via written instruction, downloadable audio guidance and exercise self-monitoring forms. Lisa also accessed some of the additional resources in the Panic Online programme (on assertiveness and time management). During the two weeks, Lisa reported back how she went with the online and offline activities, i.e. continuation with self-monitoring panic and mood, breathing control exercises and PMR practice sessions. As many of the Panic Online participants reported during the trials, Lisa also talked about how the breathing control method was the most control enabling and enjoyable technique she learnt. As discussed below, participants also reported that the exposure exercises were also very effective, but the most confronting and thus generally far less enjoyable.

Module 4

The fourth module focuses on the cognition component of panic including information about the panic cycle, understanding negative thoughts and probability over estimations, catastrophic thinking, challenging and modifying self-statements and making things more predictable. Lisa was very vigilant with the cognitive restructuring exercises and would try to catch and rate the probability of as many automatic thoughts as she could and would then generate more realistic alternatives. Lisa shared her cognitive restructuring self-monitoring forms and they were discussed via email. By the end of the programme, Lisa's scores when estimating the likelihood of her unhelpful thoughts fall from 100 to 90 % down to 1–2 %. Lisa reported feeling more and more able to generate more helpful and realistic alternative thoughts and how '*different the world looked*' once she had mastered this. Once Lisa was confident in her understanding and use of breathing control, PMR and challenging her unhelpful thoughts, she progressed to Module 5.

Module 5

The fifth module focuses on the behavioural component of panic, namely, learning about and implementing exposure techniques in a graded fashion (interoceptive, imaginal/visual and in vivo exposure). The gradual nature and timing of these exposure activities were discussed via email.

Lisa reported finding breathing through a straw and spinning in a chair the most difficult interoceptive exposure exercises. However, once Lisa successfully completed all of the exercises (distress score rating was 2/8 or lower on several occasions), she was encouraged to do some imaginal exposure exercises of real-life situations that she had been avoiding due to panic. Lisa decided to use the 'visiting the supermarket' example for her imaginal exposure exercise. Written instructions were provided within the programme, and once Lisa was able to do this on several occasions with a distress score of 2 or less, she progressed to the visual photographic representation of walking into the store, down the aisles, picking up some items and then heading back to the register and paying for the items. Lisa continued to use the pictorial visualisation exposure sequence until her distress score was 2 or less on several occasions. Other examples provided in the programme included driving a car and using public transport.

Following on from this, instructions were provided via the programme about how to do in vivo exposure exercises. Discussion of where, when, and what she would buy, use of breathing control, challenging thoughts, etc., were also communicated via email before Lisa went to the supermarket.

Lisa then proceeded to undertake the in vivo exposure task and reported back once she had completed the first exposure exercise. She admitted she felt rather overwhelmed, although she managed to stay in the supermarket and buy the items discussed. Further, email exchanges continued around encouraging and supporting Lisa with her next supermarket exposure practice sessions. After 2 weeks of continued practice, Lisa was able to enter a large shopping centre with minimal levels of anxiety. Although Lisa did report that during the sixth supermarket practice exercise, she experienced a mild panic attack; she reported that it no longer engendered the same paralysing fear that it did 2 months ago and that she was able to continue shopping without prematurely leaving the store. Lisa commented that she felt this was a '*necessary evil*' for her to experience because she was able to manage both high anxiety and a panic attack without feeling the need to escape. At the end of Module 5, Lisa also commented that doing the exposure exercises helped her to '*retrain her body and mind*' and in doing so she started to feel *'safe once again'*.

Module 6

Module 6 is a standard relapse prevention and planning module. After working though this module, Lisa mentioned that she now possessed the tools required to deal with a reoccurrence of heightened anxiety and panic. If it did, she would view this as a sign that there is something for her to address and work on, rather than a failure (and thinking… *'oh no...here we go again'*).

Lisa also reported that in her plan she would continue with PMR (Lisa reported that she found PMR far more useful than medication) and exposure exercises of more distal avoidance behaviours (e.g. Lisa had not travelled on a plane for several years due to panic, she had not played sport, etc.).

General Comments

Lisa commented that the programme and therapist email discussions helped her to realise that until she faced her thoughts and beliefs, she felt she could not move on. Instead, she felt like she was stuck in a holding pattern of *'not living'* as she was consumed by her panic and anxiety. Lisa reported gaining increasing confidence over the course of the programme, even though it was '*tough*' and '*hard bloody work*'. Lisa admitted that here were tears and fears but also much happiness. Lisa also said that doing the Panic Online programme was an amazing journey for her and that her life had changed – in that she felt she had taken back the power, felt a new sense of freedom, greater confidence, felt less depressed, was able to smile and laugh again, felt lighter and up for the challenges that life would throw her way. Lisa acknowledged that given the nature of the treatment (online, accessible 24/7, self-paced and having a therapist 'on the side' to guide and support her), she felt less overwhelmed by the ‘thought’ of therapy in the initial stages and thus more able to engage with the more challenging aspects later into the programme.

Online delivery of treatment programmes, especially self-guided ICBT, does make it easy for participants to simply switch off the computer and not interact with a programme. This may be a core reason for the high attrition rates observed early in the treatment cycle. However, at the same time, some participants report that just knowing they can ‘just switch it off’ paradoxically appears to give them the confidence to switch it on in the first critical week. Once the participants ‘expose’ themselves to the treatment programme and its process, some participants report no longer thinking about ‘switching it off’. This may suggest that first impressions count significantly with respect to continued engagement. Therefore, developers should invest considerable time thinking about how best, upon the very first log on, to positively induce, encourage and lessen participant feelings of being overwhelmed by the process of therapy. If we fail to achieve this, there appears to be a much greater likelihood that many participants will never return to the programme (especially when self-guided) following the first log on (as also illustrated in Fig. 3.1 above).

Cost-Effectiveness

There is little evidence published about the cost-effectiveness of ICBT for PD/A. However, very basic cost benefits for Panic Online were calculated in the Klein et al. (2006) study. This study compared three conditions: Panic Online with an email therapist, the provision of a structured CBT workbook with weekly telephone therapy sessions and an information control condition (psychoeducation only). Costs per person were calculated in terms of therapist time and running costs (e.g. webhosting, manual cost, telephone call costs). Costs per person were AU $350 vs. AUS $378 vs. AU $55, respectively. Although the equivalent face-to-face psychological therapy treatment costs were not calculated, delivering a standard face-to-face treatment for PD/A would have cost at least AU $800 in 2003.

The Anxiety Online/Mental Health Online international virtual psychology clinic can be cost saving as well. Comparing assessment and therapeutic costs using the Australian Psychological Society schedule of recommended fees for psychological services, human labour in a face-to-face setting would have cost AU $8.7 million for the work done to date by Anxiety Online/Mental Health Online (Klein et al. 2011). This estimation excludes the cost of developing Anxiety Online. The cost of development and ongoing maintenance of the virtual clinic from October 2009 to April 2011 has been close to AU $2.0 million, with the majority of this amount being a one-off development cost (AU $1.66 million). The labour time cost saving resulting from the Anxiety Online service in the first year and half of operation was estimated at AU $6.7 million. Given that the start-up costs would not be recurring expenses, the cost savings would be greater over time.

Cost-effectiveness for ICBT has been examined at the Internet Psychiatry Clinic in Stockholm as a secondary study aim. In a randomised controlled trial where ICBT was shown similarly effective for inpatients with PD/A symptoms compared with face-to-face group CBT, ICBT was four times more cost-effective with respect to therapist time (Bergström et al. (2010).

Clinical Implementation and Dissemination

Anxiety Online/Mental Health Online (see Klein et al. 2011 for more information) is offered to the international public for free. It currently consists of psychoeducation and service referral information, online psychological assessment, healthcare practitioner portal access and eTherapist training and self-guided ICBT treatment for PD/A, GAD, SAD, PTSD and OCD. It has also offered ICBT for depression, insomnia and bulimia nervosa and a transdiagnostic early intervention programme for young gay and lesbian adults with anxiety and/or depression, although until now only in research setting. Therapist assistance is also available, but only to Australian residents. Therapist assistance can occur via email and it has the capabilities of offering instant messaging, Internet telephony, video chat and virtual reality environment chats. From October 2009 to June 2013, Mental Health Online had received 16,999 registered clients that undertook the online psychological assessment, with 6249 commencing one of the five anxiety disorder treatment programmes.

The Internet Psychiatry Clinic in Stockholm (www.internetpsychiatry.se) has provided clinical routine-guided ICBT for PD/A for a bit more than a thousand individuals when this text is accomplished. The Stockholm County comprises more than 2.1 million individuals and the county is at present a catchment area for ICBT at the clinic. Most patients in the programme (Hedman et al. 2013) are self-referred via a web-based procedure. That selection procedure may possibly allow an advantage for individual incentive to complete the programme. However, individuals referred from other units in the healthcare systems are most welcome. Figure 3.2

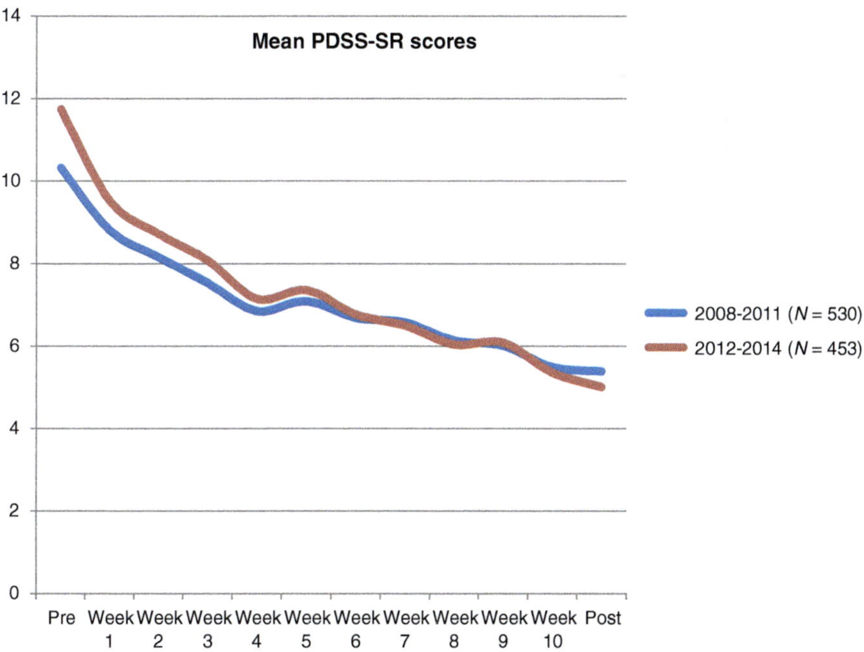

Fig. 3.2 Pre-and post-treatments and weekly self-assessments using the PDSS-SR from the first 983 patients treated for PD/A at the Internet Psychiatry Clinic in Stockholm. Results are divided in two groups with respect to treatment years

provides information from self-assessments for the first 983 treated individuals, pre- and post-treatments as well as weekly. The effect seems to be stable with a trend towards increasing within subject increase in effect size.

Analysis of predictors for ICBT at the Internet Psychiatry Clinic indicates that lower work impairment and higher anxiety sensitivity index (ASI) precede better effect, i.e. lowering of PDSS scores from pre- to post-treatment (El Alaoui et al. 2013).

Discussion and Future Challenges

In general, the literature demonstrates that guided ICBT is efficacious in research settings and it seems to be as effective as live CBT for inpatients, but evidence around its cost-effectiveness is lacking. Clinical implementation of guided ICBT for PD/A is promising, but detailed evaluations of implementation and dissemination are scarce. Unguided ICBT has been studied less often. Although the treatment adherence can be low, unguided ICBT can be disseminated on a larger scale. Research and development of both guided and unguided ICBT should be encouraged.

ICBT for PD/A Without Therapist Contact

The study on Don't Panic Online and the small difference between the adherence of the guided and the unguided group (Fig. 3.1) suggest that ICBT for PD/A with coaching instead of therapist contact entails the same problem of low adherence as unguided ICBT. A meta-analytic review of computerised CBT for depression (Richards and Richardson 2012) showed that adherence rates may be related to the type and intensity of guidance provided. On the other hand, two trials of ICBT for depression and generalised anxiety disorder that investigated types of guidance, Titov et al. (2010) and Robinson et al. (2010), found no differences in efficacy or adherence when guidance was provided by a clinician versus a technician.

While coaching by someone who is not a therapist may be sufficient, in terms of adherence, for ICBT for depression and generalised anxiety, this may not be the case for ICBT for PD/A. As described earlier, PD/A is characterised by physical symptoms and avoidance of places and situations. Important components of CBT for PD/A are interoceptive exposure and in vivo exposure. Here participants are instructed to actively confront their panic symptoms and the situations and places that they avoid, and when a panic attack occurs, attempt to gain control of their symptoms. Such exercises could be difficult to carry out with no or minimal therapist support and may result in a higher incidence rate of attrition.

Despite the indications of low adherence associated with ICBT for PD/A without therapist contact, it remains an interesting field to explore. Both require less therapist resources than ICBT with more intense guidance. It may prove profitable to place greater research efforts around what other factors may increase adherence via stronger design and technological innovations. Developers are encouraged to focus more on 'first impressions' at the commencement of ICBT, to minimise early dropout. Additionally, developers also need to consider when and how to deliver exposure exercises, so the step from the computer at home to the exposure is not too great.

Future Directions

It is reasonable to expect that ICBT for PD/A will be profitable, but more research and development is needed for success. Technological innovations may be able to increase the uptake and effect of ICBT for PD/A. These innovations may include the use of persuasive technology (i.e. technology designed to include persuasion and social influence (Kelders et al. 2012)) and the use of mobile technology and elements of virtual reality. Lindner et al. (2013) describe a trial protocol for ICBT with a smartphone app for PD/A and social anxiety disorder. The app is integrated with the exercises from the Internet-based treatment modules and was designed to keep track of the participant's behaviour and reflections on the behaviour (Lindner et al. 2013). Another ongoing study (Ebenfeld et al. 2014) applies a smartphone app as augmentation to ICBT, which consists of a diary for self-monitoring and an exposure guide that supports participants in performing exposure (Ebenfeld et al. 2014). By combining ICBT and mobile technology, the ICBT treatment is integrated in the daily life of the participants and can be taken to fearful places and situations.

Another innovation in the field of CBT for PD/A is virtual reality exposure therapy (VRET). Currently, VRET can only be used in face-to-face settings, because it involves specific hardware and software and guidance by the clinician. A systematic review (Meyerbröker and Emmelkamp 2010) describes a few small trials that show that VRET could be just as effective as CBT and exposure in vivo for PD/A and agoraphobia (Botella et al. 2007; Peñate et al. 2008; Pitti et al. 2007). However, in a later study, Meyerbröker et al. (2013) argue that VRET is not a useful substitute for in vivo exposure because it could be slightly less effective and entails more costs. At the moment, it would be difficult to apply VRET to Internet interventions due to the technological equipment and in-person support it needs (e.g. Meyerbröker et al. 2013). Attempts have been made to adapt a VRET programme to be run on a personal computer (Alcañiz et al. 2003), but there do not seem to be any studies published that tested such a programme. It is foreseeable that VRET for a personal computer could take the form of an applied game. Elements of VRET could be a valuable addition to ICBT for PD/A, where it could be a useful step before in vivo exposure. It would enable the participant to practise applying the learned skills in difficult situations, while staying in a safe and controlled place.

Besides technological innovations, future research could investigate which elements of ICBT for PD/A are especially effective and which elements may be left out. A challenge for ICBT for PD/A remains the gap between reading information and instructions on a screen and controlling the physical symptoms when confronting one's fears in vivo. Perhaps elements of VRET can bridge this gap, and mobile technology could enable the participant to take the ICBT to the places and situations where it is most needed. Continued development and investigation of ICBT for PD/A and agoraphobia are necessary to optimise the adherence and clinical effect.

References

AL-Asadi AM, Klein B, Meyer D (2014) Posttreatment attrition and its predictors, attrition bias, and treatment efficacy of the anxiety online programs. J Med Internet Res 16(10):e232

Alcañiz M, Botella C, Baños R, Perpiñá C, Rey B, Lozano JA, Guillén V, Barrera F, Gil JA (2003) Internet-based telehealth system for the treatment of agoraphobia. CyberPsychol Behav 6(4):355–358

American Psychiatric Association (2000) Diagnostic and statistical manual of mental disorders: DSM-IV-TR. 4th edition, text revision. American Psychiatric Association, Washington, DC

American Psychiatric Association (2013) Diagnostic and statistical manual of mental disorders, 5th edn. Author, Washington, DC

Andrews G, Cuijpers P, Craske MG, McEvoy P, Titov N (2010) Computer therapy for the anxiety and depressive disorders is effective, acceptable and practical health care: a meta-analysis. PLoS One 5(10):e13196

Australian Bureau of Statistics (2007) National survey of mental health and wellbeing (2007). Australian Bureau of Statistics, Canberra

Bergström J, Andersson G, Ljótsson B, Rück C, Andréewitch S, Karlsson A, Carlbring P, Andersson E, Lindefors N (2010) Internet-versus group-administered cognitive behaviour therapy for panic disorder in a psychiatric setting: a randomised trial. BMC Psychiatry 10(1):54

Botella C, García-Palacios A, Villa H, Baños RM, Quero S, Alcañiz M, Riva G (2007) Virtual reality exposure in the treatment of panic disorder and agoraphobia: a controlled study. Clin Psychol Psychother 14(3):164–175

Buist-Bouwman MA, De Graaf R, Vollebergh WA, Alonso J, Bruffaerts R, Ormel J (2006) Functional disability of mental disorders and comparison with physical disorders: a study among the general population of six European countries. Acta Psychiatr Scand 113(6): 492–500

Carlbring P, Westling BE, Ljungstrand P, Ekselius L, Andersson G (2001) Treatment of panic disorder via the Internet: a randomized trial of a self-help program. Behav Ther 32(4): 751–764

Carlbring P, Bohman S, Brunt S, Buhrman M, Westling B, Ekselius L, Andersson G (2006) Remote treatment of panic disorder: a randomized trial of internet-based cognitive behavior therapy supplemented with telephone calls. Am J Psychiatry 163(12):2119–2125

Carlbring P, Maurin L, Torngren C, Linna E, Eriksson T, Sparthan E et al (2011) Individually-tailored, Internet-based treatment for anxiety disorders: a randomized controlled trial. Behav Res Ther 49(1):18–24

De Graaf R, ten Have M, van Dorsselaer S (2010) [De psychische gezondheid van de Nederlandse bevolking. NEMESIS-2: Opzet en eerste resultaten.]. Trimbos-instituut, Utrecht

Ebenfeld L, Stegemann SK, Lehr D, Ebert DD, Jazaieri H, Van Ballegooijen W, et al (2014) Efficacy of a hybrid online training for panic symptoms and agoraphobia: study protocol for a randomized controlled trial. Trials 15(1):427

El Alaoui S, Hedman E, Ljótsson B, Bergström J, Andersson E, Rüch C, Andersson G, Lindefors N (2013) Predictors and moderators of internet- and group-based cognitive behaviour therapy for panic disorder. PLoS One 8(11):e79024

Farvolden P, Denisoff E, Selby P, Bagby RM, Rudy L (2005) Usage and longitudinal effectiveness of a Web-based self-help cognitive behavioral therapy program for panic disorder. J Med Internet Res 7(1):e7

Hedman E, Ljótsson B, Rück C, Bergström J, Andersson G, Kaldo V, Jansson L, Andersson E, Andersson E, Blom K, El Alaoui S, Falk L, Ivarsson J, Nasri B, Rydh S, Lindefors N (2013) Effectiveness of internet-based cognitive behaviour therapy for panic disorder in routine psychiatric care. Acta Psychiatr Scand 128(6):457–467

Kelders SM, Kok RN, Ossebaard HC, Van Gemert-Pijnen JE (2012) Persuasive system design does matter: a systematic review of adherence to web-based interventions. J Med Internet Res 14(6):e152

Kessler RC, Chiu WT, Demler O, Merikangas KR, Walters EE (2005) Prevalence, severity, and comorbidity of 12-month DSM-IV disorders in the National Comorbidity Survey Replication. Arch Gen Psychiatry 62(6):617–627

Kiropoulos LA, Klein B, Austin DW, Gilson K, Pier C, Mitchell J, Ciechomski L (2008) Is internet-based CBT for panic disorder and agoraphobia as effective as face-to-face CBT? J Anxiety Disord 22(8):1273–1284

Klein B, Richards JC (2001) A brief internet-based treatment for panic disorder. Behav Cogn Psychother 29(01):113–117

Klein B, Richards JC, Austin DW (2006) Efficacy of internet therapy for panic disorder. J Behav Ther Exp Psychiatry 37(3):213–238

Klein B, Shandley K, Austin D, Nordin S (2008) Pilot trial of panic online self-guided version: internet-based treatment for panic disorder. J Appl Psychol 4(2):25–30

Klein B, Austin D, Pier C, Kiropoulos L, Shandley K, Mitchell J, Gilson K, Ciechomski L (2009) Internet-based treatment for panic disorder: does frequency of therapist contact make a difference? Cogn Behav Ther 38(2):100–113

Klein B, Meyer D, Austin DW, Kyrios M (2011) Anxiety online—a virtual clinic: preliminary outcomes following completion of five fully automated treatment programs for anxiety disorders and symptoms. J Med Internet Res 13(4):e89

Lindner P, Ivanova E, Ly KH, Andersson G, Carlbring P (2013) Guided and unguided CBT for social anxiety disorder and/or panic disorder via the Internet and a smartphone application: study protocol for a randomised controlled trial. Trials 14(1):437

Meulenbeek P, Herzmanatus J, Smit F, Willemse G, van der Zanden R (2005) Cursusmap: Geen Paniek, leren omgaan met paniekklachten. Trimbos-instituut/GGNet, Utrecht

Meulenbeek P, Willemse G, Smit F, van Balkom A, Spinhoven P, Cuijpers P (2010) Early intervention in panic: pragmatic randomised controlled trial. Br J Psychiatry 196(4):326–331

Meyerbröker K, Emmelkamp PM (2010) Virtual reality exposure therapy in anxiety disorders: a systematic review of process-and-outcome studies. Depress Anxiety 27(10):933–944

Meyerbröker K, Morina N, Kerkhof GA, Emmelkamp PMG (2013) Virtual reality exposure therapy does not provide any additional value in agoraphobic patients: a randomized controlled trial. Psychother Psychosom 82(3):170–176

Peñate W, Pitti CT, Bethencourt JM, de la Fuente J, Gracia R (2008) The effects of a treatment based on the use of virtual reality exposure and cognitive-behavioral therapy applied to patients with agoraphobia. Int J Clin Health Psychol 8(1):5–22

Pier C, Austin DW, Klein B, Mitchell J, Schattner P, Ciechomski L, Wade V (2008) A controlled trial of internet-based cognitive-behavioural therapy for panic disorder with face-to-face support from a general practitioner or email support from a psychologist. Mental Health Fam Med 5(1):29

Pitti C, Peñate W, de la Fuente J, Bethencourt J, Acosta L, Villaverde M, Gracia R (2007) Agoraphobia: combined treatment and virtual reality. Preliminary results. Actas Esp Psiquiatr 36(2):94–101

Richards D, Richardson T (2012) Computer-based psychological treatments for depression: a systematic review and meta-analysis. Clin Psychol Rev 32(4):329–342

Richards JC, Klein B, Austin DW (2006) Internet cognitive behavioural therapy for panic disorder: does the inclusion of stress management information improve end-state functioning? Clin Psychologist 10(1):2–15

Robinson E, Titov N, Andrews G, McIntyre K, Schwencke G, Solley K (2010) Internet treatment for generalized anxiety disorder: a randomized controlled trial comparing clinician vs. technician assistance. PLoS One 5(6):e10942

Ruwaard J, Broeksteeg J, Schrieken B, Emmelkamp P, Lange A (2010) Web-based therapist-assisted cognitive behavioral treatment of panic symptoms: a randomized controlled trial with a three-year follow-up. J Anxiety Disord 24(4):387–396

Shandley K, Austin D, Klein B, Pier C, Schattner P, Pierce D, Wade T (2008) Therapist assisted, internet – based treatment for panic disorder: can general practitioners achieve comparable patient outcomes to psychologists? J Med Internet Res 10:e14

Silfvernagel K, Carlbring P, Kabo J, Edström S, Eriksson J, Månson L, Andersson G (2012) Individually tailored internet-based treatment for young adults and adults with panic attacks: randomized controlled trial. J Med Internet Res 14(3):e65

Smit F, Cuijpers P, Oostenbrink J, Batelaan N, De Graaf R, Beekman A (2006) Costs of nine common mental disorders: implications for curative and preventive psychiatry. J Ment Health Policy Econ 9(4):193–200

Spek V, Cuijpers P, Nyklíček I, Smits N, Riper H, Keyzer J, Pop V (2008) One-year follow-up results of a randomized controlled clinical trial on internet-based cognitive behavioural therapy for subthreshold depression in people over 50 years. Psychol Med 38(05):635–639

Svanborg P, Åsberg M (1994) A new self-rating scale for depression and anxiety states based on the Comprehensive Psychopathological Rating Scale. Acta Psychiatr Scand 89(1):21–28

Titov N, Andrews G, Davies M, McIntyre K, Robinson E, Solley K (2010) Internet treatment for depression: a randomized controlled trial comparing clinician vs. technician assistance. PLoS One 5(6):e10939

Titov N, Dear BF, Schwencke G, Andrews G, Johnston L, Craske MG et al (2011) Transdiagnostic internet treatment for anxiety and depression: a randomised controlled trial. Behav Res Ther 49(8):441–452

Van Ballegooijen W, Riper H, van Straten A, Kramer J, Conijn B, Cuijpers P (2011) The effects of an Internet based self-help course for reducing panic symptoms – Don't Panic Online: study protocol for a randomised controlled trial. Trials 12:75

Van Ballegooijen W, Riper H, Klein B, Ebert DD, Kramer J, Meulenbeek P, Cuijpers P (2013) An internet-based guided self-help intervention for panic symptoms: randomized controlled trial. J Med Internet Res 15(7):e154

Warmerdam L, van Straten A, Twisk J, Riper H, Cuijpers P (2008) Internet-based treatment for adults with depressive symptoms: randomized controlled trial. J Med Internet Res 10(4):e44

Wims E, Titov N, Andrews G, Choi I (2010) Clinician-assisted Internet-based treatment is effective for panic: a randomized controlled trial. Aust N Z J Psychiatry 44(7):599–607

World Health Organisation (2014) ICD-10 version: 2015. From: http://apps.who.int/classifications/icd10/browse/2015/en. Accessed 4th Dec 2014

Internet-Based Cognitive Behavior Therapy for Social Anxiety Disorder

4

Erik Hedman, Cristina Botella, and Thomas Berger

Abstract

Social anxiety disorder (SAD) is characterized by a marked and persistent fear of being scrutinized by others in social situations. It is highly prevalent and follows a chronic course for many affected if untreated. Treatment with cognitive behavior therapy (CBT) has been shown to be highly effective for SAD with responder rates of 50–75 %. For more than a decade, Internet-based CBT (ICBT) has been researched and evidence has been provided by four independent research groups. In essence, most forms of ICBT for SAD can generally be described as therapist-guided Internet-based self-help CBT where a named therapist guides the client through the treatment. The treatments are manualized and highly structured comprising 5–15 modules or lessons, which are the equivalent of sessions in face-to-face CBT. The existing treatments for SAD all have vital features in common including that they are based in CBT, comprise the same interventions as have been shown to be effective in face-to-face CBT, have large amount of psychoeducational material, and use asynchronous text messages as the main communication between patient and therapist. ICBT for SAD has been proven to be effective in at least 16 randomized trials and found to be non-inferior to face-to-face CBT. A few studies suggest that ICBT is a cost-effective treatment. Since SAD is known to appear at an early age in most cases, one central future challenge is

E. Hedman (✉)
Department of Clinical Neuroscience, Karolinska Institutet, Stockholm, Sweden
e-mail: kire.hedman@ki.se

C. Botella
Department of Basic, Clinical and Psichobiological Psychology,
Universitat Jaume I, Castellón, Spain
e-mail: botella@uji.es

T. Berger
Department of Clinical Psychology, University of Bern, Bern, Switzerland
e-mail: thomas.berger@ptp.unibe.ch

© Springer International Publishing Switzerland 2016
N. Lindefors, G. Andersson (eds.), *Guided Internet-Based Treatments in Psychiatry*, DOI 10.1007/978-3-319-06083-5_4

to increase the body of knowledge on ICBT for children and adolescents. For adults, ICBT for SAD is clearly an effective treatment and a promising option for increasing accessibility to evidence-based psychological treatment.

Definition and Epidemiology

According to the DSM-IV, the main diagnostic feature of social anxiety disorder (SAD) is "a marked and persistent fear of one or more social or performance situations in which the person is exposed to unfamiliar people or to possible scrutiny by others (American Psychiatric Association 1994). The individual fears that he or she will act in a way (or show anxiety symptoms) that will be humiliating or embarrassing". SAD is thus characterized by a fear of being negatively evaluated by others and the most commonly feared situation among persons with SAD is public speaking. A vast majority of affected individuals fear not just one but several social situations (Furmark et al. 1999; Ruscio et al. 2008). SAD was first viewed as a simple phobia, but several aspects of the disorder make it different compared to, for example, animal phobias. The individual with SAD not only experiences fear when in social situations but often also has high levels of anticipatory worry before entering these situations, which could increase the probability that the person avoids the social event all together or engages in safety behaviors (Clark and Wells 1995). These can be described as subtle avoidance behaviors, e.g., using anxiolytics or avoiding eye contact. After the social event, the individual with SAD often engages in postmortem processing, which means scrutinizing one's own performance and paying close attention to actions that could have been negatively perceived by others (Clark and Wells 1995). As a way of recognizing the profound impact of SAD in terms of symptom presentation and aversive consequences, the term SAD – as a complement to social phobia – was introduced in DSM-III-R (Liebowitz et al. 2000). The diagnostic criteria for SAD have remained largely the same in DSM-5 (American Psychiatric Association 2013).

SAD is one of the most common anxiety disorders with 12-month prevalence estimates of 7–8 % in large-scale community-based studies (Kessler et al. 1994; Magee et al. 1996). A stable finding from epidemiological studies on SAD is that women have a higher risk of developing the disorder (Furmark 2002). Considering sample size and methodological strengths, it is likely that the best estimate is around 1.5:1 (Furmark 2002). SAD has an early onset, usually between 11 and 13 years of age, and it is uncommon to develop the disorder in adulthood (Wittchen and Fehm 2003; Beesdo et al. 2007). More than half of persons with SAD suffer from a comorbid psychiatric disorder, often an anxiety disorder, depression, or substance abuse (Chartier et al. 2003; Ruscio et al. 2008). As the debut of SAD often precedes that of the comorbid disorders, it has been suggested that SAD may play a causal role in the development of the latter disorders. SAD is associated with functional impairment in several life domains (Fehm et al. 2005). It leads to an increased risk of unemployment (Wittchen et al. 2000; Lampe et al. 2003; Bruch et al. 2003), lower academic attainment (Furmark et al. 1999; Davidson et al. 1993), reduced quality of life (Wittchen et al. 2000; Olatunji et al. 2007), and poorer somatic health (Dahl and Dahl 2010). In clinical samples, SAD rarely remits spontaneously but is chronic for a majority of patients if untreated (Yonkers et al. 2001).

Treatment of SAD

Among psychological treatments, cognitive behavior therapy (CBT) has the most empirical support. The two most well-researched treatments are cognitive behavior group therapy (CBGT) developed by Heimberg and coworkers (2002) and individual cognitive therapy (ICT) developed by Clark and coworkers (2003). These two treatments are relatively brief (about 12–16 weeks), based on similar CBT models of social anxiety and are aimed at breaking the vicious cycle between anxiety symptoms, catastrophic interpretations, attention to internal and external threat, safety behaviors, and avoidance behaviors. Common to both CBGT and ICT is the formulation of an individual conceptualization of the patient's problem based on the CBT model. In addition, both treatments put a strong emphasis on weekly homework assignments and include exercises where exposure to social stimuli and cognitive restructuring are integrated, and finally, both entail relapse prevention. Of course, this means that both treatments are challenging for the patient as they require the patient to confront what he or she fears the most. There are however some differences between the treatments. In Heimberg's CBGT, the main component is in-session exposure to feared social situations in combination with verbal cognitive restructuring where exposure is conducted within a largely habituational framework (Heimberg and Becker 2002). In ICT, reduction of social anxiety is promoted by getting patients to make predictions and test the predictions in behavior experiments in which safety behaviors are dropped and/or feared catastrophes are intentionally enacted. The treatment also includes exercises to demonstrate the adverse effects of self-focused attention and safety behaviors, training in externally focused attention, and video feedback to correct negative self-imagery (Clark et al. 2003). The empirical evidence for these two treatments is strong as they have been tested in at least 17 randomized controlled trials and have been shown to be superior to other psychological treatments and pill placebo (Ponniah and Hollon 2008). The magnitude of effects is generally large for these two treatments. There is some empirical data suggesting that ICT may be more effective than CBGT, which could perhaps be attributable to the slightly more complex procedures per se or that the individual format allows for a more tailored treatment. Approximately two out of three patients achieve clinically significant improvement, and long-term follow-up studies have demonstrated that these two treatments yield improvements that are sustained for at least 5 years (Heimberg et al. 1993; Mörtberg et al. 2011). One study showed that a combination of pharmacological treatment (phenelzine) and CBGT produced larger improvements than CBGT alone (Blanco et al. 2010). However, the small number of studies in this field does not allow any firm conclusions that combinatorial treatment is superior to monotherapy in the treatment of SAD (Hofmann et al. 2009).

Internet-Based Treatments for SAD

SAD is one of the clinical domains where research on Internet-based treatments has been most extensive during the last decade and is likely that SAD is the disorder for which this type of treatment has the strongest empirical support. Five independent research groups in Sweden, Switzerland, Spain, Australia, and the UK have developed and tested Internet-based cognitive behavior therapy (ICBT) for SAD. In essence, most forms of ICBT for SAD can generally be described as therapist-guided Internet-based self-help CBT where a named therapist guides the client through the treatment. Common to ICBT for many other disorders, the treatments are manualized and highly structured comprising 5–15 modules or lessons, which are the equivalent of sessions in face-to-face CBT. The existing treatments for SAD all have vital features in common including that they:

- Are based on cognitive behavior therapy
- Entail treatment components that have been shown to be effective in a face-to-face format, such as exposure
- Have large amounts of psychoeducational material
- Are 8–15 weeks long
- Most often use asynchronous written text messages as the main communication form between therapist and patient
- Have integrated worksheet and assessment systems in the Internet-based treatment platform

To some extent, it could be that ICBT is especially suitable for this patient group, and it has been suggested that the absence of face-to-face contact, which can be fear provoking for persons with SAD, might actually improve learning of the psychoeducational parts of the treatment (Hedman et al. 2014a). That is, learning the relatively complex treatment models and principles underlying the treatment may be easier if not done in a social context where the patient may feel that he or she is being evaluated by the therapist. In the following, a brief description of the five different ICBT treatments is presented.

The Swedish ICBT for SAD

One of the first therapist-guided ICBT treatments was developed by Andersson and coworkers (2006). This treatment is primarily based on Clark et al.'s individual cognitive treatment for SAD and thus comprises components such as behavior experiments, manipulation of safety behaviors, and attention training. It also entails exposure exercises and social skills training. The treatment is structurally based on 9–15 so-called modules, which are text chapters that correspond to therapy sessions and are designed to provide the patient with the same knowledge and tools as he or she would obtain in face-to-face CBT. Table 4.1 displays an example of the contents of modules in ICBT for SAD. To each module belongs a set of homework exercises and the patient is granted

Table 4.1 Example of module contents in Internet-based cognitive behavior therapy for social anxiety disorder

Module	Contents	Main homework exercises	No. of pages
1	Introduction and information about social anxiety and the treatment	Reading text about social anxiety, answering questions to show that one understands the rationale for treatment	19
2	Psychoeducation about Clark and Wells model of social anxiety	Mapping one's own cognitive, affective, and behavior responses in accordance with the model	20
3	Cognitive restructuring	Identifying and disputing negative automatic thoughts	30
4	Behavior experiments	Testing negative predictions in social situations	23
5	Exposure, part I	Systematic exposure to social events	21
6	Training in shifting attention	Exercises in shifting focus of attention	19
7	Exposure, part II	Systematic exposure to social events	17
8	Social skill training	Assertiveness training	19
9	Exposure, part III	Systematic exposure to social events	10
10	Relapse prevention	Designing individual plan to prevent relapse	21
			Total: 199

gradual access to the modules contingent on completion of homework exercises. The patient has access to an identified and personal therapist throughout the treatment and the contact is almost exclusively through written text messages. The patient also has access to a discussion forum where he or she anonymously can post messages to other patients that receive treatment. Generally, this treatment has few complex technical features, is heavily text based, and could essentially be described therapist-guided online bibliotherapy. Although most conducted studies have used on beforehand fixed modules, i.e., all participants regardless of symptom profiles have been exposed to the same modules, a more recent development has been to tailor the treatment content to the patient's characteristics (e.g., Carlbring 2011a). This could, for example, be that a patient with SAD who has comorbid sleep difficulties is granted access to additional insomnia modules containing information about how to improve sleep.

The Swiss ICBT for SAD

The Swiss treatment, developed by Berger and coworkers (2009), is also explicitly based on individual cognitive therapy and therefore shares many basic components with the Swedish treatment program. The treatment is 10 weeks long and comprises five lessons, and the patient has access to a named therapist as well as to a discussion forum. In contrast to the Swedish program, this treatment includes more interactive features and is less like a self-help book. For instance, participants are asked to use online diaries or to make an exposure hierarchy online. In addition, it uses the video format as a phobic stimulus in the sense that patients are encouraged to conduct exposure exercises and behavior experiments in front of, e.g., a virtual video audience. The program does not only include a discussion forum but also other collaborative online group elements such as the possibility to anonymously share work sheets and diaries with other participants. The program can be used in an unguided and guided format (Berger et al. 2011) and in a tailored approach in which the self-help guide is individually tailored to comorbid other anxiety disorders (panic disorder with or without agoraphobia, generalized anxiety disorder) (Berger et al. 2014).

The Spanish ICBT for SAD

Botella and coworkers developed the first ICBT for SAD (Botella et al. 2000, 2004). This ICBT includes several components: psychoeducation, cognitive restructuring, attention training, and exposure. Figure 4.1 presents the structure and contents of the different modules of this ICBT. To each module belongs a set of homework exercises and the patient is granted gradual access to the module contingent on completion of homework exercises. The treatment can be fully automated; this means that potential patients go through an online self-report assessment and are granted access to treatment if predefined criteria for eligibility are met. In this case, the patient has no therapist contact but is asked to complete questions and is not allowed to go through the program if the answers indicate that he or she has not understood the main aspects of the treatment and/or if the level of anxiety confronting the feared situation has not decreased. In these cases, the patient is asked to look over the treatment material once more. It is possible also to deliver the program in a blended form, that is, the online program can be combined with therapist's contact (by phone or face to face). The main component of the treatment is virtual exposure, and the program entails six different typical scenarios that evoke social anxiety in persons with SAD, e.g., "The class" or "The job interview." For each scenario there is a set of video films that constitute the phobic stimulus and the patient is asked to conduct oral presentations in front of these video audiences. The program organizes a hierarchy created during the initial assessment, and the specific scenarios are presented based on levels of fear, progressing from those less feared to those more feared. The program provides different advice to users depending on their level of fear upon finishing the exposure, encourages the users to continue working, and congratulates them for their effort. The program also recommends completing daily homework assignments.

The Australian ICBT for SAD

Titov, Andrews, and coworkers have developed and tested an Internet-based treatment for SAD often referred to as The Shyness Program (Titov et al. 2008a). This ICBT for SAD is based on the previously developed CLIMATEGP online lessons

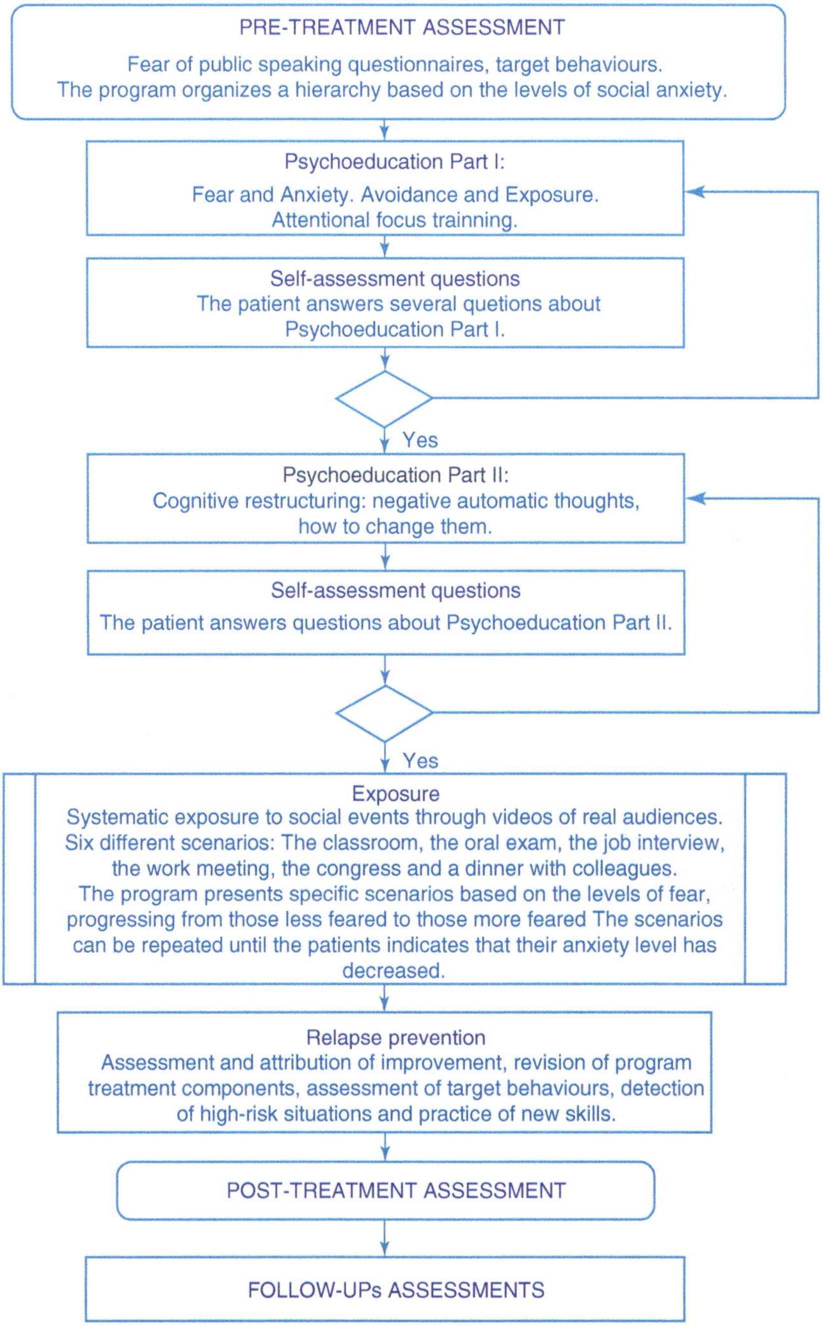

Fig. 4.1 Example of the structure and contents of an Internet-based cognitive behavior treatment for social anxiety disorder

for SAD. This treatment comprises six lessons over 10 weeks where the main components are psychoeducation about CBT and social anxiety, exposure exercises, and cognitive restructuring. The main message of each lesson is illustrated in part through a treatment story where a fictive person with SAD learns to overcome social anxiety through CBT. Structurally, the treatment is similar to the Swedish and Swiss treatments meaning that patients have access to an identified therapist who provide asynchronous written feedback on homework exercises. Integrated in the treatment is also an online discussion forum where patients can share experiences and provide support to each other anonymously.

The British ICBT for SAD

This type of ICBT for SAD (Stott et al. 2013) is fully based on the individual cognitive therapy developed by Clark and coworkers. It is designed to incorporate all central components of individual cognitive therapy while using less therapist time and has largely the same structure as the Swedish, Swiss, and Australian treatments. That is, the patient has email-like contact with a named therapist, the treatment is comprised of several Internet-based modules, and patients spend about the same time in treatment as in face-to-face treatment. Nine core modules are obligatory for all patients, but if the therapist judges it to be helpful, he or she can assign additional modules to the patient that address common obstacles in treatment or problem-specific aspects that may not be applicable for all persons with SAD. This treatment is relatively advanced from a technical view; it entails several psychoeducational video clips and uses web-cam linked communication. Recordings from webcam interactions are also used in video-feedback exercises where patients can learn to discriminate between self-perceptions and actual social performance. An instruction video describing the treatment is available on the following URL: http://youtu.be/rXXOOSkA0qg.

Studies on Internet-Based CBT for SAD

Independent researchers in different countries (Australia, Sweden, Switzerland, Spain, and United Kingdom) have tested several ICBT programs for SAD. The existing empirical evidence is quite strong with at least 16 conducted RCTs demonstrating the treatment's efficacy. Data from a meta-analysis (Andrews et al. 2010) showed that the overall effect size of ICBT for SAD compared to control group was large ($g = 0.92$, 95 % CI 0.74–1.09), and the results indicate both short- and long-term improvements. Furthermore, the findings showed that treatment adherence was good and that patients were satisfied with the treatment despite the relatively limited therapist contact. ICBT appears to be a promising way to overcome treatment barriers for persons suffering from SAD. Here we present the most relevant research conducted in the field of ICBT for SAD.

Efficacy and Long-Term Outcomes

In a case study using an ICBT program for SAD, Botella and coworkers in Spain found initial empirical support for the treatment efficacy (Botella et al. 2004). This same program was further tested in a series of case studies (Botella et al. 2007) presenting efficacy data from 12 social phobia patients with good results. The Swedish team (Carlbring et al. 2006) published an open trial in which 26 participants were treated with an ICBT program plus weekly therapist contact via email. The results showed that the participants improved significantly on all outcomes and the treatment gains were maintained or improved at the 6-month follow-up. All these studies provided preliminary evidence supporting the use of ICBT programs for people diagnosed with SAD.

Table 4.2 presents an overview of randomized clinical trials investigating the effect of Internet-based CBT. Andersson and coworkers published the first RCT (Andersson et al. 2006) on the efficacy of ICBT for SAD which was then followed by several trials with the same ICBT program (see below). In this first RCT, 64 participants were randomly assigned to the ICBT program supported by email contact of a named therapist plus two in vivo exposure sessions in a group format, or a waiting list control condition. The results revealed that the ICBT condition was significantly more efficacious than the control condition with treatment gains maintained at 1-year follow-up. The authors also published results on long-term outcome (30-month follow-up) which suggested that the long-term effects seen in previous live treatment CBT for SAD trials also occur in Internet-delivered treatment (Carlbring et al. 2009). Using largely the same treatment but without in vivo exposure sessions, Hedman and coworkers found that treatment gains were sustained 5 years after treatment (Hedman et al. 2011a). The efficacy of ICBT for SAD has also been demonstrated in several trials conducted in Australia. Titov and colleagues (2008b) carried out an RCT in which 105 participants with SAD were randomly assigned to an ICBT program or to a waiting list control group. The results showed significant differences between treatment and waiting list participants. As in the trials conducted in Sweden, effects were comparable with those obtained in face-to-face treatment. In Switzerland, Berger and coworkers conducted an RCT (Berger et al. 2009) including 52 individuals with SAD who were randomly assigned either to an ICBT program with minimal therapist contact via email or to a waiting list control group. Significant differences between the two groups were found at post-treatment on all primary outcome measures. The results provided additional support to the hypothesis that ICBT interventions with minimal therapist contact are a promising treatment for SAD. Gallego, Emmelkamp, van der Kooj, and Mees (2011) presented an RCT in which the effects of a Dutch version of the Spanish ICBT for SAD were investigated. Forty-one participants suffering from SAD were randomly assigned to either the ICBT program combined with minimal therapist contact via email or a waiting list control group. The group treated with ICBT was significantly improved from pretest to posttest on all SAD measures, and this condition was significantly more effective than the control group. This study as well as a

Table 4.2 Randomized controlled trials investigating the effect of Internet-based cognitive behavior therapy for social anxiety disorder

Country [reference]	Treatment arms	*N**	Outcome	Effect sizes (*d*) in active treatment arms (pre-post) (note: *d* according to label under "treatment arms")	Year
Australia (Titov et al. 2008a)	(a) ICBT	105	SIAS	(a) 1.24	2008
Australia (Titov et al. 2008b)	(a) ICBT	88	SIAS	(a) 1.21	2008
Australia (Titov et al. 2008c)	(a) ICBT (b) Unguided ICBT	98	SIAS	(a) 1.47 (b) 0.36	2008
Australia (Titov et al. 2009a)	(a) Unguided ICBT (b) Unguided ICBT+telephone support	168	SIAS	(a) 1.41 (b) 0.98	2009
Australia (Titov et al. 2009b)	(a) ICBT+support by "technician" (b) ICBT	85	SIAS, SPS	(a) 1.47 (SIAS) and 1.15 (SPS) (b) 1.56 (SIAS) and 1.15 (SPS)	2009
Australia (Titov et al. 2010a)	(a) ICBT (b) ICBT+motivational support	113	SIAS, SPS	(a) 1.16 (SIAS) and 1.04 (SPS) (b) 1.15 (SIAS) and 0.75 (SPS)	2010
Australia (Andrews et al. 2011b)	(a) ICBT (b) Live CBT	37	SIAS, SPS	(a) 0.74 (SIAS) and 0.58 (SPS) (b) 0.89 (SIAS) and 0.82 (SPS)	2011
Germany/Switzerland (Boettcher et al. 2012a)	(a) Unguided+SCID interview (b) Unguided – SCID interview	109	SIAS, SPS	(a) 1.63 (SIAS) and 1.39 (SPS) (b) 1.28 (SIAS) and 1.00 (SPS)	2012
The Netherlands (Gallego et al. 2011)	(a) ICBT	41	FPSQ	(a) 1.13	2011
Spain (Botella et al. 2010)	(a) ICBT (b) Live CBT	98	FPSQ	(a) 0.91 (b) 0.90	2010
Sweden (Andersson et al. 2006)	(a) ICBT+exposure	64	LSAS-SR	(a) 0.91	2006
Sweden (Carlbring et al. 2007)	(a) ICBT+telephone support	60	LSAS-SR	(a) 1.00	2007

Sweden (Tillfors et al. 2008)	(a) ICBT + exposure (b) ICBT	38	LSAS-SR	(a) 0.82 (b) 1.01	2008
Sweden (Furmark et al. 2009a)	(a) ICBT	120	LSAS-SR	(a) 0.93 (b) 0.78	2009
Sweden (Furmark et al. 2009a)	(a) ICBT (d) IAR	115	LSAS-SR	(a) 1.35 (d) 0.99	2009
Sweden (Hedman et al. 2011b)	(a) ICBT (b) Live CBT	126	LSAS	(a) 1.42 (b) 0.97	2011
Switzerland (Berger et al. 2009)	(a) ICBT	52	LSAS-SR	(a) 0.82	2009
Switzerland (Berger et al. 2011)	(a) ICBT (b) Unguided ICBT (c) ICBT with flexible support	81	LSAS-SR	(a) 1.53 (b) 1.48 (c) 1.41	2011

Abbreviations: *ICBT* Internet-based cognitive behavior therapy, *LSAS* Liebowitz social anxiety scale, *SIAS* social interaction anxiety scale, *SPS* social phobia scale, *SR* self-report, *FPSQ* fear of public speaking questionnaire pilot study of the British team (Stott et al. 2013) provides additional evidence for the efficacy of ICBT for SAD and shows that an ICBT program can be adapted and used with maintained effects in different cultural frameworks.

ICBT Compared to Face-to-Face CBT

ICBT has also been compared to traditional face-to-face CBT for SAD. Hedman et al. (2011b) carried out an RCT to investigate whether ICBT was at least as effective as traditional CBT group therapy when treatments are delivered in a psychiatric setting. One hundred and twenty-six individuals with SAD were randomly assigned to one of these two treatment conditions. The results revealed that both conditions made large and similar improvements and it was concluded that ICBT can be as effective as traditional CBT group therapy in the treatment of SAD. Botella and coworkers (2010) conducted an RCT in which 127 participants with a diagnosis of SAD were randomly assigned to three experimental conditions: an ICBT self-administered program, the same CBT treatment applied by a therapist, and a waiting list control group. The data showed that both treatment formats (self-administered and therapist administered) were equally efficacious and superior to the waiting list condition. The treatment gains were maintained at 1-year follow-up. In a study conducted in Australia, Titov et al. (Andrews et al. 2011b) also compared the effectiveness of ICBT with face-to-face CBT group therapy for SAD in an RCT including 75 participants. Both treatment formats yielded significant improvements and there were no significant differences between them. All these results provide evidence showing that both forms of delivering the treatment (face-to-face CBT and ICBT) can be equally effective while the difference in therapist time required is substantial. The results are also consistent with previous findings obtained in ICBT for panic disorder (e.g., Carlbring et al. 2005).

Studies Investigating Therapist Support

An important line of research has focused on studying the degree of support and guidance needed during the treatment. Tillfors and coworkers (Tillfors et al. 2008) carried out an RCT specifically targeting university students and investigating whether the ICBT self-help program would be more effective if five live group exposure sessions were added. Thirty-eight participants meeting the diagnostic of SAD were randomized into two different treatment groups: ICBT combined with five group exposure sessions or the same ICBT program alone. Both treatment conditions showed significant improvements from pre- to posttest and from pretest to 1-year follow-up on all measured SAD dimensions. The results suggest that adding group exposure sessions did not improve the outcome significantly.

Berger and coworkers (Berger et al. 2011) studied the role and necessity of therapist guidance in an RCT comparing the benefits of a 10-week unguided treatment, with the same intervention complemented with minimal weekly therapist support via email. The study included a third condition, in which the level of support was flexibly stepped up from no support to email or telephone support on demand of the participants. Eighty-one individuals with SAD were randomly assigned to one of the three conditions. Results showed significant improvements in all three treatment groups and no differences between the conditions regarding clinical outcomes, dropout rates, and adherence to treatment. These results provided additional evidence showing that ICBT for SAD is an effective treatment option when therapist guidance is provided but also when no support is provided.

The Australian team also contributed to this line of research carrying out several RCTs. For instance, in a trial by Titov and coworkers (2008c), 98 participants suffering from SAD were randomly assigned to a clinician-assisted ICBT program (email contact with a therapist and participation in an online discussion forum), the same ICBT program but without contact with a clinician, or to a wait list control group. The therapist-guided condition was superior to the self-guided condition, but a subgroup of participants who completed the program benefited considerably from the latter. In a subsequent study, Titov and colleagues (2009a) compared the self-guided treatment with a self-guided plus weekly telephone reminder condition in which participants were called once a week by a research assistant. Results showed that adherence and outcome were better in the condition that included reminders.

Overall, results on unguided treatments for SAD are still inconclusive. However, it is quite surprising that some studies (Berger et al. 2011), including a trial by Furmark and coworkers (Furmark et al. 2009b) in which an unguided treatment for SAD delivered in the form of bibliotherapy with no therapist support was as efficacious as guided ICBT, found no difference between unguided and guided treatments. Data from meta-analyses on ICBT for several disorders indicate better results of guided versus unguided treatments regarding improvements and dropout rates (Richards and Richardson 2012; Spek et al. 2007). It may be that guidance is less important in ICBT for SAD than for other disorders such as depression. However, it may also be that unguided treatments only achieve good therapeutic outcome under specific conditions. In the two studies mentioned above, a proper diagnosis was established and there was a contact with a clinician or the study team during the diagnostic phase. In one uncontrolled study in which there was no contact at all with the researchers, dropout was substantial (Klein et al. 2011). In another study in which the effects of clinician contact in the diagnostic phase was evaluated in an unguided treatment, participation in the structured diagnostic interview did not influence primary outcome but had a beneficial effect on adherence and secondary outcomes (Boettcher et al. 2012a). Clearly, more research is needed with regard to the role of support and contact before and during ICBT for SAD.

Another line of research that addresses questions on the role of support is related to therapists in guided ICBT. Does it matter who provides the support? Titov and coworkers (2009b) found that ICBT for SAD with guidance given by non-clinicians resulted in good outcomes. Andersson and coworkers (Andersson et al. 2012) evaluated the role of therapist experience and found no differences between experienced therapists and therapists with no previous experience in ICBT. However, inexperienced therapists needed more time to provide guidance than experienced therapists.

Overall, the findings suggest that ICBT does not require experienced therapists to be effective which is plausible given that (a) the treatment is highly structured and (b) the main component is a self-help program which also incorporates clinical expertise. In addition, it is important to note that non-clinicians and inexperienced therapists were under careful clinical supervision in all studies that included support by inexperienced therapists/coaches.

Another issue that has been examined is the possible role of including additional strategies for enhancing clinical results. For instance, Titov and coworkers (2010a) added motivational enhancement strategies to their ICBT program (understanding and exploring ambivalence about change, enhancing self-efficacy, etc.). Results of an RCT showed that ICBT with or without this additional component was efficacious. Although more participants in the motivational treatment condition completed the treatment lessons (75 % versus 56 %, respectively), no differences between the two conditions were found at posttreatment and at 3-month follow-up.

It is also possible that adding collaborative online group elements such as discussion groups could enhance treatment effects. There is at least indirect evidence that integrating collaborative elements into ICBT could be beneficial. Titov and colleagues could improve small within-group effect sizes for unguided ICBT for SAD (Titov et al. 2008c) by adding a clinician-moderated online discussion forum in a subsequent study. As mentioned previously, in the study by Furmark and coworkers (2009a), an intervention consisting of a self-help guide delivered in the form of bibliotherapy with no therapist support but with access to an online discussion forum was as effective as guided ICBT. Moreover, qualitative analyses of the content of discussions in integrated forums showed that therapeutic mechanisms of change may come into play that are known from research on group psychotherapies (e.g., normalization, altruism, instillation of hope, development of socializing techniques, imitative behavior, cohesiveness (Berger 2011)). However, since to the best of our knowledge there are no studies directly comparing the same internet-based treatment with and without collaborative elements, it is not possible to draw firm conclusions on the effects of integrated online discussion boards.

Addressing Comorbidity in ICBT for SAD

Still another arena of research explores whether addressing the high comorbidity rates in patients with SAD is beneficial. This was done with unified transdiagnostic treatments (Titov et al. 2010b, 2011; Johnston et al. 2011) and tailored approaches in which the self-help guide is individually tailored to the symptom profile of a patient by providing modules on comorbid problems and disorders such as mood disorders, other anxiety disorders, or insomnia (Berger et al. 2014; Carlbring et al. 2011b; Andersson et al. 2011). Both approaches seem to be effective, but it is not clear whether patients with SAD would benefit more from a transdiagnostic or tailored approach than from a treatment that targets SAD only. There is one study directly comparing a tailored versus standardized disorder-specific approach finding no differences between the two approaches, but this trial included patients with various anxiety disorders and levels of comorbidity (Berger et al. 2014). It is possible that a tailored approach is especially beneficial for subgroups of SAD patients such as individuals with high levels of comorbidity. This could not be tested in the trial mentioned above as the subgroup of SAD patients with high comorbidity rates was too small for appropriate subgroup analyses (Berger et al. 2014). Indeed, in a controlled trial comparing standard ICBT versus a tailored intervention in depression with comorbid problems, it was found that the tailored treatment was better suited to handle more severe disorders (Johansson et al. 2012).

Predictors and Mediators

As shown before, guided and unguided ICBT have shown to be effective treatments and may increase access to evidence-based psychological treatment for SAD. However, as at least a third of patients do not respond sufficiently to treatment, it is important to identify specific predictors and mediators that can guide the clinician in making treatment decisions. Knowledge on predictors and mediators can lead to more effective implementation of ICBT and ultimately to a larger proportion of patients that respond to treatment (Kraemer et al. 2002).

In their RCT comparing ICBT with group therapy, Hedman et al. (2012a) investigated possible clinical and genetic predictors and moderators of outcome. The results showed that the most stable predictors of better treatment outcomes were working full time, having children, suffering from less depressive symptoms, treatment expectancy and credibility, and better adherence to treatment. There were no significant results regarding gene polymorphisms that have also been tested. As for moderators, it was found that lower levels of comorbid anxiety and depression were associated with a better treatment response in the ICBT condition but not in the face-to-face CBT group therapy. Nordgreen et al. (2012) evaluated a series of pretreatment symptoms (including baseline SAD symptoms and comorbid depressive symptoms) and program factors (e.g., credibility and adherence) as potential predictors of treatment adherence and outcome in the context of guided and unguided self-help for SAD. The study included 245 patients who received either guided or unguided self-help for SAD. The results were in the same line than those obtained in the face-to-face CBT literature treatment for SAD (Eskildsen et al. 2010), namely, the intensity of SAD symptoms before treatment predicted treatment outcomes in both unguided and guided ICBT conditions, and the results were similar, regardless of whether participants had a diagnosis of generalized or specific SAD. The findings partly contrasted to those in the study by Hedman et al. (2012a) as treatment expectancy and credibility was unrelated to outcome. Nordgreen et al. (2012) also investigated predictors of adherence and found that in the guided ICBT condition, neither pretreatment symptoms nor credibility predicted treatment adherence. For the unguided ICBT group, higher credibility ratings of the treatment program were associated with increased treatment adherence with no group differences in credibility ratings between guided and unguided ICBT. That is, patients in the unguided intervention who perceived the program as a highly credible treatment, showing high expectations, had similar adherence rates as patients in the guided ICBT. Taking into account their findings, Nordgreen and coworkers (2012) recommended to provide the patients information about the potential effects of guided and unguided ICBT for SAD in order to promote positive expectations. In this same line, Boettcher and colleagues (2013a) hypothesized the relevance of patient expectations as an important mechanism to explain the change. They conducted a study including 109 participants that went through an unguided ICBT program for SAD. The results confirmed that positive outcome expectations were a significant predictor of change and treatment adherence, and this effect was mediated by early symptom change. These authors concluded that patient expectations could be a useful factor for guiding clinical decisions about possible treatments for SAD.

Globally, the results of all these studies highlight the importance of conducting further research to examine the predictors and mediators of outcomes in various clinical settings and populations to guide future dissemination efforts in ICBT for SAD.

Case Description

Hanna, 32 years old, suffers from social fears since childhood. She has become aware of the Internet-based guided self-help treatment, which is provided by the University of Bern in Switzerland, through a newspaper article. Hanna gets in touch by email and is then asked to answer different online questionnaires about anxiety, depression, well-being, and other aspects. From the answers, it becomes apparent that Hanna lives alone, has no children, has never been in psychotherapy, is not suicidal, and exceeds the cutoff criteria for SAD on various social phobia questionnaires. In a following diagnostic interview by phone, the diagnosis of SAD is confirmed. During the phone call, Hanna says that she is a teacher and lives in a village in the Swiss mountains where no psychotherapeutic treatment is available. She has decided to take advantage of the Internet-based approach because she does not want to drive to the next town for traditional therapy and is also afraid that someone in the small village would find out that she – the small village teacher – is in psychotherapy.

Hanna receives access to the first session of the Internet-based password-protected program, and she is told that a psychologist named Simon Weber will support her during her work with the program by a secure integrated email system. The psychologist will write her a feedback on her progress once a week and will be at her disposal if there are any questions. In a therapist cockpit, in which therapists/coaches can track participants' program use and symptomatic progress, Simon Weber observes that Hanna is working through the first self-help session, which contains many psychoeducational elements and an online anxiety diary. In his first weekly feedback, he writes in the integrated email system: "Dear Hanna, I see that you have worked through the first session. That's great! Your entries in the anxiety diary are very understandable. You describe a teacher's meeting in which you sat quietly in the corner and had thoughts like 'I won't be able to say anything because I'm so nervous'. These are behaviours and thoughts which are very typical for people suffering from social anxiety. We can assume that this program fits very well to your needs. In the course of the program we will work towards changing the behaviours and thoughts you have noted. You may start with the second session now."

Hanna instantly writes back that she has read the first session with great interest and is now very motivated to start with the second session. In this second session, she is asked to develop an individual explanatory model of her social anxieties on the basis of the cognitive-behavior model. Hanna writes that she was teased in primary school because she could not pronounce the letter R properly. Later her teachers made a fool of her in front of the class. Furthermore, she recognizes several of the described safety behaviors. Before parent-teacher conferences, she always takes a sedative tablet and practices her statements with great care. In these situations, she also focuses her attention very strongly toward herself in hopes of controlling bodily symptoms such as blushing. Now she understands that this behavior only reinforces and preserves her fears.

After a short and motivating feedback from the psychologist, Hanna begins with the third session. She is instructed to question her negative thoughts that she has noted in the anxiety diary and to find more realistic thoughts. Hanna seems to succeed in this task. However, in a message to the psychologist, she writes that her realistic thoughts collapse like a house of cards and the negative thoughts take over in real-life situations. The psychologist reassures her that she has already done a great job by not avoiding the situation and that it needs time and effort to change the negative thought patterns she has developed over the years.

In the fourth session, Hanna is instructed to conduct various exercises on self-focused attention in which she learns to focus her attention toward the task and the environment and not toward herself. In a message to the psychologist, Hanna writes that the exercises have helped her a lot because she could apply all that she has learned in a social small-talk situation in which she succeeded to focus on the environment and not on herself. She writes that the exercise had broadened her horizon and that she had not felt so helpless toward her fears anymore.

In session five, the exposure rationale and a diary are introduced in which fear-evoking situations are noted. Hanna is told that it is especially important that she write down situations that are important to her in a sense that they hinder her from living the life she wants and also that it should be likely to expose to the situations within a few weeks. The expected level of anxiety and safety behavior, which should be reduced, are noted in the diary. During the 10-week intervention, Hanna notes a total of 30 situations of which she finally exposes herself to 24. In most cases after experiencing the situation, she reports that the actual fear was much less than anticipated. From the entries, it becomes evident that with time she finds it easier to seek social situations and to refrain from safety behaviors.

After 10 weeks, Hanna does not fulfill the criteria of SAD anymore which becomes clear in a final diagnostic interview. The same pattern of improvement emerges in different disorder-specific questionnaires. Hanna writes a concluding message to her therapist: "I can only say that I am doing well. The social anxiety symptoms bother me considerably less and I hope that it will stay that way. I have started the school year probably just as motivated as my new first graders and I also enjoy my free time. I reread all the messages we sent each other and you deserve a huge compliment on your work! You and the program have accompanied me competently on a piece of my journey. During that time I always felt as though I was in good hands. I could venture on things that I had remained silent for years. Thank you so much." In a 6-month follow-up, it becomes apparent that the positive change has been maintained.

Cost-Effectiveness

SAD is associated with a great individual burden (Stein and Stein 2008; Kessler et al. 2012) and the majority of patients with SAD also suffer from other comorbid mental disorders (e.g., depression, other anxiety disorders, or substance abuse) (Fehm et al. 2005; Lipsitz and Schneier 2000). Besides the suffering of the affected individuals, SAD is associated with an important economic burden for the society in terms of direct and indirect costs (Stuhldreher et al. 2014). Also, this condition is characterized by an increased risk of unemployment and disability; the annual societal costs of SAD have been estimated to more than \$350 million per 1 million inhabitants (Hedman et al. 2014b). However, while costs incurred by healthcare utilization of patients suffering SAD (direct costs) are rather low, the societal burden resulting from lost productivity (indirect costs) is considerable. This might indicate that most patients had not sought for sufficient treatment yet (Stuhldreher et al. 2014).

As noted above, guided ICBT has shown to be a promising treatment for SAD. In addition, ICBT has the potential to dramatically increase availability of traditional face-to-face CBT for SAD (Hedman et al. 2012b). However, a key question before the dissemination of ICBT programs can be massively recommended is to know more about their health economic effects. Studies on the cost-effectiveness of SAD treatment are scarce. In fact, Lewis, Pearce, and Bisson (2012) carried out a systematic review to determine the efficacy and cost-effectiveness of self-help interventions for anxiety disorders. The results showed that self-help interventions appear to be an effective treatment for individuals diagnosed with SAD, but it was not possible to conclude anything about cost-effectiveness because none of the studies included in the review conducted a concurrent economic evaluation of the self-help intervention. Here we will try to summarize the most important contributions on cost-effectiveness of ICBT for SAD.

Titov and coworkers (2009d) carried out a study trying to determine cost-effectiveness of an ICBT program for SAD. One hundred and ninety-three participants were randomly assigned to an ICBT program or a waiting list condition. Cost-effectiveness was calculated to determine the cost per year gained living with disability (YLD). The results showed better results in the ICBT group treatment. The authors concluded that the ICBT program appears to be cost-effective. However, an important limitation of this study was that the effect sizes and estimates of staff time were derived from published results of a benchmarking study of face-to-face group treatment for SAD (McEvoy 2007).

In their RCT comparing ICBT with face-to-face group CBT, Hedman et al. (2011c) conducted the first prospective RCT investigating the cost-effectiveness of ICBT from a societal perspective; that is, both direct and indirect costs were analyzed. Results revealed that the total costs were significantly reduced in both treatment conditions. Furthermore, both treatments were equivalent in reducing SAD symptoms and gross total costs. The authors concluded that both treatments are useful in reducing societal costs for SAD, but ICBT can be considered more cost-effective than CBGT due to lower intervention costs regarding therapist time required. On average, in ICBT, the therapist spent 5.5 min weekly per patient; in CBGT, the corresponding estimate was 50 min (2.5 h sessions with two therapists and six patients). Recently, the same group presented the 4-year follow-up data (Hedman et al. 2014b). Results revealed that, at long term, ICBT for SAD is as effective as CBGT and that the interventions have similar longer-term health economic effects.

Hedman and coworkers (2012b) also conducted a systematic review on the efficacy and cost-effectiveness of ICBT. The results showed large effects for ICBT, and combining this data with the limited therapist time required by ICBT, the authors suggested that this kind of intervention may be highly cost-effective. However, it is important to underscore that of the 108 studies included in the review, only eight provided data regarding cost-effectiveness, and only two of these studies were focused on SAD.

Finally, Nordgreen et al. (2014) conducted an RCT to investigate the effectiveness and cost-effectiveness of ICBT when tailoring the treatment to address comorbidities and preferences for primary-care patients with a principal diagnosis of anxiety disorder. The authors were interested in studying whether treatment could lower direct and indirect societal costs in this population. The trial included one hundred participants that were recruited through their primary-care contact and randomized to an ICBT condition with scheduled guidance (7–10 weekly individually assigned modules guided by online therapists) or an active waiting list control group ("attention control"). Thirty-two percent of participants in both groups had a primary diagnosis of SAD. Costs were assessed at pretreatment, posttreatment, and at 12-month follow-up. The control condition was crossed over to treatment after posttreatment, then between-group comparisons were made only for the posttreatment data. The cost analysis results showed significant reduction of total costs for the tailored ICBT group. The results were maintained at 1-year follow-up, and the incremental cost-effectiveness ratio favored tailored ICBT compared to the control group. That is, from a societal perspective, the treatment constitutes a win-win situation as patients make large improvements while society makes a substantial net reduction of costs. This study provides evidence of cost savings without compromising clinical effectiveness. Given that evidence-based psychological treatments often are lacking in primary care, this kind of intervention may be an excellent treatment alternative.

In summary, it is possible to conclude that although the studies on cost-effectiveness of SAD are scarce, the results are quite encouraging. The available data show that ICBT is a cost-effective and well-established alternative to traditional CBT for SAD. However, research is needed to further evaluate the long-term cost-effectiveness of SAD treatment.

Clinical Implementation and Dissemination

Most of the studies mentioned above are efficacy trials conducted under controlled conditions with participants recruited via advertisement. There are, however, at least three studies examining the effectiveness of ICBT for SAD delivered in regular clinical services: one larger study conducted in a regular clinic in Stockholm, in which ICBT is delivered regularly to patients from the Stockholm county region (Hedman et al. 2011c), and two smaller studies conducted with patients referred to an anxiety disorder clinic in Australia (Andrews et al. 2011b; Aydos et al. 2009). The results of these studies, but also clinical experience and unpublished findings from the clinics mentioned above, show that the promising effects found in efficacy trials can be replicated in routine clinical practice.

However, the small number of studies and involved clinics also illustrates that ICBT for SAD is not yet implemented into clinical services on a larger scale. This may change in the future since data on aspects that are important to consider in the dissemination of a treatment such as patient preferences and cost-effectiveness may support efforts for the sustained implementation: Hedman and colleagues (2011c) as well as Andrews and colleagues (2011b) report that about half of the patients treated in a regular clinical setting prefer ICBT over face-to-face therapy. Moreover, and as described above, ICBT for SAD has been shown to be more cost-effective when compared with a cognitive behavior group therapy, mainly because ICBT was associated with less treatment costs (Hedman et al. 2011c). Of course, one of the strongest arguments for implementation on a larger scale is that the body of knowledge indicates that ICBT increases accessibility by a factor of four while producing large improvement in social anxiety.

As in ICBT for other conditions, the clinical implementation may be hindered by negative clinician attitudes toward Internet-based interventions (Mohr et al. 2010). Regarding ICBT for SAD, it may be especially important to inform and educate clinicians about these interventions because it is not obvious that ICBT should work for patients with social phobia. Indeed, it has been found that persons with social phobia do use the Internet extensively (Erwin et al. 2004), and it could be argued that ICBT reinforces their avoidance of contact with people. It is important to understand that Internet interventions do not direct patients to stay at home in front of their computer, but encourage participants to conduct real-life exposures. Our experience is that many patients manage to seek outside exposure with the guidance of a self-help program and the limited support of a clinician.

Finally, it is important to note that the implementation into routine clinical practice is only one pathway through which ICBT can and should be disseminated. Given that treatment rates among individuals suffering from SAD are particularly low (Kessler 2003), presumably also because of the increased fear and embarrassment in social situations, the development of low-threshold services providing direct online access to evidence-based ICBT for SAD should also be considered. However, such services should also include good referral methods to traditional treatments when ICBT does not result in sufficient improvement.

Discussion and Future Challenges

SAD is one of the most researched disorders in field of ICBT. More than 20 studies have consistently produced outcomes that are in line with results found in studies on face-to-face CBT, making ICBT one of the most evidence-based treatments for SAD. Effects tend to be stable over long-term follow-up, and there are indications that ICBT also works under clinically representative conditions.

On the basis of this extensive evidence, research on ICBT for SAD has already moved beyond a legitimation phase, i.e., research that basically addresses the question whether a treatment works. There is already a considerable amount of research on questions such as "What works better?," though results are not always conclusive. For example, the available evidence does not clearly answer important questions regarding the role of therapist support. More research is needed to establish the type and amount of support that is optimal in ICBT for SAD, and it should be underscored that power has been rather limited in the studies investigating the role of the therapist.

Further research regarding "What works better in IBCT for SAD" is important since a considerable number of patients do not benefit or recover fully from traditional or Internet-based treatments for SAD (Heimberg et al. 1993; Boettcher et al. 2013b). Because studies on Internet interventions can be conducted faster and more efficiently than trials on face-to-face treatments, it is likely that research on ICBT for SAD will also contribute to the overall development of new or optimized interventions for SAD in the future.

Another way of optimizing treatments for SAD is to understand better for whom and how treatments work. As outlined above, research on predictors of ICBT for SAD is still rather scarce and few findings are stable across studies. The only finding that seems to be relatively consistent is that baseline social anxiety levels and patient expectations are related to outcome. Future directions in this line of research should also be to take advantage of the fact that ICBT confers the possibility to easily monitor patients' behavior. Assessing early process predictors, such as program usage, could be used to inform therapeutic decisions on an ongoing basis.

More research is also necessary regarding moderators of outcome in face-to-face therapy versus ICBT because it is likely that patients may be more or less suitable for either format. As described above, it may be that patients with comorbid general anxiety and depression are somewhat more suitable for face-to-face CBT, but results need to be replicated before any strong clinical recommendations can be made concerning when a patient should receive ICBT and when face-to-face CBT is preferable.

When it comes to treatment mechanisms, it is likely that ICBT partly achieve its effects through the same mechanisms as face-to-face CBT. But there may also be working mechanisms of change that are unique or realized to a larger extent in Internet interventions. For instance, there are indications that in comparison with usual care, web-based interventions may have a positive effect on patient empowerment, self-efficacy, and mastery (Samoocha et al. 2010). This is plausible since ICBT aims at improving self-management and self-help capabilities. Another aspect previously mentioned is that especially SAD patients may be more relaxed when learning about their condition at home in a "safe" environment. Thus, the increase of knowledge about SAD through psychoeducation may be larger in Internet-based than face-to-face treatments and may play a more important role in ICBT. While there is no data to support this notion, there is at least one study showing that knowledge about SAD increased during ICBT, and that knowledge gain was significantly, although modestly, associated with outcome (Andersson et al. 2012).

Overall, ICBT for SAD is clearly an effective treatment and a promising treatment option for increasing accessibility to evidence-based psychological treatment. Since SAD is known to appear at an early age in most cases, one central future challenge is to increase the body of knowledge on ICBT for children and adolescents. Blended treatments combining face-to-face sessions with internet-based interventions should also be considered and researched in the future. And finally, more research is needed on how Internet-based treatments work and for whom they are indicated.

References

American Psychiatric Association (1994) Diagnostic and statistical manual of mental disorders: DSM-IV, 4th edn. American Psychiatric Association, Washington

American Psychiatric Association (2013) Diagnostic and statistical manual of mental disorders, 5th edn. American Psychiatric Publishing, Arlington

Andersson G, Carlbring P, Holmström A, Sparthan E, Furmark T, Nilsson-Ihrfelt E, Buhrman M, Ekselius L (2006) Internet-based self-help with therapist feedback and in vivo group exposure for social phobia: a randomized controlled trial. J Consult Clin Psychol 74:677–686

Andersson G, Estling F, Jakobsson E, Cuijpers P, Carlbring P (2011) Can the patient decide which modules to endorse? An open trial of tailored internet treatment of anxiety disorders. Cogn Behav Ther [Research Support, Non-U.S. Gov't] 40:57–64

Andersson G, Carlbring P, Furmark T, Group SOFIER (2012) Therapist experience and knowledge acquisition in internet-delivered CBT for social anxiety disorder: a randomized controlled trial. PLoS One [Randomized Controlled Trial Research Support, Non-U.S. Gov't] 7:e37411

Andrews G, Cuijpers P, Craske MG, McEvoy P, Titov N (2010) Computer therapy for the anxiety and depressive disorders is effective, acceptable and practical health care: a meta-analysis. PLoS One 5, e13196

Andrews G, Davies M, Titov N (2011b) Effectiveness randomized controlled trial of face to face versus internet cognitive behaviour therapy for social phobia. Aust N Z J Psychiatry [Randomized Controlled Trial] 45:337–340

Aydos L, Titov N, Andrews G (2009) Shyness 5: the clinical effectiveness of internet-based clinician-assisted treatment of social phobia. Australas Psychiatry 17:488–492

Beesdo K, Bittner A, Pine DS, Stein MB, Hofler M, Lieb R, Wittchen HU (2007) Incidence of social anxiety disorder and the consistent risk for secondary depression in the first three decades of life. Arch Gen Psychiatry 64:903–912

Berger T (2011) Web 2.0 – soziale netzwerke und psychotherapie. Psychother Dialog 12:118–122

Berger T, Hohl E, Caspar F (2009) Internet-based treatment for social phobia: a randomized controlled trial. J Clin Psychol 65:1021–1035

Berger T, Caspar F, Richardson R, Kneubuhler B, Sutter D, Andersson G (2011) Internet-based treatment of social phobia: a randomized controlled trial comparing unguided with two types of guided self-help. Behav Res Ther 49:158–169

Berger T, Boettcher J, Caspar F (2014) Internet-based guided self-help for several anxiety disorders: a randomized controlled trial comparing a tailored with a standardized disorder-specific approach. Psychotherapy [Research Support, Non-U.S. Gov't] 51:207–219
Blanco C, Heimberg RG, Schneier FR, Fresco DM, Chen H, Turk CL, Vermes D, Erwin BA, Schmidt AB, Juster HR, Campeas R, Liebowitz MR (2010) A placebo-controlled trial of phenelzine, cognitive behavioral group therapy, and their combination for social anxiety disorder. Arch Gen Psychiatry 67:286–295
Boettcher J, Berger T, Renneberg B (2012a) Does a pre-treatment diagnostic interview affect the outcome of internet-based self-help for social anxiety disorder? A randomized controlled trial. Behav Cogn Psychother 40:513–528
Boettcher J, Berger T, Renneberg B (2012b) Does a pre-treatment diagnostic interview affect the outcome of internet-based self-help for social anxiety disorder? A randomized controlled trial. Behav Cogn Psychother [Randomized Controlled Trial] 40:513–528
Boettcher J, Renneberg B, Berger T (2013a) Patient expectations in internet-based self-help for social anxiety. Cogn Behav Ther 42:203–214
Boettcher J, Carlbring P, Renneberg B, Berger T (2013b) Internet-based interventions for social anxiety disorder – an overview. Verhaltenstherapie 23:160–168
Botella C, Banos RM, Guillén V, Perpina C, Alcaniz M, Pons A (2000) Telepsychology: public speaking fear treatment on the internet. Cyber Psychol Behav 3:959–968
Botella C, Hofmann S, Moscovitz D (2004) A self-applied internet-based intervention for fear of public speaking. J Clin Psychol 60:1–10
Botella C, Guillen V, Banos RM, García-Palacios A, Gallego MJ, Alcaniz M (2007) Telepsychology and self-help: the treatment of fear of public speaking. Cogn Behav Pract 14:46–57
Botella C, Gallego MJ, Garcia-Palacios A, Guillen V, Banos RM, Quero S, Alcaniz M (2010) An internet-based self-help treatment for fear of public speaking: a controlled trial. Cyberpsychol Behav Soc Netw 13:407–421
Bruch MA, Fallon M, Heimberg RG (2003) Social phobia and difficulties in occupational adjustment. J Counc Psychol 50:109–117
Carlbring P, Furmark T, Steczko J, Ekselius L, Andersson G (2006) An open study of internet-based bibliotherapy with minimal therapist contact via email for social phobia. Clin Psychol 10:30–38
Carlbring P, Gunnarsdottir M, Hedensjo L, Andersson G, Ekselius L, Furmark T (2007) Treatment of social phobia: randomised trial of internet-delivered cognitive-behavioural therapy with telephone support. Br J Psychiatry 190:123–128
Carlbring P, Bergman Nordgren L, Furmark T, Andersson G (2009) Long-term outcome of internet-delivered cognitive-behavioural therapy for social phobia: a 30-month follow-up. Behav Res Ther 47:848–850
Carlbring P, Maurin L, Torngren C, Linna E, Eriksson T, Sparthan E, Straat M, Marquez von Hage C, Bergman-Nordgren L, Andersson G (2011a) Individually-tailored, internet-based treatment for anxiety disorders: a randomized controlled trial. Behav Res Ther 49:18–24
Carlbring P, Maurin L, Torngren C, Linna E, Eriksson T, Sparthan E, Straat M, Marquez von Hage C, Bergman-Nordgren L, Andersson G (2011b) Individually-tailored, internet-based treatment for anxiety disorders: a randomized controlled trial. Behav Res Ther [Randomized Controlled Trial Research Support, Non-U.S. Gov't] 49:18–24
Chartier MJ, Walker JR, Stein MB (2003) Considering comorbidity in social phobia. Soc Psychiatry Psychiatr Epidemiol 38:728–734
Clark DM, Wells A (1995) A cognitive model of social phobia. In: Heimberg RG, Leibowitz M, Hope DA, Schneider FR (eds) Social phobia: diagnosis, assessment and treatment. Guilford press, New York
Clark DM, Ehlers A, McManus F, Hackmann A, Fennell M, Campbell H, Flower T, Davenport C, Louis B (2003) Cognitive therapy versus fluoxetine in generalized social phobia: a randomized placebo-controlled trial. J Consult Clin Psychol 71:1058–1067
Dahl AA, Dahl CF (2010) Are there gender differences in impairment associated with high social anxiety? A community-based study. J Anxiety Disord 24:487–493

Davidson JR, Hughes DL, George LK, Blazer DG (1993) The epidemiology of social phobia: findings from the duke epidemiological catchment area study. Psychol Med 23:709–718

Erwin BA, Turk CL, Heimberg RG, Fresco DM, Hantula DA (2004) The internet: home to a severe population of individuals with social anxiety disorder? J Anxiety Disord 18:629–646

Eskildsen A, Hougaard E, Rosenberg NK (2010) Pre-treatment patient variables as predictors of drop-out and treatment outcome in cognitive behavioural therapy for social phobia: a systematic review. Nord J Psychiatry 64:94–105

Fehm L, Pelissolo A, Furmark T, Wittchen H-U (2005) Size and burden of social phobia in europe. Eur Neuropsychopharmacol 15:453–462

Furmark T (2002) Social phobia: overview of community surveys. Acta Psychiatr Scand 105:84–93

Furmark T, Tillfors M, Everz P, Marteinsdottir I, Gefvert O, Fredrikson M (1999) Social phobia in the general population: prevalence and sociodemographic profile. Soc Psychiatry Psychiatr Epidemiol 34:416–424

Furmark T, Carlbring P, Hedman E, Sonnenstein A, Clevberger P, Bohman B, Eriksson A, Hallen A, Frykman M, Holmstrom A, Sparthan E, Tillfors M, Ihrfelt EN, Spak M, Ekselius L, Andersson G (2009a) Guided and unguided self-help for social anxiety disorder: randomised controlled trial. Br J Psychiatry J Ment Sci [Randomized Controlled Trial Research Support, Non-US Gov't] 195:440–447

Furmark T, Carlbring P, Hedman E, Sonnenstein A, Clevberger P, Bohman B, Eriksson A, Hallen A, Frykman M, Holmstrom A, Sparthan E, Tillfors M, Ihrfelt EN, Spak M, Eriksson A, Ekselius L, Andersson G (2009b) Guided and unguided self-help for social anxiety disorder: randomised controlled trial. Br J Psychiatry J Ment Sci [Randomized Controlled Trial Research Support, Non-U.S. Gov't] 195:440–447

Gallego M, Emmelkamp P, van der Kooj M, Mees H (2011) The effects of a Dutch version of an internet based treatment program for fear of public speaking: a controlled study. Int J Clin Health Psychol 11:459–472

Hedman E, Furmark T, Carlbring P, Ljotsson B, Ruck C, Lindefors N, Andersson G (2011a) A 5-year follow-up of internet-based cognitive behavior therapy for social anxiety disorder. J Med Internet Res 13, e39

Hedman E, Andersson G, Ljótsson B, Andersson E, Rück C, Mörtberg E, Lindefors N (2011b) Internet-based cognitive behavior therapy vs cognitive behavioral group therapy for social anxiety disorder: a randomized controlled non-inferiority trial. PLoS ONE 6, e18001

Hedman E, Andersson E, Ljotsson B, Andersson G, Ruck C, Lindefors N (2011c) Cost-effectiveness of internet-based cognitive behavior therapy vs. cognitive behavioral group therapy for social anxiety disorder: results from a randomized controlled trial. Behav Res Ther 49:729–736

Hedman E, Andersson E, Ljótsson B, Andersson G, Andersson E, Schalling M, Lindefors N, Ruck C (2012a) Clinical and genetic outcome determinants of internet- and group-based cognitive behavior therapy for social anxiety disorder. Acta Psychiatr Scand 126:126–136

Hedman E, Ljótsson B, Lindefors N (2012b) Cognitive behavior therapy via the internet: a systematic review of applications, clinical efficacy and cost-effectiveness. Expert Rev Pharmacoecon Outcomes Res 12:745–764

Hedman E, Carlbring P, Ljótsson B, Andersson G (2014a) Internetbaserad psykologisk behandling: evidens, indikation och praktiskt genomförande. Natur & Kultur, Stockholm

Hedman E, El Alaoui S, Lindefors N, Andersson E, Ruck C, Ghaderi A, Kaldo V, Lekander M, Andersson G, Ljotsson B (2014b) Clinical effectiveness and cost-effectiveness of internet- vs. group-based cognitive behavior therapy for social anxiety disorder: 4-year follow-up of a randomized trial. Behav Res Ther 59:20–29

Heimberg RG, Becker RE (2002) Cognitive-behavioral group therapy for social phobia. Basic mechanisms and clinical strategies. Guilford Press, New York

Heimberg RG, Salzman DG, Holt CS, Blendell KA (1993) Cognitive-behavioral group treatment for social phobia: effectiveness at five-year follow up. Cogn Ther Res 17:325–339

Hofmann SG, Sawyer AT, Korte KJ, Smits JA (2009) Is it beneficial to add pharmacotherapy to cognitive-behavioral therapy when treating anxiety disorders? A meta-analytic review. Int J Cogn Ther 2:160–175

Johansson R, Sjoberg E, Sjogren M, Johnsson E, Carlbring P, Andersson T, Rousseau A, Andersson G (2012) Tailored vs. standardized internet-based cognitive behavior therapy for depression and comorbid symptoms: a randomized controlled trial. PLoS One [Clinical Trial Randomized Controlled Trial Research Support, Non-U.S. Gov't] 7:e36905

Johnston L, Titov N, Andrews G, Spence J, Dear BF (2011) A RCT of a transdiagnostic internet-delivered treatment for three anxiety disorders: examination of support roles and disorder-specific outcomes. PLoS One 6, e28079

Kessler RC. The impairments caused by social phobia in the general population: implications for intervention. Acta Psychiatr Scand Suppl [Research Support, Non-U.S. Gov't Review] 2003:19–27

Kessler RC, McGonagle KA, Zhao S, Nelson CB, Hughes M, Eshleman S, Wittchen HU, Kendler KS (1994) Lifetime and 12-month prevalence of dsm-iii-r psychiatric disorders in the United States. Results from the national comorbidity survey. Arch Gen Psychiatry 51:8–19

Kessler RC, Petukhova M, Sampson NA, Zaslavsky AM, Wittchen HU (2012) Twelve-month and lifetime prevalence and lifetime morbid risk of anxiety and mood disorders in the United States. Int J Methods Psychiatr Res 21:169–184

Klein B, Meyer D, Austin DW, Kyrios M (2011) Anxiety online: a virtual clinic: preliminary outcomes following completion of five fully automated treatment programs for anxiety disorders and symptoms. J Med Internet Res [Clinical Trial Research Support, Non-U.S. Gov't]. 13:e89

Kraemer HC, Wilson GT, Fairburn CG, Agras WS (2002) Mediators and moderators of treatment effects in randomized clinical trials. Arch Gen Psychiatry 59:877–883

Lampe L, Slade T, Issakidis C, Andrews G (2003) Social phobia in the Australian national survey of mental health and well-being (NSMHWB). Psychol Med 33:637–646

Lewis C, Pearce J, Bisson JI (2012) Efficacy, cost-effectiveness and acceptability of self-help interventions for anxiety disorders: systematic review. Br J Psychiatry 200:15–21

Liebowitz MR, Heimberg RG, Fresco DM, Travers J, Stein MB (2000) Social phobia or social anxiety disorder: what's in a name? Arch Gen Psychiatry 57:191–192

Lipsitz JD, Schneier FR (2000) Social phobia. Epidemiology and cost of illness. Pharmacoeconomics 18:23–32

Magee WJ, Eaton WW, Wittchen HU, McGonagle KA, Kessler RC (1996) Agoraphobia, simple phobia, and social phobia in the national comorbidity survey. Arch Gen Psychiatry 53:159–168

McEvoy PM (2007) Effectiveness of cognitive behavioural group therapy for social phobia in a community clinic: a benchmarking study. Behav Res Ther 45:3030–3040

Mohr DC, Siddique J, Ho J, Duffecy J, Jin L, Fokuo JK (2010) Interest in behavioral and psychological treatments delivered face-to-face, by telephone, and by internet. Ann Behav Med Publ Soc Behav Med [Comparative Study Research Support, N.I.H., Extramural] 40:89–98

Mörtberg E, Clark DM, Bejerot S (2011) Intensive group cognitive therapy and individual cognitive therapy for social phobia: sustained improvement at 5-year follow-up. J Anxiety Disord 25:994–1000

Nordgreen T, Havik OE, Ost LG, Furmark T, Carlbring P, Andersson G (2012) Outcome predictors in guided and unguided self-help for social anxiety disorder. Behav Res Ther 50:13–21

Nordgren LB, Hedman E, Etienne J, Bodin J, Kadowaki A, Eriksson S, Lindkvist E, Andersson G, Carlbring P (2014) Effectiveness and cost-effectiveness of individually tailored internet-delivered cognitive behavior therapy for anxiety disorders in a primary care population: a randomized controlled trial. Behav Res Ther 59:1–11

Olatunji BO, Cisler JM, Tolin DF (2007) Quality of life in the anxiety disorders: a meta-analytic review. Clin Psychol Rev 27:572–581

Ponniah K, Hollon SD (2008) Empirically supported psychological interventions for social phobia in adults: a qualitative review of randomized controlled trials. Psychol Med 38:3–14

Richards D, Richardson T (2012) Computer-based psychological treatments for depression: a systematic review and meta-analysis. Clin Psychol Rev [Meta-Analysis] 32:329–342

Ruscio AM, Brown TA, Chiu WT, Sareen J, Stein MB, Kessler RC (2008) Social fears and social phobia in the USA: results from the national comorbidity survey replication. Psychol Med 38:15–28

Samoocha D, Bruinvels DJ, Elbers NA, Anema JR, van der Beek AJ (2010) Effectiveness of web-based interventions on patient empowerment: a systematic review and meta-analysis. J Med Internet Res [Meta-Analysis Review] 12:e23

Spek V, Cuijpers P, Nyklicek I, Riper H, Keyzer J, Pop V (2007) Internet-based cognitive behaviour therapy for symptoms of depression and anxiety: a meta-analysis. Psychol Med [Comparative Study Meta-Analysis Research Support, Non-U.S. Gov't] 37:319–328

Stein MB, Stein DJ (2008) Social anxiety disorder. Lancet 371:1115–1125

Stott R, Wild J, Grey N, Liness S, Warnock-Parkes E, Commins S, Readings J, Bremner G, Woodward E, Ehlers A, Clark DM (2013) Internet-delivered cognitive therapy for social anxiety disorder: a development pilot series. Behav Cogn Psychother 41:383–397

Stuhldreher N, Leibing E, Leichsenring F, Beutel ME, Herpertz S, Hoyer J, Konnopka A, Salzer S, Strauss B, Wiltink J, Konig HH (2014) The costs of social anxiety disorder: the role of symptom severity and comorbidities. J Affect Disord 165:87–94

Tillfors M, Carlbring P, Furmark T, Lewenhaupt S, Spak M, Eriksson A, Westling BE, Andersson G (2008) Treating university students with social phobia and public speaking fears: internet delivered self-help with or without live group exposure sessions. Depress Anxiety 25:708–717

Titov N, Andrews G, Schwencke G, Drobny J, Einstein D (2008a) Shyness 1: distance treatment of social phobia over the internet. Aust N Z J Psychiatry 42:585–594

Titov N, Andrews G, Schwencke G (2008b) Shyness 2: treating social phobia online: replication and extension. Aust N Z J Psychiatry 42:595–605

Titov N, Andrews G, Choi I, Schwencke G, Mahoney A (2008c) Shyness 3: randomized controlled trial of guided versus unguided internet-based CBT for social phobia. Aust N Z J Psychiatry 42:1030–1040

Titov N, Andrews G, Choi I, Schwencke G, Johnston L (2009a) Randomized controlled trial of web-based treatment of social phobia without clinician guidance. Aust N Z J Psychiatry 43:913–919

Titov N, Andrews G, Schwencke G, Solley K, Johnston L, Robinson E (2009b) An RCT comparing effect of two types of support on severity of symptoms for people completing internet-based cognitive behaviour therapy for social phobia. Aust N Z J Psychiatry 43:920–926

Titov N, Andrews G, Johnston L, Schwencke G, Choi I (2009c) Shyness programme: longer term benefits, cost-effectiveness, and acceptability. Aust N Z J Psychiatry 43:36–44

Titov N, Andrews G, Schwencke G, Robinson E, Peters L, Spence J (2010a) Randomized controlled trial of internet cognitive behavioural treatment for social phobia with and without motivational enhancement strategies. Aust N Z J Psychiatry 44:938–945

Titov N, Andrews G, Johnston L, Robinson E, Spence J (2010b) Transdiagnostic internet treatment for anxiety disorders: a randomized controlled trial. Behav Res Ther [Randomized Controlled Trial Research Support, Non-U.S. Gov't] 48:890–899

Titov N, Dear BF, Schwencke G, Andrews G, Johnston L, Craske MG, McEvoy P (2011) Transdiagnostic internet treatment for anxiety and depression: a randomised controlled trial. Behav Res Ther [Randomized Controlled Trial Research Support, Non-U.S. Gov't] 49:441–452

Wittchen HU, Fehm L (2003) Epidemiology and natural course of social fears and social phobia. Acta Psychiatr Scand Suppl 4–18

Wittchen HU, Fuetsch M, Sonntag H, Müller N, Liebowitz M (2000) Disability and quality of life in pure and comorbid social phobia. Findings from a controlled study. Eur Psychiatry 15:46–58

Yonkers KA, Dyck IR, Keller MB (2001) An eight-year longitudinal comparison of clinical course and characteristics of social phobia among men and women. Psychiatr Serv 52:637–643

ICBT in Psychiatry: Generalised Anxiety Disorder

5

Nickolai Titov, Gerhard Andersson, and Björn Paxling

Abstract

Generalised anxiety disorder (GAD) is a common anxiety disorder characterised by excessive and uncontrollable worry. It is a chronic disorder associated with considerable disability. Historically, GAD has been considered one of the least successfully treated anxiety disorders. In recent years, more than ten published studies have described outcomes of Internet-delivered cognitive behavioural therapy (ICBT) for GAD. These include research trials and reports of use in clinics. The results of research trials consistently reveal that large effect sizes are obtained during therapist-guided ICBT, with gains sustained up to 2 years post-treatment. Reports of use of ICBT for GAD from clinics are also highly promising and indicate that those who complete the interventions obtain outcomes similar to those reported in clinical trials. To date, most reports from clinics using ICBT for GAD have been limited to analyses of outcomes from those who have completed the ICBT intervention. This limits the conclusions that can be drawn about the effectiveness of existing ICBT interventions for GAD at this time. It is expected, however, that future reports will confirm the potential of ICBT interventions for treating GAD.

N. Titov (✉)
Department of Psychology, Macquarie University,
Nickolai Titov, Room 723, Building C3A, Sydney NSW 2109, Australia
e-mail: nick.titov@mq.edu.au

G. Andersson
Department of Behavioural Sciences and Learning, Linköping University,
Linköping, Sweden

Department of Clinical Neuroscience, Psychiatry, Karolinska Institutet,
Stockholm, Sweden

B. Paxling, PhD
Psykologpartners, Private Practice, Malmö, Sweden

© Springer International Publishing Switzerland 2016

N. Lindefors, G. Andersson (eds.), *Guided Internet-Based Treatments in Psychiatry*, DOI 10.1007/978-3-319-06083-5_5

Description of the Disorder

Generalised anxiety disorder (GAD) is a common anxiety disorder described as a condition characterised by excessive, frequent and uncontrollable worry (American Psychiatric Association, 2000), or by persistent, generalised and *free-floating* anxiety (World Health Organization 1992). Common foci of worry include minor and daily hassles, worry about health, employment, finances and the future of self and loved ones (Breitholtz et al. 1998) and even fear that worrying will lead to further emotional or physical illness. In addition to cognitive symptoms, people with GAD frequently experience psychological and somatic complaints, including irritability, problems with concentrating, autonomic arousal, sleep problems, muscle tension and restlessness and fatigue.

Similar to other anxiety disorders (Kessler and Greenberg 2002), GAD is often chronic and associated with low levels of remission without treatment (Noyes et al. 1996; Yonkers et al. 2003). GAD is highly co-morbid with other anxiety disorders and in particular with major depressive disorder. GAD is highly disabling and is associated with levels of disability comparable to depression (Hoffman et al. 2008). People with GAD make considerable use of general healthcare facilities (Spitzer et al. 2006; Wittchen 2002), visiting their doctor twice as frequently as patients with comparable chronic physical conditions and similar demographic characteristics (Kessler and Wittchen 2002). Although people with GAD frequently utilise healthcare facilities, they often report somatic rather than psychological symptoms, making diagnosis and therefore treatment difficult. Moreover, treatment may also be complicated by changes in the content of the worry over time (Constans et al. 2002).

Estimates of the 12-month prevalence rate of GAD range between 1.0 and 4.1 % (Gale and Davidson 2007; Kessler et al. 2008) and estimates of lifetime prevalence range between 4.3 and 5.9 % (Tyrer and Baldwin 2006). GAD is more prevalent in females, and nationally representative data from the USA and from the World Health Organization World Mental Health Surveys indicates the age of onset to be approximately 30 years (Kessler et al. 2007). It should be noted, however, that the onset of GAD may be subtle with many individuals experiencing chronic symptoms before meeting full diagnostic criteria for a disorder (Rapee and Bryant 2009).

Treatment

Historically, GAD was considered the least successfully treated anxiety disorder (Brown et al. 1994). However, meta-analyses now indicate that both pharmacological and psychological treatments are effective in the treatment of GAD (Cuijpers et al. 2014).

A wide range of pharmacotherapies are used for treating GAD including selective serotonin reuptake inhibitors (SSRIs), serotonin/norepinephrine reuptake inhibitors, tricyclic antidepressants and monoamine oxidase inhibitors, benzodiazepines, anticonvulsants and antipsychotics (Ravindran and Stein 2009). SSRIs are a recommended medication for the treatment of GAD (NICE 2007) and are generally preferred over other pharmacotherapies due to their favourable side-effect profile, tolerability to consumers and superior efficacy (Stein 2006). Meta-analyses of double-blind placebo-controlled trials for GAD (Hidalgo et al. 2007) have demonstrated significant improvement in response to SSRI treatment.

A broad range of psychological therapies have been used to treat GAD including non-directive supportive therapy (Stanley et al. 1996) and psychodynamic therapies (Leichsenring et al. 2009; Levy Berg et al. 2009). The majority of psychological therapies are based on principles of cognitive and behavioural therapy (CBT). Cognitive behavioural therapy (CBT) is a psychotherapeutic approach that addresses maladaptive behaviours, dysfunctional emotions and cognitive processes and contents. This is done through a number of goal-oriented, systematic procedures. Early treatments were based on the cognitive model of Beck (Beck et al. 1985), amongst others, who proposed that anxiety and depressive disorders including GAD were associated with disorder-specific maladaptive beliefs, judgments and memories influencing how an individual perceived themselves, their world and future (Beck 1991; Beck et al. 1985). More recent CBT models of GAD have proposed a relationship between cognitions, avoidance and escape behaviours and physical arousal. Such models include those described by Borkovec et al. (2004) and Dugas et al. (1997, 1998); (Wells 1995; Wells and Carter 1999). A common focus in recent CBT treatments for GAD is for the patient to analyse and understand how his/her voluntary behaviours affect their experienced problems with worry and to explore ways of acting differently. Despite similarities between the above-mentioned models of CBT treatments, differences exist in the relative importance and role of uncertainty and problem orientation (Dugas et al. 1997, 1998), cognitive avoidance (Borkovec et al. 2004), intolerance of uncertainty, beliefs about worry and meta-worry (Wells 1995; Wells and Carter 1999). More recent extensions of CBT for GAD include acceptance-based therapy (Roemer and Orsillo 2002; Treanor et al. 2011) and metacognitive therapy (Wells and King 2006).

Psychological therapies for GAD have mostly been administered as individual face-to-face treatments, although several have been administered as self-help therapies (Bowman et al. 1997) or group treatments (Dugas et al. 2003). More recently, several Internet-delivered cognitive behavioural treatments (ICBT) for GAD have been reported and evaluated. The general benefits of ICBT are described in Chap. 1 and will not be repeated here. Current ICBT psychological treatments typically include a combination of several of the following components: cognitive restructuring, graded exposure, problem-solving and relaxation skills. Additional details about the characteristics and evidence for ICBT interventions for GAD are described below.

Existing ICBT Programmes for GAD

To date, at least 11 ICBT interventions for GAD have been developed and evaluated in published research trials (Carlbring et al. 2011; Dear et al. 2011a; Draper et al. 2008; Johnston et al. 2011; Klein et al. 2011; Newby et al. 2013; Paxling et al. 2011; Titov et al. 2009a, 2013, 2011). Several of these interventions have also been evaluated in clinical settings with clinical populations as part of routine clinical practice.

The majority of Internet-delivered interventions for GAD are based on principles of CBT; however, at least one intervention based on psychodynamic therapy has been developed and evaluated (Andersson et al. 2012). Moreover, there is currently one intervention based on acceptance, and commitment therapy that has been evaluated but not yet published.

The duration of ICBT interventions for GAD typically ranges between 8 and 12 weeks. However, most ICBT interventions allow patients to continue to log on and access treatment materials beyond the formal end point of the intervention. For example, Draper et al. (2008) reported one patient took 22 weeks to complete the intervention. Patients sometimes terminate their treatments in advance, and reasons for this have been examined in one study (Johansson et al. 2015).

ICBT interventions for GAD also differ in their level of attention to treating other disorders in addition to GAD. For example, some are primarily concerned with treating symptoms specific to GAD (*disorder-specific* interventions), while others target symptoms of GAD in addition to symptoms of other anxiety disorders and/or depression (*transdiagnostic interventions* or *tailored interventions*). This point is particularly important given the high rates of co-morbidity between GAD and depression and between GAD and other anxiety disorders. It should be noted that although an intervention may be *disorder specific* with respect to targeting one disorder, given the overlap in symptoms between anxiety disorders and depression, improvement in one domain is often associated with improvement in other disorders (Andersson and Titov 2014; Titov et al. 2012; Titov et al. 2009b).

Another important difference between ICBT interventions for GAD is whether they are administered by a therapist, that is, *therapist guided*, or without a therapist, that is, *self-guided*. To date, the majority of Internet-delivered treatments for GAD have been administered with therapist support, although self-guided versions have also been evaluated (Klein et al. 2011; Titov et al. 2013, 2014). Those utilising therapist support have used either text-based communication, or a combination of text and telephone support. Such interventions typically utilise scripts or guidelines for therapist contact, which facilitate attention to key messages in the intervention while also reducing therapist drift.

Treatment Components and Strategies

ICBT interventions for GAD comprise highly structured materials that target three core symptoms believed to be problematic in GAD and other anxiety disorders. These core symptoms include maladaptive cognitions, maladaptive behaviours including avoidance behaviours and physiological arousal. Similar to face-to-face CBT, in ICBT, these core symptoms are treated using generic CBT strategies that target each of these symptom groups including cognitive challenging and restructuring, imaginal and graded exposure and applied relaxation and de-arousal strategies.

Teaching of these strategies is usually preceded by educational material which provides a conceptual framework for helping the participant recognise the core symptoms and the factors that trigger and maintain these symptoms. This framework, or *formulation*, also provides the rationale for learning and applying the core CBT strategies. Typically, each strategy is taught in isolation, with increasing emphasis on applying the skill regularly and across a broad range of situations. However, it should be noted that in latter phases of treatment once a participant has learned the key components of each strategy, the person is often encouraged to use the strategies at the same time. For example, in latter phases of treatment, participants may be encouraged to use de-arousal strategies such as controlled breathing in combination with cognitive skills for challenging unhelpful thoughts and beliefs about worry.

Additional strategies and skills taught in such interventions often include strategies for managing intolerance of uncertainty, managing unhelpful metacognitive beliefs and strategies associated with acceptance and mindfulness models of psychological therapy. Scheduled worry time (Borkovec and Costello 1993; Borkovec et al. 1983) is an intervention in which the patient is encouraged to postpone worry to a specific period each day which helps to increase discriminative control regarding stimuli that trigger worrying. Practical problem solving is another commonly used intervention, which helps patients to separate worry topics so they can do something practical about them and gives patients a concrete framework for acting accordingly. To facilitate the process of learning, patients are usually provided with homework assignments which may be reviewed by their therapist. Finally, most ICBT interventions provide information and recommendations about increasing resilience and reducing risk of relapse. A list of interventions used in different treatment programmes is presented in Table 5.1.

Effects in Research and Clinic: Results of Research Trials and Clinical Use

The studies described below report published outcomes for ICBT interventions for GAD (see Table 5.2). Studies were included if they evaluated interventions that were designed specifically for treating GAD or designed to target symptoms of GAD in addition to symptoms of other anxiety disorders or depression. All studies included were conducted in either Sweden or Australia. Before discussing the results of these studies, it is helpful to consider issues in diagnosis and measurement of symptoms of GAD.

Diagnosis and Measurement of GAD

It should be noted that several strategies have been used in studies of ICBT for GAD to identify people with clinical or subclinical levels of GAD. These include manually administered clinical interviews, automated structured diagnostic interviews, or

Table 5.1 Treatment strategies included in studies of Internet-delivered cognitive behavioural treatments for GAD

	Educational material	Applied relaxation or other relaxation/ de-arousal intervention	Cognitive restructuring for thoughts, beliefs and meta-cognitive beliefs	Scheduled worry time	Problem solving	Worry exposure/ behavioural experiments	Interpersonal problem solving and/or communication skills training	Sleep management	Behavioural activation/ activity scheduling	Mindfulness	Relapse prevention
Carlbring et al. (2011)	x	(x)*	x	x	x	x		(x)*	(x)*		x
Dear et al. (2011a)	x	x	x	(x)*	(x)*	X	(x)*	(x)*	x		x
Draper et al. (2008)	x	x	x		x	x				x	x
Johnston et al. (2011)	x	x	x	(x)*	(x)*	x	(x)*	(x)*	x		x
Newby et al. (2013)	x	x	x		x	x			x		x
Paxling et al. (2011)	x	x	x	x	x	x	x	x			x
Titov et al. (2013)	x	x	x	(x)*	(x)*	x	(x)*	(x)*	x		x
Titov et al. (2011)	x	x	x	(x)*	(x)*	x	(x)*	(x)*	x		x
Titov et al. (2009a)	x	x	x	(x)*	(x)*	x	(x)*	(x)*	x		x

*(x)** Indicates the treatment strategy was administered to participants who the therapist thought would benefit from them

Table 5.2 Studies of Internet-delivered cognitive behavioural treatments for GAD

Authors (country)	Design					Sample		Results			
	Design conditions (n)	Primary outcome measures	Intervention components	Treatment duration	Guidance	*N*	Diagnostic tool/criteria	Analysis	Total therapist contact	Within-group ES (pre-post *d*)	Within-group ES (pre-follow-up *d*) (duration)
Draper et al. (2008) (Australia)	Research open trial 1. TG ICBT	(a) GADQ-IV, (b) PSWQ	11 CBT-based online lessons; occasional telephone calls	11 weeks	Self-guided	3	SCID-IV	ITT/completer	Occasional phone calls to facilitate engagement	–	–
Titov et al. (2009a) (Australia)	Research RCT 1. TG ICBT 2. WLC	(a) GAD-7, (b) PSWQ	6 CBT-based online lessons; homework assignments; additional written resources; weekly secure messaging or telephone calls; online discussion forum	8 weeks	Therapist guided	45	MINI	ITT	130 min	1. (a) 1.67; (b) 0.98 2. (a) 0.34; (b) 0.02	–
Robinson et al. (2010) (Australia)	Research RCT 1. TG ICBT 2. CG ICBT 3. WLC	(a) GAD-7, (b) PSWQ	6 CBT-based online lessons; homework assignments; additional written resources; weekly secure messaging or telephone calls; automated emails; online discussion forum	10 weeks	Therapist guided	145	MINI	ITT	TG ICBT 81 min; CG ICBT 75 min	1. (a) 1.55; (b) 1.16 2. (a) 1.73; (b) 1.07 3. (a) 0.38; (b) 0.14	1. a) 1.48; b) 1.42 2. a) 1.61; b) 0.97 – (3 months)

(continued)

Table 5.2 (continued)

Au thors (country)	Design					Sample		Results			
	Design conditions (n)	Primary outcome measures	Intervention components	Treatment duration	Guidance	*N*	Diagnostic tool/criteria	Analysis	Total therapist contact	Within-group ES (pre-post *d*)	Within-group ES (pre-follow-up *d*) (duration)
Titov et al. (2010) (Australia)	Research RCT 1. TD TG ICBT 2. WLC	(a) GAD-7, (b) PSWQ	6 CBT-based online lessons; homework assignments; additional written resources; weekly secure messaging or telephone calls; online discussion forum	8 weeks	Therapist guided	78	MINI	ITT	46 min	1. a) 0.81; b) 0.60 2. a) -0.01; b) 0.21	1. (a) 0.73; (b).79 (3 months)
Johnston et al. (2010) (Australia)	Research RCT 1. TG ICBT 2. CG ICBT 3. WLC	(a) GAD-7, (b) PSWQ	8 CBT-based online lessons; homework assignments; additional written resources; weekly secure messaging or telephone calls; automated emails; online discussion forum	10 weeks	Therapist guided	131	MINI	ITT	TG ICBT 70 min; CG ICBT 69 min	1. (a) 0.71; (b) 0.81 2. (a) 1.06; (b) 1.17 3. (a) 0.15; (b) 0.02	1. (a) 0.57; (b) 0.81 2. (a) 1.18; (b) 1.12 – (3 months)
Carlbring et al. (2011) (Sweden)	Research RCT 1. IT TG ICBT 2. AC	(a) BAI, (b) MADRS-S	Participants prescribed 6 to 10 CBT-based online modules based on existing ICBT interventions for panic disorder, social phobia, GAD and depression	10 weeks	Therapist guided	54	SCID-I	ITT	85 min	1. (a) 1.12; (b) 1.21 2. (a) 0.44; (b) 0.46	1. (a) 1.23; (b) 1.31 (Entire sample 2 years)

Titov et al. (2011) (Australia)	Research RCT 1. TD TG ICBT 2. WLC	(a) GAD-7, (b) PSWQ	8 CBT-based online lessons; homework assignments; additional written resources; weekly secure messaging or telephone calls; online discussion forum	10 weeks	Therapist guided	74	MINI	ITT	85 min	1. (a) 0.92; (b) 0.68 2. (a) 0.22; (b) -0.08	1. (a) 0.94; (b) 0.63 (3 months)
Dear et al. (2011a) (Australia)	Research open trial 1. TD TG ICBT	(a) GAD-7, (b) PSWQ	5 CBT-based online lessons; homework assignments; additional written resources; weekly secure messaging or telephone calls; online discussion forum	8 weeks	Therapist guided	32	MINI	ITT	45 min	1. (a) 1.06; (b) 0.84	1. (a) 0.95; (b) 0.90 (3 months)
Paxling et al. (2011) (Sweden)	Research RCT 1. TG ICBT 2. WLC	(a) PSWQ	8 online treatment modules based on Paxling et al. (2011), weekly homework assignments, weekly secure messaging with therapist	8 weeks	Therapist guided	89	GADQ-IV	ITT	113 min	1. (a) 1.08 2. (a) -0.01	1. (a) 1.66 (12 months); (a) 1.40 (3 years)
Klein et al. (2011) (Australia)	Clinical open trial 1. SG ICBT	(a) GAD-CDSR	12 CBT-based online lessons; homework tasks, delivered in a fully automated system	12 weeks	Self-guided	88	Online diagnostic system/at least subclinical levels of GAD	Completers (88/704)	Nil	(a) 1.22	–

(continued)

Table 5.2 (continued)

Au thors (country)	Design					Sample		Results			
	Design conditions (n)	Primary outcome measures	Intervention components	Treatment duration	Guidance	*N*	Diagnostic tool/criteria	Analysis	Total therapist contact	Within-group ES (pre-post *d*)	Within-group ES (pre-follow-up *d*) (duration)
Andersson et al. (2012) (Sweden)	Research RCT 1. TG ICBT 2. TG IPDT 3. WLC	(a) PSWQ	1. 8 online treatment modules based on Paxling et al. (2011), weekly homework assignments, weekly secure messaging with therapist 2. 8 online chapters based on Make the Leap, self-help book and recommended writing assignments, weekly assignments, weekly secure messaging with therapist	8 weeks	Therapist guided	81	SCID-I	ITT	TG ICBT 92 min; IPDT 113 min	1. (a) 0.87 2. (a) 1.16 3. (a) 0.72	1. (a) 1.88 2. (a) 1.92 3. – (18 months)
Mewton et al. (2012) (Australia)	Clinical open trial 1. TG ICBT	(a) GAD-7	6 CBT-based online lessons; homework tasks, unspecified support from external health professional	11 weeks	Therapist guided	588	N/A	Completers (324/588)	Not described	(a) 0.91	–
Kirkpatrick et al. (2013) (Australia)	Clinical open trial 1. TG ICBT	(a) GAD-7, (b) PHQ-9	5 CBT-based online lessons; homework assignments; additional written resources; weekly telephone calls	8 weeks	Therapist guided	10	GAD-7 $\geq$ 5	ITT	Not described	1. (a) 1.07; (b) 1.76	1. (a) 1.61; (b) 2.17 (2 months)

Newby et al. (2013) (Australia)	Research RCT 1. TD TG ICBT 2. WLC	(a) GAD-7, (b) PSWQ	6 CBT-based online lessons; homework assignments; additional written resources; weekly secure messaging or telephone calls	8 weeks	Therapist guided	99	MINI	ITT	24 min	1. (a) 0.96; (b) 0.87 2. (a) 0.07; (b) 0.01	Not reported (3 months)
Newby et al. (2013) (Australia)	Clinical open trial 1. TD TG ICBT	(a) GAD-7, (b) PHQ-9	6 CBT-based online lessons; homework tasks, unspecified support from external health professional	8 weeks	Therapist guided	136	N/A	ITT	Not described	1. (a) 1.05; (b) 0.94	–
Titov et al. (2013, 2014) (Australia)	Research RCT 1. SGE ICBT 2. SG ICBT 3. WLC	(a) GAD-7, (b) PHQ-9	5 CBT-based online lessons; homework assignments; additional written resources; weekly secure messaging or telephone calls	8 weeks	Self-guided	257	GAD-7 $\geq$ 8, or PHQ-9 > 10, or MINI-SPIN $\geq$5, or ANSQ $\geq$1	ITT	Nil	1. (a) 1.08; (b) 0.96 2. (a) 0.76; (b) 0.68 3. (a) 0.14; (b) 0.02	1. (a) 1.08; (b) 1.10 2. (a) 1.01; (b) 0.98 (12 months)

AC Attention Control, *ANSQ* Autonomic Nervous System Questionnaire, *CG IPDT* Coach-Guided IPDT: Internet-Based Psychodynamic Treatment Group, *Completer* Analysis restricted to completers only, *ES* Effect Size, *GAD-7* Generalized Anxiety Disorder Scale, 7-Item Scale, *GAD-CDSR* GAD Clinical Disorder Severity Rating for Online Diagnostic System, *GADQ-IV* Generalized Anxiety Disorder Questionnaire, *IT TG ICBT* Individually Tailored Therapist-Guided ICBT, *MINI* Mini International Neuropsychiatric Interview Version 5.0.0, *MINI-SPIN* MINI Social Phobia Inventory, *PHQ-9* Patient Health Questionnaire-9-Item, *PSWQ* Penn State Worry Questionnaire, *SCID-I* Structured Clinical Interview for DSM-IV Axis 1 Disorders Research Version, *SCID-IV* Structured Clinical Interview for DSM-IV, *SG ICBT* Self-Guided ICBT, *SGE ICBT* Self-Guided ICBT with Automated Email Reminders, *TD* Transdiagnostic, *TG ICBT* Therapist-Guided Internet-Based Cognitive Behaviour Therapy, *IPDT* Internet-Based Psychodynamic Treatment Group, *ITT* Intention to Treat, *WLC* Waitlist Control Group cut-off scores based on responses to standardised questionnaires which are usually administered online. Where possible, these different criteria are noted below.

With respect to measurement of symptoms and severity of GAD in trials of ICBT, most studies have reported the use of the Penn State Worry Questionnaire (PSWQ) (Meyer et al. 1990) or the Generalized Anxiety Disorder 7-Item Scale (GAD-7) (Spitzer et al. 2006). The PSWQ consists of 16 items and is considered a valid clinical measure of worry characteristic of GAD. Early psychometric evaluations revealed the PSWQ had high internal consistency and temporal stability (Meyer et al. 1990) and was able to differentiate patients with GAD from those with other anxiety disorders (Brown et al. 1992). The GAD-7 is an increasingly popular measure of symptoms of GAD, which comprises seven items from the DSM-IV criteria for GAD. Psychometric evaluations of the GAD-7 indicate it is sufficiently sensitive to detect GAD, panic disorder, social phobia and post-traumatic stress disorder. A recent psychometric comparison of the PSWQ and GAD-7 revealed a moderate correlation between the two scales, and both were sensitive to change, although the GAD-7 appeared to be more sensitive and may, therefore, confer some advantages in clinical work (Dear et al. 2011b).

Outcomes of Disorder-Specific ICBT for GAD

The first report of disorder-specific ICBT for GAD was described by Draper et al. (2008) who reported results of an open trial using an 11-module intervention. This study included a small sample of three people who met DSM-IV criteria for GAD as determined by clinical interview. This ICBT intervention was administered as a self-guided intervention, although participants received occasional telephone calls to facilitate engagement and remind them to complete and return symptom questionnaires. Results were positive for all three patients with large clinically significant change observed from pre- to post-treatment which was maintained at 5-month follow-up in the two participants who provided data at that time point.

The first randomised controlled trial evaluating an ICBT intervention for GAD was reported by Titov and colleagues (2009a), who randomly allocated 48 participants who met DSM-IV criteria for GAD to a therapist-guided treatment condition or to a waitlist control condition. The ICBT intervention evaluated in this RCT comprised six online lessons, printable summary and homework assignments, automated emails and additional resource documents, with weekly support from a therapist via telephone or secure email. The intervention was completed over 10 weeks, and large pre- and post-treatment effect sizes were found on both the GAD-7 and PSWQ. The therapist spent an average of 130 min with each participant over the duration of the trial; however, a follow-up was not conducted.

The intervention used by Titov and colleagues was tested in a subsequent RCT by the same research group who replicated and extended the earlier results. This extension study (Robinson et al. 2010) explored whether the same ICBT intervention could be successfully and safely administered by a coach, or non-mental health professional who was supervised by a mental health professional. One hundred and fifty adults who met DSM-IV criteria for GAD were randomly allocated to either a therapist-guided group, a coach-guided group or to a waitlist control condition. Large (≥0.80) within-group effect sizes were found for each treatment condition on both the PSWQ and GAD-7, which were sustained at 3-month follow-up. In this RCT, the therapist and coach spent an average of less than 90 min during treatment in contact with patients.

An RCT evaluating the efficacy of a Swedish ICBT intervention for GAD was reported by Paxling et al. (2011) who randomly allocated 89 participants diagnosed with GAD to receive either an eight-module therapist-guided ICBT intervention delivered over 8 weeks, or to a waitlist control condition. Consistent with the RCTs described above, large within-group effect sizes were found for the treatment group between pre- and post-treatment on the PSWQ. Importantly, and representing an extension of previous findings, this study reported that treatment gains were sustained at 1- and 3-year follow-up. As with the previously reported studies, the therapists in the study by Paxling and colleagues spent an average of 97 min during treatment in contact with patients.

In a rather unique study, the ICBT intervention evaluated by Paxling et al. (2011) was subsequently compared with an eight-module psychodynamically informed Internet-delivered treatment (IPDT) using an RCT design (Andersson et al. 2012). In this study, a total of 81 participants diagnosed with GAD were randomly allocated to receive therapist-guided ICBT, therapist-guided IPDT or to a waitlist control condition. No statistical differences were found on the PSWQ between the treatment groups and the control group, although moderate to large within-group effect sizes were found at 3- and 18-month follow-up in a completer analysis.

The first description of outcomes from a disorder-specific ICBT intervention for GAD at an online clinic was reported by Klein et al. (2011). These results were obtained from an Australian national and publically accessible website offering ICBT interventions for a range of anxiety disorders. Potential participants were required to register at the website and complete an online and automated diagnostic tool. Those who were subsequently diagnosed with at least subclinical levels of GAD were provided with logins to the 12-week 12-module fully automated intervention. Of the 704 people who started the intervention, 88 (13 %) provided post-treatment results. Analyses using data from completers indicated significant reductions in clinical disorder severity ratings and decreases in the total number of clinical diagnoses. Unfortunately, while these results are encouraging, the lack of standardised clinical measures of GAD limits ability to compare results with the other studies.

Results of clinical use of a disorder-specific ICBT intervention for GAD at another online clinic were reported by Mewton, Wong and Andrews (2012) who described results of using the ICBT intervention previously reported (Robinson et al. 2010; Titov et al. 2009a). No diagnostic measures or exclusion criteria were used in this study. Of 588 patients who began the six-lesson therapist-guided ICBT intervention, 324 completed the intervention (324/588 = 55 %). Based on completers, a large within-group effect size was reported for the GAD-7, although follow-up results were not reported.

Outcomes of Transdiagnostic and Tailored ICBT for GAD

As indicated above, several ICBT interventions for GAD have also been developed to target symptoms of other anxiety disorders and/or depression, that is, transdiagnostic or tailored interventions. Given the high rates of comorbidity between GAD and other anxiety disorders and between GAD and depression (Hoffman et al. 2008), interventions that can effectively treat more than one target disorder are of both theoretical and pragmatic importance. Both transdiagnostic and tailored approaches have resulted in encouraging results in both research and clinical results, attesting to their potential implementation. Studies evaluating transdiagnostic and tailored ICBT interventions for GAD are discussed below.

Results of the first transdiagnostic ICBT intervention which targeted symptoms of three anxiety disorders (GAD, panic disorder and social anxiety disorder) were reported by Titov et al. (2010). Seventy-eight participants were randomly allocated to receive a therapist-guided transdiagnostic ICBT intervention, or to a waitlist control condition. All participants met diagnostic criteria for a principal diagnosis of GAD, panic disorder and social anxiety disorder. A clinically and statistically significant difference was found on the GAD-7 between the treatment groups and the control group at post-treatment, but not on the PSWQ. This transdiagnostic ICBT intervention was subsequently revised and extended before further evaluation in a second RCT (Johnston et al. 2011). This study explored whether the transdiagnostic ICBT intervention could be successfully and safely administered by a coach, or non-mental health professional supervised by a mental health professional. The 131 participants who met diagnostic criteria for a principal diagnosis of GAD, panic disorder and social anxiety disorder were randomly allocated to either a therapist-guided group, a coach-guided group or to a waitlist control condition. Large effect sizes were found for each treatment condition on both the PSWQ and GAD-7 at post-treatment, which were sustained at 3-month follow-up. In this RCT, the therapist and coach spent an average of approximately 70 min during treatment in contact with patients.

The same research team subsequently created an eight-lesson transdiagnostic ICBT intervention which targeted symptoms of depression and of three anxiety disorders (GAD, panic disorder and social anxiety disorder) (Titov et al. 2011). This intervention was initially tested in an RCT in which 74 participants were randomly allocated to receive the therapist-guided transdiagnostic ICBT intervention, or to a waitlist control condition. All participants met diagnostic criteria for a principle diagnosis of depression, GAD, panic disorder or social anxiety disorder. The intervention was administered over 10 weeks and the therapist spent approximately 85 min in total with each participant during treatment. A clinically and statistically significant difference was found on the PSWQ between the treatment groups and the control group at post-treatment, with gains in the treatment group sustained at 3-month follow-up. A brief five-lesson version of this intervention administered over 8 weeks was developed and evaluated in an open trial (Dear et al. 2011a) with 32 participants. Large within-group effect sizes were found for both the GAD-7 and PSWQ at post-treatment, which were maintained at follow-up. In this open trial, the therapist spent an average of approximately 45 min during treatment in contact with patients.

Another Australian research team created a six-lesson transdiagnostic ICBT intervention which targeted symptoms of GAD and depression, which was evaluated in both an RCT and in an online clinic (Newby et al. 2013). In the RCT, 99 participants were randomly allocated to receive the therapist-guided transdiagnostic ICBT intervention, or to a waitlist control condition. All participants met diagnostic criteria for a principle diagnosis of depression or GAD. The intervention was administered over 8 weeks and the therapist spent approximately 24 min with each participant during treatment. A clinically and statistically significant difference was found on the PSWQ between the treatment and the control group at post-treatment, with gains in the treatment group sustained at 3-month follow-up. This intervention was then evaluated in an online clinic with 136 patients of which 41 % completed the intervention and provided post-treatment data compared to 89 % in the RCT. Large effect sizes were found on the GAD-7 and PHQ-9 at post-treatment, although interpretation of results is difficult given the large amount of missing data.

Recent developments in ICBT interventions for GAD include a five-lesson transdiagnostic ICBT intervention that targets symptoms of depression, GAD, panic disorder and social anxiety disorder (Titov et al. 2013, 2014). This intervention has been evaluated as a self-guided and as a therapist-guided intervention. In one study, 257 people with elevated symptoms of GAD, panic disorder, social anxiety disorder or depression were randomly allocated to the 8-week self-guided version of the course either with or without automated emails, or to a waitlist control group (Titov et al. 2013). Completion rates of questionnaires at post-treatment and at 12-month follow-up were 85 and 80 %, respectively. At post-treatment, both treatment groups obtained superior outcomes relative to the control group, with the treatment group who received the automated emails obtaining larger within-group effect sizes on measures of anxiety (GAD-7) and depression (Patient Health Questionnaire-9-Item Scale; PHQ-9) compared to the treatment group who did not receive the automated emails. These gains were sustained at 12-month follow-up (Titov et al. 2014). This intervention was subsequently tested in a small open trial by a community mental health service (Kirkpatrick et al. 2013) with therapist guidance. Consistent with the previous trial, large effect sizes were found on both the GAD-7 and PHQ-9, which were sustained at 2-month follow-up.

Results of the first tailored ICBT intervention which targeted symptoms of depression, GAD, panic disorder and social anxiety disorder were reported by Carlbring et al. (2011). Fifty-four participants, all of whom met diagnostic criteria for depression, GAD, panic disorder or social anxiety disorder, were randomly allocated to receive a therapist-guided tailored ICBT intervention, or to an attention control condition. All participants were prescribed 6–10 modules to work on over 10 weeks. These modules were from existing ICBT interventions for depression, GAD, panic disorder and social anxiety disorder. All participants were prescribed an introduction module and a module on relapse prevention, but other modules were prescribed based on their specific symptoms. Significant differences were found between treatment and control groups at post-treatment on the Beck Anxiety

Inventory (BAI) (Beck et al. 1988), the Montgomery-Åsberg Depression Rating Scale (MADRS-S) (Svanborg and Åsberg 1994) and the Quality in Life Inventory (QOLI) (Frisch et al. 1992). These results were sustained at 2-year follow-up, by which time the attention control group had also completed treatment.

More recently, a Swedish effectiveness study was conducted in a primary care setting which tested the effects of tailored ICBT for anxiety disorders including GAD (Nordgren et al. 2014). One hundred participants were recruited through their primary care contact and randomised to either treatment or an active control group. The treatment consisted of 7–10 weekly individually assigned modules guided by online therapists. At post-treatment, 46 % of the treatment group had achieved clinically significant improvement on the primary outcome measure (CORE-OM) and between-group effect sizes at ranged from $d=0.20$–0.86, with a mean effect of $d=0.59$. At one-year follow-up, within-group effect sizes varied between $d=0.53$–1.00.

Case Study

Carol, a 44-year-old Australian woman, was referred by her primary care physician to the MindSpot Clinic for treatment of generalised anxiety disorder (GAD) and co-morbid depression. The MindSpot Clinic is a national Australian treatment service that provides telephone or Internet-delivered psychological assessment and treatment services for people with anxiety disorders or depression. Assessment indicated Carol was presenting with high levels of GAD and was moderately depressed. She reported a history of excessive worry since childhood, followed by bouts of depression since her late teens. The MindSpot Clinic therapist discussed with Carol the nature and content of the Internet-delivered treatment, and she consented to treatment.

Carol was assigned to a 10-week therapist-guided Internet treatment that targeted symptoms of both GAD and depression. Carol's physician received an assessment report from the MindSpot Clinic, which included details about Carol's symptoms and about the treatment course.

Carol logged in weekly and read all five of the assigned lessons during the 10-week course. She received automated emails at the start of each week providing details about the recommended reading and homework for that week. Carol was also provided with homework tasks in PDF format. These summarised the key points for each lesson and provided examples of how to apply the skills described in that lesson. Each week, new resources were made available that addressed symptoms frequently experienced by people with anxiety and depression including managing difficulties with sleep, relationships and communication.

Carol completed online symptom measures each week which helped her assigned online MindSpot therapist monitor her progress and safety. Carol had weekly telephone contact with her therapist at the same time each week for between 10 and 20 min. The therapist reviewed Carol's progress over the previous week, answered questions, reinforced progress and helped Carol resolve difficulties that could affect her progress. The therapist also encouraged Carol to take the antidepressant medication prescribed by her primary care physician.

At post-treatment, Carol's symptoms had reduced to the mild and asymptomatic ranges for depression and generalised anxiety, respectively. Carol's therapist assisted her to develop goals for the next 6 months and provided Carol with ongoing access to the online materials. Carol's primary care physician received a report from the MindSpot Clinic summarising her activity and progress.

Cost-Effectiveness

A review of cost-effectiveness and cost of illness in anxiety disorders (Konnopka et al. 2009) concluded that GAD and panic disorder were the most costly anxiety disorders per identified case, although the reported direct excess costs varied greatly, from $625 (Smit et al. 2006) to $20,184 (Olfson and Gameroff 2007). The Swedish effectiveness study described above (Nordgren et al. 2014) included a cost analysis which revealed a significant reduction of total costs for the ICBT group, with the incremental cost-effectiveness ratio favouring ICBT compared to control group. To date, no other ICBT studies have reported cost-effectiveness or health economic analyses of ICBT for GAD.

Discussion and Future Challenges

The overall pattern of results of studies evaluating ICBT interventions for GAD is encouraging. Large treatment effects have been consistently reported in both research trials and in evaluations of ICBT for GAD in clinical practice. Importantly, in addition to improvements in symptoms of GAD, large improvements have also typically been reported in other domains, including depression and disability, indicating the gains generalised to other aspects of the person's life.

These results may be further summarised as follows. First, the results of therapist-guided research trials examining the efficacy of ICBT interventions designed specifically for treating GAD have consistently demonstrated large clinical effects on measures of GAD. These results have been replicated across several research groups and have been demonstrated as robust for periods of up to 3 years post-treatment.

Second, the results of therapist-guided research trials examining the efficacy of transdiagnostic or tailored ICBT interventions that are designed to target symptoms of GAD and other anxiety disorders and/or depression have also produced consistent and positive results, although the magnitude of improvement has not consistently been as large as for the disorder-specific interventions. This apparent difference may reflect a sampling artefact, in that participants in studies evaluating transdiagnostic ICBT interventions may not meet diagnostic criteria for GAD, but may meet diagnostic criteria for another anxiety disorder or for depression. Thus, the baseline scores on measures of GAD for the entire sample are likely to be lower than for participants included in trials of disorder-specific interventions for GAD.

Third, the results of evaluations of ICBT for GAD in clinical settings are encouraging, with studies indicating that those who complete the interventions obtain large effect sizes. However, the robustness of these findings is currently limited because with few exceptions (e.g. Bergman Nordgren et al. 2014; Titov et al. 2015), there has been reliance on data limited to people who have completed the intervention, that is, completer analyses. It is likely that future reports based on complete data sets will confirm these positive preliminary results.

Fourth, the preliminary results of evaluations of self-guided ICBT for GAD are also encouraging. Although one study relied on completer analyses (Klein et al. 2011), those who did complete appeared to obtain considerable benefits. The studies by Titov et al. (2013, 2014) which included data from approximately 80 % of participants at post-treatment and 1-year follow-up provided further evidence that a self-guided model of intervention can result in significant levels of clinical change. While further studies of self-guided ICBT for GAD are required, these preliminary results are highly encouraging and indicate the potential of the self-guided model of intervention as a public health tool.

Notwithstanding these promising outcomes, there a several limitations which future reports should address. These include the need for independent replications across more countries. In addition, and in contrast to other disorders such as social anxiety disorder and depression, there are no direct comparisons of ICBT for GAD against face-to-face treatment (see Chap. 1 for review of these trials). Finally, more information about the longer-term effects of disorder-specific, transdiagnostic and tailored ICBT will help inform therapists about optimal models of care for their patients.

In conclusion, guided ICBT for GAD is a promising new treatment. While more work is needed to address the current gaps in knowledge, the results to date have been consistently positive and encouraging. We conclude that it is likely that ICBT for GAD is ready for dissemination.

References

American Psychiatric Association (2000) Diagnostic criteria from DSM-IV-TR. American Psychiatric Association, Washington, D.C

Andersson G, Titov N (2014) Advantages and limitations of Internet-based interventions for common mental disorders. World Psychiatry 13:4–11

Andersson G, Paxling B, Roch-Norlund P, Ostman G, Norgren A, Almlov J, Georen L, Breitholtz E, Dahlin M, Cuijpers P, Carlbring P, Silverberg F (2012) Internet-based psychodynamic versus cognitive behavioral guided self-help for generalized anxiety disorder: a randomized controlled trial. Psychother Psychosom 81:344–355

Beck AT (1991) Cognitive therapy. A 30-year retrospective. Am Psychol 46:368–375

Beck A, Emery G, Greenberg R (1985) Anxiety disorders and phobias: a cognitive approach. Basic, New York

Beck AT, Epstein N, Brown G, Steer RA (1988) An inventory for measuring clinical anxiety: psychometric properties. J Consult Clin Psychol 56:893

Borkovec T, Costello E (1993) Efficacy of applied relaxation and cognitive-behavioral therapy in the treatment of generalized anxiety disorder. J Consult Clin Psychol 61:611

Borkovec TD, Wilkinson L, Folensbee R, Lerman C (1983) Stimulus control applications to the treatment of worry. Behav Res Ther 21:247–251

Borkovec TD, Alcaine O, Behar E (2004) Avoidance theory of worry and generalized anxiety disorder. In: Heimberg RG, Turk CL, Mennin DS (Eds) Generalized anxiety disorder: advances in research and practice. The Guildford Press, New York.

Bowman D, Scogin F, Floyd M, Patton E, Gist L (1997) Efficacy of self-examination therapy in the treatment of generalized anxiety disorder. J Couns Psychol 44:267

Breitholtz E, Westling BE, Ost LG (1998) Cognitions in generalized anxiety disorder and panic disorder patients. J Anxiety Disord 12:567–577

Brown TA, Antony MM, Barlow DH (1992) Psychometric properties of the Penn State Worry Questionnaire in a clinical anxiety disorders sample. Behav Res Ther 30:33–37

Brown TA, Barlow DH, Liebowitz MR (1994) The empirical basis of generalized anxiety disorder. Am J Psychiatry 151(9):1272–1280

Carlbring P, Maurin L, Torngren C, Linna E, Eriksson T, Sparthan E, Straat M, Marquez Von Hage C, Bergman-Nordgren L, Andersson G (2011) Individually-tailored, internet-based treatment for anxiety disorders: a randomized controlled trial. Behav Res Ther 49:18–24

Constans JI, Barbee JG, Townsend MH, Leffler H (2002) Stability of worry content in GAD patients: a descriptive study. J Anxiety Disord 16:311–319

Cuijpers P, Sijbrandij M, Koole S, Huibers M, Berking M, Andersson G (2014) Psychological treatment of generalized anxiety disorder: a meta-analysis. Clin Psychol Rev 34:130–140

Dear BF, Titov N, Schwencke G, Andrews G, Johnston L, Craske MG, Mcevoy P (2011a) An open trial of a brief transdiagnostic internet treatment for anxiety and depression. Behav Res Ther 49:830–837

Dear BF, Titov N, Sunderland M, Mcmillan D, Anderson T, Lorian C, Robinson E (2011b) Psychometric comparison of the generalized anxiety disorder scale-7 and the Penn State Worry Questionnaire for measuring response during treatment of generalised anxiety disorder. Cogn Behav Ther 40:216–227

Draper M, Rees CS, Nathan PR (2008) Internet-based self-management of generalised anxiety disorder: a preliminary study. Behav Chang 25:229–244

Dugas MJ, Freeston MH, Ladouceur R (1997) Intolerance of uncertainty and problem orientation in worry. Cogn Ther Res 21:593–606

Dugas MJ, Gagnon F, Ladouceur R, Freeston MH (1998) Generalized anxiety disorder: a preliminary test of a conceptual model. Behav Res Ther 36:215–226

Dugas MJ, Ladouceur R, Leger E, Freeston MH, Langlois F, Provencher MD, BOISVERT JM (2003) Group cognitive-behavioral therapy for generalized anxiety disorder: treatment outcome and long-term follow-up. J Consult Clin Psychol 71:821–825

Frisch MB, Cornell J, Villanueva M, Retzlaff PJ (1992) Clinical validation of the Quality of Life Inventory. A measure of life satisfaction for use in treatment planning and outcome assessment. Psychol Assess 4:92

Gale C, Davidson O (2007) Generalised anxiety disorder. BMJ 334:579–581

Hidalgo RB, Tupler LA, Davidson JR (2007) An effect-size analysis of pharmacologic treatments for generalized anxiety disorder. J Psychopharmacol 21:864–872

Hoffman DL, Dukes EM, Wittchen HU (2008) Human and economic burden of generalized anxiety disorder. Depress Anxiety 25:72–90

Johansson O, Michel T, Andersson G, Paxling B (2015) Experiences of non-adherence to internet-delivered cognitive behavior therapy: a qualitative study. Internet Interventions 2:137–142

Johnston L, Titov N, Andrews G, Spence J, Dear BF (2011) A RCT of a transdiagnostic internet-delivered treatment for three anxiety disorders: examination of support roles and disorder-specific outcomes. PLoS One 6:e28079

Kessler RC, Greenberg PE (2002) The economic burden of anxiety and stress disorders. Neuropsychopharmacology 67:982–992
Kessler RC, Wittchen H-U (2002) Patterns and correlates of generalized anxiety disorder in community samples. J Clin Psychiatry 63:4–10
Kessler RC, Angermeyer M, Anthony JC, De Graaf R, Demyttenaere K, Gasquet I, De Girolamo G, Gluzman S, Gureje O, Haro JM (2007) Lifetime prevalence and age-of-onset distributions of mental disorders in the World Health Organization's World Mental Health Survey Initiative. World Psychiatry 6:168
Kessler RC, Berglund PA, Chiu WaiTat, Demler O, Glantz M, Lane MA, Jin R, Merikangas KR, Nock M, Olfson M, Pincus HA, Walters EE, Wang PS, Wells KB (2008) The National Comorbidity Survey Replication (NCS-R): cornerstone in improving mental health and Mental Health Care in the United States. The WHO world mental health surveys: global perspectives on the epidemiology of mental disorders 165–210
Kirkpatrick T, Manoukian L, Dear BF, Johnston L, Titov N (2013) A feasibility open trial of internet-delivered cognitive-behavioural therapy (ICBT) among consumers of a non-governmental mental health organisation with anxiety. PeerJ 1:e210
Klein B, Meyer D, Austin DW, Kyrios M (2011) Anxiety online—a virtual clinic: preliminary outcomes following completion of five fully automated treatment programs for anxiety disorders and symptoms. J Med Internet Res 13:e89
Konnopka A, Leichsenring F, Leibing E, König H-H (2009) Cost-of-illness studies and cost-effectiveness analyses in anxiety disorders: a systematic review. J Affect Disord 114:14–31
Leichsenring F, Salzer S, Jaeger U, Kächele H, Kreische R, Leweke F, Rüger U, Winkelbach C, Leibing E (2009) Short-term psychodynamic psychotherapy and cognitive-behavioral therapy in generalized anxiety disorder: a randomized, controlled trial. Am J Psychiatry 166:875–881
Levy Berg A, Sandell R, Sandahl C (2009) Affect-focused body psychotherapy in patients with generalized anxiety disorder: Evaluation of an integrative method. J Psychother Integr 19:67
Meyer TJ, Miller ML, Metzger RL, Borkovec TD (1990) Development and validation of the penn state worry questionnaire. Behav Res Ther 28:487–495
Mewton L, Wong N, Andrews G (2012) The effectiveness of internet cognitive behavioural therapy for generalized anxiety disorder in clinical practice. Depression and Anxiety 29(10):843–849
Newby JM, Mackenzie A, Williams AD, Mcintyre K, Watts S, Wong N, ANDREWS G (2013) Internet cognitive behavioural therapy for mixed anxiety and depression: a randomized controlled trial and evidence of effectiveness in primary care. Psychol Med 43:2635–2648
Nice 2007 Management of anxiety (panic disorder, with or without agoraphobia, and generalized anxiety disorder) in adults in primary, secondary, and community care. In: Health (ed) Clinical Guideline 22 (amended)
Nice 2011 Generalised Anxiety Disorder and Panic Disorder (With Or Without Agoraphobia) in Adults: Management in Primary, Secondary and Community Care. NICE clinical guideline 113. Available at www.nice.org.uk/CG113 [NICE guideline].
Nordgren LB, Hedman E, Etienne J, Bodin J, Kadowaki Å, Eriksson S, Lindkvist E, Andersson G, Carlbring P (2014) Effectiveness and cost-effectiveness of individually tailored internet-delivered cognitive behavior therapy for anxiety disorders in a primary care population: a randomized controlled trial. Behav Res Therapy 59:1–11
Noyes R, Holt CS, Woodman CL (1996) Natural course of anxiety disorders. In: Mavissakalian M, Prien R (eds) Long-term treatments of anxiety disorders. American Psychiatric Press, Washington, DC
Olfson M, Gameroff MJ (2007) Generalized anxiety disorder, somatic pain and health care costs. Gen Hosp Psychiatry 29:310–316
Paxling B, Almlov J, Dahlin M, Carlbring P, Breitholtz E, Eriksson T, Andersson G (2011) Guided internet-delivered cognitive behavior therapy for generalized anxiety disorder: a randomized controlled trial. Cogn Behav Ther 40:159–173
Rapee RM, Bryant RA (2009) Stress and psychosocial factors in onset of fear circuitry disorders. In: Andrews G, Charney D, Sirovatka P, Regier D (eds) Stress-induced and fear circuitry disor-

ders: advancing the research agenda for DSM-V. American Psychiatric Publishing, In, Arlington
Ravindran LN, Stein MB (2009) Anxiety disorders: somatic treatment. In: Sadock BJ, Sadock VA (eds) Kaplan and Sadock comprehensive textbook of psychiatry. Lippincott Williams & Wilkins, Philadelphia
Robinson E, Titov N, Andrews G, Mcintyre K, Schwencke G, Solley K (2010) Internet treatment for generalized anxiety disorder: a randomized controlled trial comparing clinician vs technician assistance. PLoS One 5:e10942
Roemer L, Orsillo SM (2002) Expanding our conceptualization of and treatment for generalized anxiety disorder: Integrating mindfulness/acceptance-based approaches with existing cognitive-behavioral models. Clin Psychol 9:54–68
Smit F, Cuijpers P, Oostenbrink J, Batelaan N, De Graaf R, Beekman A (2006) Costs of nine common mental disorders: implications for curative and preventive psychiatry. J Ment Health Policy Econ 9:193–200
Spitzer RL, Kroenke K, Williams JB, Löwe B (2006) A brief measure for assessing generalized anxiety disorder: the GAD-7. Arch Intern Med 166:1092–1097
Stanley MA, Beck JG, Glassco JD (1996) Treatment of generalized anxiety in older adults: a preliminary comparison of cognitive-behavioral and supportive approaches. Behav Ther 27:565–581
Stein DJ (2006) Evidence-based treatment of anxiety disorders. Int J Psychiatry Clin Pract 10:16–21
Svanborg P, Åsberg M (1994) A new self-rating scale for depression and anxiety states based on the Comprehensive Psychopathological Rating Scale. Acta Psychiatr Scand 89:21–28
Titov N, Andrews G, Robinson E, Schwencke G, Johnston L, Solley K, Choi I (2009a) Clinician-assisted Internet-based treatment is effective for generalized anxiety disorder: randomized controlled trial. Aust N Z J Psychiatry 43:905–912
Titov N, Gibson M, Andrews G, Mcevoy P (2009b) Internet treatment for social phobia reduces comorbidity. Aust N Z J Psychiatry 43:754–759
Titov N, Andrews G, Johnston L, Robinson E, Spence J (2010) Transdiagnostic Internet treatment for anxiety disorders: A randomized controlled trial, Behaviour Research and Therapy 48: 890–899. doi:10.1016/j.brat.2010.05.014
Titov N, Dear BF, Schwencke G, Andrews G, Johnston L, Craske MG, Mcevoy P (2011) Transdiagnostic internet treatment for anxiety and depression: a randomised controlled trial. Behav Res Ther 49:441–452
Titov N, Dear B, Johnston L, Terides M (2012) Transdiagnostic internet treatment for anxiety and depression. Revista de Psicopatologia y Psicologia Clinica (RPPC) 17:237–260
Titov N, Dear BF, Johnston L, Lorian C, Zou J, Wootton B, Spence J, Mcevoy PM, Rapee RM (2013) Improving adherence and clinical outcomes in self-guided internet treatment for anxiety and depression: randomised controlled trial. PLoS One 8:e62873
Titov N, Dear BF, Johnston L, Mcevoy PM, Wootton B, Terides MD, Gandy M, Fogliati V, Kayrouz R, Rapee RM (2014) Improving adherence and clinical outcomes in self-guided internet treatment for anxiety and depression: a 12-month follow-up of a randomised controlled trial. PLoS One 9:e89591
Titov N, Dear BF, Staples LG, Bennett-Levy J, Klein B, Rapee RM, Shann C, Richards D, Andersson G, Ritterband L, Purtell C, Bezuidenhout G, Johnston L, Nielssen O (2015) MindSpot Clinic: an accessible, efficient and effective online treatment service for anxiety and depression. Psychiatr Serv 66(10):1043–1050
Treanor M, Erisman SM, Salters-Pedneault K, Roemer L, Orsillo SM (2011) Acceptance-based behavioral therapy for GAD: effects on outcomes from three theoretical models. Depress Anxiety 28:127–136
Tyrer P, Baldwin D (2006) Generalised anxiety disorder. Lancet 368:2156–2166
Wells A (1995) Meta-cognition and worry: a cognitive model of generalized anxiety disorder. Behav Cogn Psychother 23:301–320

Wells A, Carter K (1999) Preliminary tests of a cognitive model of generalized anxiety disorder. Behav Res Ther 37:585–594

Wells A, King P (2006) Metacognitive therapy for generalized anxiety disorder: an open trial. J Behav Ther Exp Psychiatry 37:206–212

Wittchen HU (2002) Generalized anxiety disorder: prevalence, burden, and cost to society. Depress Anxiety 16:162–171

World Health Organization. The ICD-10 classification of mental and behavioural disorders: clinical descriptions and diagnostic guidelines. Geneva: World Health Organization; 1992

Yonkers KA, Bruce SE, Dyck IR, Keller MB (2003) Chronicity, relapse, and illness—course of panic disorder, social phobia, and generalized anxiety disorder: findings in men and women from 8 years of follow-up. Depress Anxiety 17:173–179

Internet-Delivered Cognitive Behavior Therapy (ICBT) for Obsessive-Compulsive Disorder

6

Bethany M. Wootton, Erik Andersson, and Christian Rück

Abstract

Obsessive-compulsive disorder (OCD) is a common and disabling condition. Efficacious treatments have been developed, but many patients have difficulty accessing such treatments and the rate of untreated individuals with OCD is high. Internet-delivered cognitive behavior therapy (ICBT) for OCD has been investigated by a number of research groups over the past 5 years with the aim to improve access to evidence-based treatment for this disorder. Results to date are promising for both guided and unguided treatments, and while ICBT is a promising treatment format, there are a number of important future directions that remain unstudied. While investigating these unanswered questions is an important next step, it is hoped that the research conducted to date can be adapted and will lead to similar research in other underserved OCD-related disorders such as body dysmorphic disorder, hoarding disorder, trichotillomania, and excoriation (skin picking) disorder.

Description of the Disorder

What Is OCD?

Obsessive-compulsive disorder (OCD) has been described in the literature for several hundred years (Burton 1989) and is characterized by the presence of anxiety eliciting obsessions and anxiety reducing compulsions (American Psychiatric Association 2013). OCD is a heterogeneous disorder and contemporary

B.M. Wootton (✉)
Discipline of Psychology, University of Tasmania, Hobart, Australia
e-mail: bethany.wootton@utas.edu.au

E. Andersson • C. Rück
Division of Psychiatry, Department of Clinical Neuroscience, Karolinska Institutet, Stockholm, Sweden

© Springer International Publishing Switzerland 2016

N. Lindefors, G. Andersson (eds.), *Guided Internet-Based Treatments in Psychiatry*, DOI 10.1007/978-3-319-06083-5_6

conceptualizations of OCD generally include four main symptom domains: (1) contamination obsessions and washing and cleaning compulsions, (2) responsibility for harm and checking or repeating behaviors, (3) unwanted sexual, aggressive, or religious thoughts with mental rituals, and (4) ordering and arranging obsessions and compulsions (Williams et al. 2011). OCD has a 12-month prevalence of approximately 2 % (Australian Bureau of Statistics 2007; Kessler et al. 2012) and recent research indicates that the age of onset in OCD appears to be bimodal (mean onset at ages 13 and 25), and those with the younger onset appear to have more severe symptoms (Anholt et al. 2014). Research into sex differences in OCD demonstrates that the disorder is more prevalent in females (Kessler et al. 2012; Ruscio et al. 2010). It is well known that there is a strong genetic component to the disorder (Mataix-Cols et al. 2013; Monzani et al. 2014); however, the exact etiology of the disorder is unknown.

The symptoms of OCD often result in a considerable impact on quality of life and have a significant societal cost. For instance, individuals with OCD tend to be impaired in social, work, and home life responsibilities (Ruscio et al. 2010) and there is some evidence to suggest that compulsions rather than obsessions cause the largest impact on quality of life (Stengler-Wenzke et al. 2007). The impact on functioning appears to be directly related to the severity of the symptoms (Ruscio et al. 2010) and those with the most severe symptoms have impairments that are similar to those seen in patients with severe mental illnesses, such as schizophrenia (Calvocoressi et al. 1998). The burden of the disease appears to also extend to family members (Grover and Dutt 2011) and the societal costs are significant, with an estimated total cost of US$8.4 billion per annum (DuPont et al. 1995).

Traditionally, OCD was classified as an anxiety disorder; however, in DSM-5 OCD was moved from the anxiety disorders to a newly created section of the manual, termed the obsessive-compulsive and related disorders (OCRD) (American Psychiatric Association 2013). OCD is located in the OCRD section along with body dysmorphic disorder (BDD), trichotillomania (TTM), hoarding disorder (HD), and excoriation (skin picking) disorder (SPD) (American Psychiatric Association 2013). Despite the commonality of engaging in repetitive behaviors, many experts in the field do not support the reclassification (Mataix-Cols et al. 2007) and OCD differs from other OCRD in terms of clinical features and treatment response to evidence-based treatment for OCD (Abramowitz et al. 2009). However, a recent study has shown that OCD, BDD, and HD do seem to share a significant part of the genetic variance of the OCRD category, whereas SPD and TTM do not seem to fit genetically with the rest of the disorders (Monzani et al. 2014).

Individuals with OCD often present with a variety of comorbidities and the most common comorbid conditions include anxiety, mood, impulse control, and substance use disorders (Ruscio et al. 2010). However, it is difficult to ascertain the true level of comorbidity in individuals with OCD, as all investigations conducted to date include individuals who would now be diagnosed with HD, which is characterized by significant co-occurring psychopathology (Frost et al. 2011). For this reason, the comorbidity statistics for OCD require reevaluation with the new DSM-5 structure.

Exposure and Response Prevention for OCD

The psychological treatment with the strongest evidence base is a cognitive behavior therapy (CBT) technique called exposure and response prevention (ERP), which has been used successfully to treat OCD since the 1960s (Meyer 1966). ERP aims to address the maintaining factors of OCD and involves four components: (1) exposure in vivo, (2) imaginal exposure, (3) response prevention (eliminating compulsions), and (4) a processing component, which includes discussing with the client the outcome of the exposure and what they learned from it (usually that their feared event is unlikely to occur) (Foa 2010). In order to complete ERP, the patient will develop a hierarchy of feared situations and will gradually expose themselves to those situations without allowing themselves to engage in their compulsions.

Barriers to Accessing Evidence-Based Treatment

Despite the efficacy of CBT for OCD, it remains an undertreated condition (Blanco et al. 2006; Kohn et al. 2004; Torres et al. 2007) and the median rate of untreated individuals from epidemiological studies is estimated to be as high as 60 % (Kohn et al. 2004). Significant treatment barriers include direct and indirect costs of treatment, difficulty accessing a trained therapist due to the low numbers of therapists experienced in delivering CBT for OCD or issues related to geographical isolation, and stigma (Baer and Minichiello 2008; Belloch et al. 2009; Goodwin et al. 2002; Marques et al. 2010). These barriers are likely to contribute to the high rates of untreated patients with this disorder and addressing these barriers has become a considerable focus of research in the last decade. Remote treatments, including internet-delivered CBT (ICBT), may be beneficial in reducing these barriers to treatment as it requires less therapist time (resulting in savings to treatment providers) and treatment information can be accessed remotely, overcoming geographical isolation or the need to locate an expert therapist.

Overview of the Current ICBT Programs for OCD

Over the past 5 years, a number of research groups have investigated the efficacy of ICBT in the treatment of OCD for adult populations. The review provided below is limited only to those programs with outcome data that was obtained as part of a clinical trial and used a standardized OCD outcome measure. It is not an exhaustive description of all current ICBT programs that are available for OCD.

Karolinska Institutet, Sweden

The Karolinska Institutet (KI) was the first to publish results of a clinical trial of ICBT for OCD in the literature (E. Andersson et al. 2011). The KI ICBT program follows the "Swedish model" (Andersson 2009), which can be described as therapy that in its content mirrors face-to-face treatment, is time limited, has consecutive access to each treatment modules (chapters), and is guided by a therapist. The program involves reading online self-help text (approximately 100 A4 pages) and the patient then works online with homework assignments that are subsequently examined by a therapist. The program uses interactive features including treatment text that adjusts itself based on the patient's primary symptom subtype (i.e., washing, checking, symmetry, violent thoughts). The patient proceeds consecutively through the treatment and knowledge of each module is examined by answering questions about the module. The therapist and the patient focus on adapting the psychological model of OCD to his/her OCD symptoms via email correspondence. The patient makes an online exposure hierarchy and starts ERP after module 4. The treatment content is outlined in Table 6.1. The KI ICBT program for OCD is also supported by high-frequency proactive therapist support (i.e., the therapist sends an email in the treatment platform if the patient has not logged in for 3 days and the therapist

Table 6.1 Summary of the content of the KI OCD treatment manual

Module 1 *Psycho-education on CBT and OCD*	The treatment rationale is presented and includes a description of OCD symptoms (obsessions and compulsions), prevalence, and main principles of conducting online CBT treatment. Different fictional patient characters are introduced (each example represents a specific OCD symptom dimension). The participant has the opportunity to follow one or all four characters (washing, checking, symmetry, or violent thoughts). *Homework: Register OCD symptoms in the Internet platform diary.*
Module 2 *Assessing OCD symptoms with the CBT model*	The autonomic nervous system and its interaction with OCD symptoms is explained. Participants begin to link obsessions and compulsions to the OCD cycle and learn how to conduct a functional analysis of their OCD problems. Each OCD cycle is presented visually for each example character. *Homework: Continue OCD diary registrations and apply these to the OCD cycle.*
Module 3 *Cognitive restructuring*	Common OCD meta-cognitions are explained, such as inflated responsibility, absolute need for certainty, thought-action fusion and exaggerated need to control thoughts. The focus is to register and discuss meta-cognitions with the psychologist from a functional perspective. *Homework: Continue OCD diary registrations and use these registrations to analyze meta-cognitions associated with obsessions.*
Module 4 *Establish treatment goals and exposure hierarchy*	Introduction to exposure with response prevention (ERP). Different strategies for conducting ERP are explained and examples given of treatment goals and different ways of constructing exposure hierarchies for each example character. *Homework: Register treatment goals and then construct an exposure hierarchy with the information from these goals.*

Table 6.1 (continued)

Module 5 *Exposure with response prevention (ERP)*	Different aspects of ERP are highlighted, along with common obstacles associated with ERP and how to overcome them. The participant then chooses an ERP exercise at the bottom of the exposure hierarchy. *Homework: Start ERP and report to the psychologist after 2 days.*
Modules 6–9 *ERP exercises*	Each module focuses on certain ERP exercises with examples from each treatment character. The text for each module is short (1–2 pages), as the focus is reporting and planning the weekly exposures. *Homework: Conduct daily ERP and report to the psychologist at least once per week.*
Module 10 *ERP exercises. Establishing valued directions for further improvements*	The modules focus on daily ERP with further exercises added that are adopted from acceptance and commitment therapy. These include establishing valued based goals and how they are applied in daily exposure tasks. The treatment is summarized, and the participant learns the distinction between relapse and setback and further treatment strategies. The participant establishes a relapse prevention program based on his/her valued based goals. *Homework: Continue ERP. Establish valued based goals and apply them in daily exposure exercises. Summarize the treatment and establish a relapse prevention plan.*

always respond to the patient within 24 h on weekdays). A text message is also sent to the patient's cell phone each time the therapist sends an email. The time spent for each participant in the trials has been about 92–129 min for the whole treatment and the duration of each communication is generally short (i.e., short messages to the patient) but with high frequency (i.e., several times per week).

eCentreClinic, Australia

The eCentreClinic is a research clinic located at Macquarie University that aims to develop and evaluate ICBT programs for a variety of mental health conditions. The eCentreClinic OCD Course uses both cognitive and behavioral treatment techniques (including ERP) that are based on best-practice face-to-face treatment for OCD. The treatment techniques are described from the perspective of both a clinician and fictional characters. The course is hosted on a secure website and the lessons are released according to a set timetable to ensure that participants adhere to the structure of the program and participants are not able to read ahead. Automated emails are programmed into the system and are sent to participants (1) when a lesson becomes available, (2) to remind the participant to complete a lesson, and (3) when the participant completes a lesson. When a participant completes a lesson, they then download an overview of the lesson and this overview includes their homework tasks; however, homework tasks are not submitted to the therapist for review. Participants generally obtain brief (i.e., 5–10 min) but regular

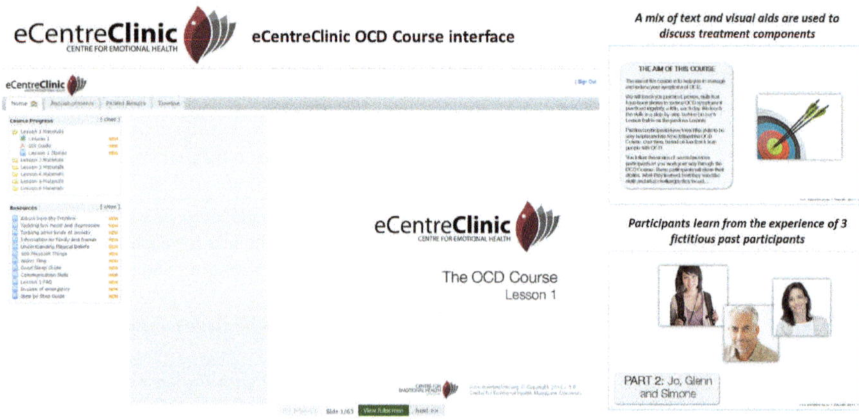

Fig. 6.1 Overview of the eCentreClinic OCD Course Content

(i.e., twice per week) therapist support via the telephone; however, self-guided interventions have also been studied. Due to the high comorbidity rates of mood and other anxiety disorders, the eCentreClinic OCD Course also makes available additional self-help materials to address these comorbidities. An overview of the eCentreClinic OCD Course interface and examples of treatment information can be seen in Fig. 6.1.

"Internet-Based Therapist-Guided Writing Therapy," Germany

This treatment was developed by Herbst and colleagues and is referred to as "Internet-based therapist-guided writing therapy" (Herbst et al. 2014). In this treatment, the patient and the therapist have two sessions per week, where they communicate synchronously in a treatment platform through text alone. There is no standardized self-help text, as in the Swedish and Australian ICBT protocols, and the treatment is, as in face-to-face CBT, provided by the therapist. Content wise, this treatment is similar as the other ICBT and face-to-face protocols as the main intervention is ERP.

"OCFighter™," USA

OCFighter is an Internet adaptation of the BTSteps program, which is a 9-step computerized treatment that utilizes a touch-tone telephone to deliver information related to the treatment of OCD. OCFighter is hosted on a secure website and consists of a number of interactive videos that are narrated by a therapist. The therapist explains how to use the program and provides psychoeducation on OCD and

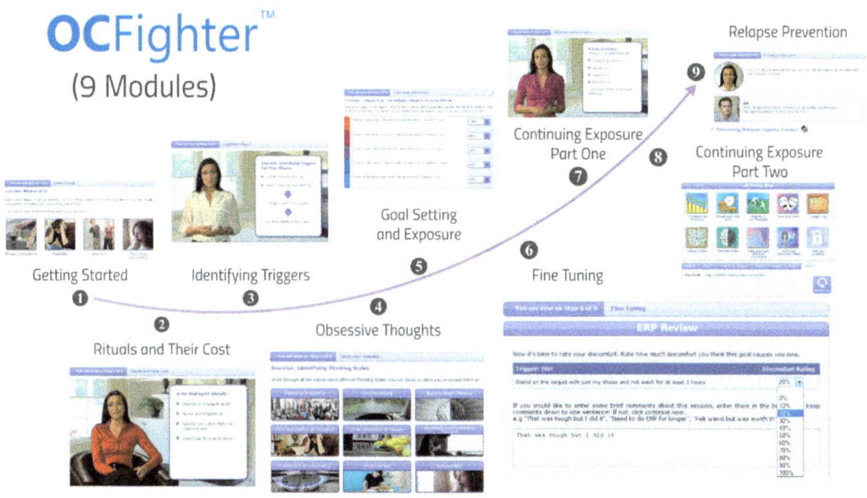

Fig. 6.2 Overview of the OCFighter Program Content

ERP. The program assists participants to develop their own relevant exposure hierarchy and allows participants to track their progress via interactive logging of exposure tasks and subjective units of distress. The 9 steps are not completed according to any specific timeline; however, participants must generally wait 24 h before commencing the next step in the program. An overview of the OCFighter program and examples of the interface are displayed in Fig. 6.2. While BTSteps has been demonstrated to be efficacious in several RCTs (Greist et al. 2002; Kenwright et al. 2005), the efficacy of the Internet-administered version (OCFighter) has been demonstrated in only one open trial to date.

Effects in Research and Clinic

The KI Program

Pilot Study

The ICBT treatment at the KI was first tested in an open pilot study where 23 adult OCD patients received 15 weeks of treatment (Andersson et al. 2011). Mean OCD symptom duration was 13 years, most had received previous OCD treatment, and the majority of participants had a high school education or above. The Y-BOCS was administered by a psychiatrist at pre- and posttreatment (there was no data loss), and a large within-group effect size was observed ($d = 1.56$), with 61 % classified as responders and 41 % classified as being in remission at posttreatment.

Randomized Controlled Trial

The results of the pilot study were later replicated and extended in a randomized controlled trial (RCT) where 101 OCD participants were randomized either to 10 weeks of ICBT or to a control condition, which consisted of online supportive therapy (basic attention control) (Andersson et al. 2012). Most subjects were self-referred and blind assessors conducted the Y-BOCS at posttreatment and at 4-month follow-up. All subjects were started in treatment on the same day and were treated simultaneously. The attrition rate was low (1 %) in this study and results showed a significant interaction effect with a large between-group effect size ($d=1.12$) favoring ICBT, and results were sustained at follow-up. The within-group effect size in the ICBT group (pre to post: $d=1.55$) was similar to that seen in the pilot study. The therapists in this study were psychology students in their final year of training. We concluded that the treatment was promising, despite the long-standing symptoms, previous treatment failures, and small amount of therapist contact required (approximately 13 min per week per patient).

Long-Term Efficacy and Relapse Prevention by Adding a Booster Program

Although both the pilot study and the RCT showed promising results, the long-term efficacy of ICBT required investigation. This subsequent study aimed to (1) investigate the long-term effects of ICBT and (2) test if an Internet-based booster program could further enhance the treatment effects (Andersson et al. 2014). Half of the sample was randomized to a 3-week Internet-based booster program 6 months after receiving ICBT and follow-up data from the RCT was obtained at 7, 12, and 24 months. Assessors were blind to treatment allocation. The booster treatment in this study followed the same procedure as in the RCT (i.e., written self-help material, consecutive access to materials, integrated therapist contact, etc.), but the treatment content differed significantly. In our previous trial, we regarded the therapist as an external stimulus with the main function to reinforce ERP behaviors. In the booster treatment developed in this study, the main aim was to get the patient to develop external stimuli in his/her natural environment that could reinforce further ERP (i.e., a partner, friend, or family member). Thus, instead of coaching the patient several times per week to do ERP, the therapists in this study instead coached the patient to utilize a support person that he/she could use to facilitate weekly check-ups with and plan the upcoming exposure exercises.

Results from this study showed that the effect of ICBT was sustained at follow-up for the completer sample across the different assessment points using the Y-BOCS ($d=1.58$–2.09) (Andersson et al. 2014). The booster treatment group had a significant improvement at 7 months but not at 12 or 24 months on the Y-BOCS. The booster group also had better general functioning at 7, 12, and 24 months, with fewer relapses, and the booster group appeared to have a slower relapse rate. We concluded that the effects of ICBT is sustained up to 2 years after completed treatment and that adding an Internet-based booster program can prevent relapse.

The eCentreClinic Program

Pilot Study

The eCentreClinic OCD Course was initially tested in a feasibility study, which consisted of 22 individuals in an open trial format[1] (Wootton et al. 2011a). In this study, participants completed 8 modules over an 8-week period and received twice weekly phone calls from a registered clinical psychologist. Overall, 81 % of the participants completed the program within the 8 weeks and participants improved significantly on the Y-BOCS from pretreatment to posttreatment and from pretreatment to 3-month follow-up. Within-group effect sizes were large from pretreatment to posttreatment (d= 1.52) and from pretreatment to 3-month follow-up (d= 1.28). The intervention required on average 86 min of clinician time per participant across the 8 weeks (approximately 10 min per week). Similar to the KI program, most participants (96 %) had received a previous treatment for OCD in the past. This study provided preliminary evidence for the efficacy of the eCentreClinic OCD Course.

Randomized Controlled Trial

The initial feasibility study was later replicated and extended in a 3-group RCT comparing ICBT, bibliotherapy-based CBT (bCBT), and a waitlist control group (Wootton et al. 2013). In this study, 56 participants completed 5 modules over an 8-week period and received twice weekly phone calls from a registered clinical psychologist. The mean number of modules completed within the 8 weeks was 4.30 in the ICBT group and 4.33 in the bCBT group. Participants in both of the active treatment groups demonstrated significant reduction on the Y-BOCS at both posttreatment and 3-month follow-up, and there were no significant differences between the groups. Within-group effect sizes were large from pretreatment to posttreatment for both the ICBT and bCBT groups at posttreatment (ICBT, d=2.16; bCBT, d= 1.65) and 3-month follow-up (ICBT, d= 1.28; bCBT, d= 1.29). At posttreatment, effect sizes between the active treatment groups and the control group were large (ICBT, d =1.57; bCBT, d= 1.40) and there was a small nonsignificant between-group effect size between the ICBT and bCBT group (d=0.17). Forty-seven percent of participants in the ICBT group and 40 % of participants in the bCBT group met conservative criteria for clinically significant change at posttreatment, which reduced to 27 % in the ICBT group and 20 % in the bCBT group at 3-month follow-up. The ICBT intervention required 89 min of clinician time and the bCBT program 102 min of clinician time on average (a nonsignificant difference) (Wootton et al. 2013). This study provided further evidence for the efficacy of ICBT for OCD and demonstrated that therapist-guided remote treatments, delivered via the Internet or bibliotherapy, appeared equally efficacious.

[1] The initial feasibility study was conducted as part of a research team at the University of New South Wales. The team later moved to Macquarie University and conducted all subsequent trials.

Reduced Clinician Contact

At the conclusion of the active treatment in the abovementioned RCT, the waitlist control group commenced active treatment. Participants in this group completed the same ICBT program (5 lessons over 8 weeks); however, the clinician contact was reduced to once a week in order to test the efficacy of reduced clinician contact. In this study, 59 % of the 17 participants completed the program within the 8 weeks and effect sizes were large from pre- to posttreatment ($d = 1.11$) and pretreatment to 3-month follow-up ($d = 1.50$). Thirty-three percent met conservative criteria for clinically significant change at both posttreatment and 3-month follow-up. The reduced contact meant that only 57 min of therapist time was required on average to complete the intervention across the 8 weeks (approximately 7 min per week per client) (Wootton et al. 2013); however, the outcomes were similar to the more intensive treatment. This study demonstrated that weekly contact also resulted in significant and clinically meaningful gains.

Self-Guided Treatments

While it is hypothesized that ICBT reduces barriers to accessing treatment, many patients may be reluctant to engage with therapist-guided treatments, as stigma is a major barrier to accessing treatment for individuals with OCD (Belloch et al. 2009; Marques et al. 2010). For this reason, the eCentreClinic team has commenced an investigation of the efficacy of self-guided ICBT for OCD and we have now completed two open trials demonstrating the efficacy of self-guided administration of the eCentreClinic OCD program (Wootton et al. 2014). In the first self-guided study, we used the same protocol as the previous RCT (5 lessons delivered over 8 weeks). There was no pretreatment clinician contact and participants were entered into the study based on scores on the self-report Y-BOCS (a score of ≥16 was required for study entry). Forty-four percent of the 16 participants completed the program and there was a significant decrease in symptoms from pretreatment to posttreatment (effect size, $d = 1.05$) and from pretreatment to 3-month follow-up (effect size, $d = 1.34$). In addition, 19 % of participants met criteria for clinically significant change at posttreatment and 29 % at 3-month follow-up. While these results were promising, the completer rates were lower than that seen in our previous studies (e.g., 81 % in the first open trial) (Wootton et al. 2011a) and the number of participants meeting criteria for clinically significant change was slightly lower than our guided studies (33–47 %) (Wootton et al. 2014; Wootton et al. 2013; Wootton et al. 2011).

We hypothesized that participants may benefit from additional time to complete the program and practice their ERP tasks. For this reason, in the second self-guided study, we extended the treatment to 6 lessons delivered over 10 weeks. Again, there was no pretreatment clinical contact and participants were accepted into the study based on their responses on the self-report Y-BOCS (a score of ≥16). The results appeared improved over the first open trial with 64 % of the 33 participants completing the program within the study timeframe and a within-group pretreatment to posttreatment effect size of $d = 1.37$ and pretreatment to 3-month follow-up effect size of $d = 1.17$. In addition, 36 % met criteria for clinically significant change at posttreatment and 32 % met criteria at 3-month follow-up (Wootton et al. 2014). While replication and extension in an RCT are required and currently underway, it appears that self-guided treatments may be acceptable and efficacious for some individuals with OCD, especially those who cite stigma as their major barrier to commencing treatment.

Long-Term Outcomes in Self-Guided Treatment

Finally, the eCentreClinic team has recently obtained preliminary 12-month follow-up results from the second self-guided open trial. Results from this study indicate a large effect size on the Y-BOCS from pretreatment to 12-month follow-up ($d = 1.08$) for people who returned their questionnaires, and a moderate effect size when carrying forward the participants' last available observation for those who did not return their questionnaires ($d = 0.65$). However, only 43 % of original participants returned questionnaires and further research is required to understand the long-term outcomes of self-guided ICBT for OCD (Wootton et al. 2015).

"Internet-Based Therapist-Guided Writing Therapy," Germany

Pilot RCT

The Internet-based therapist-guided writing therapy program was initially studied in an RCT comparing active treatment with a waitlist control group (Herbst et al. 2014). Thirty-four participants were randomized and a large between-group effect size ($d = 0.82$) was found at posttreatment (Herbst et al. 2014). When all results were pooled (after the waitlist group commenced treatment), large within-group effect sizes at posttreatment ($d = 0.83$) and follow-up ($d = 0.89$) (Herbst et al. 2014).

The OCFighter ™ Program

Pilot Study

In the only trial conducted to date, 26 participants completed the OCFighter program in an open trial, and participants were contacted nine times across the 17 weeks of the study. The clinician contact in this study mirrored that reported in the previous Kenwright et al. (2005) BTSteps study. Two participants did not commence the treatment and a total of 17/24 (71 %) completed the 17-week program. Results indicated clinically significant reductions in symptoms on the Y-BOCS from pretreatment to posttreatment and large effect sizes on the clinician-administered Y-BOCS were seen ($d = 1.15$) (Diefenbach et al. 2015). This study demonstrates the preliminary efficacy of the OCFighter program; however, further controlled trials are needed.

Case Description

Mr J. was a 45-year old man who participated in one of the KI trials in Sweden. Mr J. presented with severe OCD (31/40 on the Y-BOCS) and presented with anxiety eliciting obsessions about becoming contaminated from germs and washing/cleaning compulsions (he washed his hands up to 100 times per day). Mr J. reported that he had been on a disability pension for the last 10 years due to OCD, depression, and severe alcohol abuse. However, at the time, he commenced treatment he did not meet criteria for depression and had been sober the past 2 years. Mr J. was currently living in a group home with daily support from personnel (e.g., taking walks outside, planning daily activities). Mr J. applied to our study after seeing a newspaper advertisement and, when considering the history of alcohol abuse and depression and his social situation in general, we first hesitated to include him in the ICBT study. However, he did not fulfill any exclusion criteria and was thus included in the study. Mr J. had no difficulties reading and writing and he was familiar with the use of the Internet. He completed modules 1–4 within 2 weeks and he decided to work with what he referred to "the cold turkey method" (i.e., completely refraining from all rituals). He did this for 1 week and had daily email correspondence with his therapist during this time. The therapist contact was intensive with about 3–4 emails being sent per week. At week two, Mr J. also conducted planned exposures in his apartment and at other places in addition to his complete response prevention. At mid-treatment, Mr J. felt he had made some substantial progress and the rest of the treatment focused on higher level exposure tasks such as dating and meeting with friends, which he had previously avoided because of both contamination concerns and low mood. Mr J. had a Y-BOCS score of 3 at posttreatment, 1 at the 3-month follow-up, and 0 at the 12-month follow-up. Although this may not be the typical patient in ICBT, it demonstrates that anyone can potentially benefit from ICBT even those patients who, at first sight, may not seem appropriate for remote treatment.

Cost-Effectiveness of ICBT

The cost-effectiveness of ICBT was analyzed using data from cost-assessment questionnaires that were obtained in the Swedish waitlist controlled trial (Andersson et al. 2012). Results showed that, when including all societal costs (i.e., health-care visits, time off work, medications, etc.), one additional remission in ICBT can be achieved for a price of <$1300 when compared to support therapy (i.e., online support therapy) (Andersson et al. 2015). When narrowing the perspective to include only the direct treatment costs, the price for one additional remission was even lower (preliminary findings). Thus, it seems that ICBT is not only effective but may also be a cost-effective treatment. An important next step in understanding the cost-effectiveness of ICBT for OCD is to compare the cost of ICBT when compared to face-to-face CBT.

Clinical Implementation and Dissemination

While ICBT has demonstrated efficacy, effectiveness studies are still lacking and ICBT for OCD has not yet been disseminated and tested within the regular health-care system. This is unfortunate as there are many promising practical advantages of this treatment format. For instance, and as mentioned above, ICBT can help to overcome geographical barriers to treatment, and those patients who avoid seeking help, or who experience shame because of their symptoms, may be more likely to seek help via the Internet; thus, ICBT likely improves access to evidence-based care. Secondly, ICBT increases treatment capacity and uses about 25 % of therapist time required in traditional individual therapy. This is likely to reduce the costs of treatment significantly and result in considerable savings for both the individual and society. Thirdly, the ICBT treatment format is highly controlled which minimizes the risk of therapist drift (Waller 2009) allowing patients to receive optimal care and full access to the evidence-based intervention. Finally, self-report measures can be automatically administered and activated in the treatment platform; thus, symptom severity and safety can be collected in a systematic way, with little room for data loss and with full traceability. This allows the clinician to intervene if the client is not responding or may be at risk of harm. Thus, a next step in this line of research is to test the feasibility of ICBT for OCD in the regular health-care system.

In addition to the dissemination of ICBT in the health-care system, ICBT can also benefit future research into OCD more generally because of its high level of accessibility and relative ease of recruiting participants. The use of ICBT may allow researchers to recruit the sample sizes required for important research studies such as meditational analyses and inferiority trials. One example of how researchers have achieved large sample sizes using the ICBT format is the work by Ljotsson et al. (2011) who managed to recruit and randomize 195 patients with irritable bowel syndrome to two active treatments (exposure treatment vs. stress management) and, in a subsequent study, randomized 311 patients to systematic exposure + mindfulness training vs. mindfulness training only (Ljotsson et al. 2014) within a short period of time. Thus, it seems that ICBT can enhance participant recruitment and make it possible to test hypotheses that demand large sample sizes, making the research results more reliable.

Discussion and Future Challenges

Results from multiple research groups across the world now demonstrate the efficacy of both guided and self-guided ICBT for OCD. There is also evidence to suggest that this format of treatment is cost-effective and can assist researchers investigating OCD more generally, due to the possibility of recruiting larger sample sizes than is typically seen in face-to-face studies. Despite the promising findings to date, there are some limitations to the existing literature and some important future directions that require further study.

Limitations of the Literature

While it appears that ICBT is efficacious and cost-effective in the treatment of OCD, there are some important limitations to the existing ICBT literature that need to be addressed as the field moves forward. Firstly, the psychometric properties of Internet-administered measures require further investigation as the self-report outcome measures that are commonly used as dependent variables in ICBT studies (including the Y-BOCS, OCI-R, and DOCS) were originally developed as paper and pencil tests. At this stage, we currently lack sufficient data on the psychometric properties of these assessment questionnaires when they are administered via the Internet. Some studies have indicated that responses on these questionnaires are equivalent when administered in paper and pencil or online format (Coles et al. 2007; Enander et al. 2012); however, further research should focus on this issue.

Secondly, in the ICBT studies conducted to date, the majority of participants typically self-refer and are generally highly educated. This potential selection bias can affect the generalizability of the results and further attempts need to be made to make the samples more representative in future studies. Additionally, in many of the ICBT studies conducted to date, blinding was not used when administering the Y-BOCS, which may have introduced bias. The exception to this is two of the KI trials (Andersson et al. 2012, 2014) that used blinded interviewers. Future studies that include a clinician assessment prior to treatment should ideally use blinded interviewers moving forward in order to decrease the potential for bias in the results.

Future Directions

There are several important future directions in the field of ICBT for OCD. These include comparing ICBT with traditional face-to-face treatment, exploring alternative platforms for delivery of the interventions, investigating optimal levels of therapist contact, understanding treatment preferences, and investigating moderators and mediators of outcome.

Comparisons Between ICBT and Traditional Face-to-Face CBT

A number of studies have compared ICBT with traditional face-to-face treatment for diagnostic groups including depression, social anxiety disorder, and chronic pain, and these studies have shown that outcomes from ICBT programs are equivalent to face-to-face treatment (Andrews et al. 2011; De Boer et al. 2014; Wagner et al. 2014). However, such a comparison has not yet been conducted in OCD and further research is required to ascertain whether the outcomes from ICBT studies are equivalent to standard face-to-face treatment for OCD. This is an important question as it will help the field to understand whether ICBT can be delivered as an alternative to face-to-face treatment or whether it should be a lower step in a stepped care model of treatment.

Alternative Treatment Platforms

ICBT programs to date have focused on programs that can be delivered on a desktop computer. An obvious future direction would be to expand this treatment to mobile platforms such as smartphones, thereby further increasing the possibility to influence the patients to initiate and maintain ERP behaviors. Smartphones have been tested in recent trials in depression with promising results (Ly et al. 2014), and this modality has also the potential to collect larger amounts of data with high precision pertaining to both cognitive- and ERP-based interventions (i.e., daily registrations on obsessive beliefs, ERP frequency, duration, within- and between-session habituation, etc.). By expanding ICBT to smartphones, we can possibly enhance the treatment effects further and also conduct research on process outcome such as emotional processing and habituation.

Investigating the Role of Therapist Contact

Generally, ICBT for OCD is provided with some therapist contact; however, as discussed above, self-guided treatments have also been investigated. The intensity of the contact in the therapist-guided studies has also differed quite significantly. Some studies have contacted the participant several times per week (Andersson et al. 2011, 2012; Wootton et al. 2013), others once per week (Wootton et al. 2013), and others less than once per week (Diefenbach et al. 2015). Therefore, another important future research area would be to compare the frequency of therapist contact within a single study to ascertain the optimum level of contact required.

Understanding Treatment Preferences

At this stage, we do not understand treatment preferences of individuals with OCD. Previous research informs us that many individuals with OCD and other health disorders find ICBT to be acceptable (Ferwerda et al. 2013; Wootton et al. 2011a, b); however, we do not yet know what proportion of the treatment-seeking population with OCD may prefer ICBT over face-to-face treatment or vice versa. This is an important question from a treatment delivery perspective, and therefore, further research is required into treatment preferences for individuals with OCD.

Moderators and Mediators of Outcome

As mentioned above, ICBT studies are a potential avenue for testing hypotheses that are difficult to test in face-to-face treatment due to the length of time and cost it takes to recruit large enough sample sizes. One important area of such research is investigating differential outcome of CBT for different OCD symptom clusters and investigating predictors, moderators and mediators. Thus, future ICBT research should also focus on designing well-powered studies that can further explore the active treatment mechanisms and progress the field further.

Therapist Training

ICBT may serve as a tool to train therapists in protocol-based therapy and requires further investigation. Most of the Swedish ICBT trials have used psychology students in their final year of training as therapists and our experience is that ICBT can serve as a good basis for junior therapist to learn the CBT treatment components for OCD and other disorders. The therapist can practice in front of a computer to provide efficient and concise communication with a patient, and this could potentially improve the general therapist skills. Additionally, it is easy for the supervisor to monitor the therapist feedback, and this also decreases the risk of therapist drift. The clinical psychology program at the KI now has a mandatory course in ICBT where the students treat real patients and receive supervision via the Internet. Thus, ICBT may be a promising education tool for novice therapists in the future. This is an important issue as there is evidence that inexperienced therapists at master level can be as capable as experienced therapists given that proper supervision is provided (van Oppen et al. 2010). Thus, ICBT has the potential to serve as a secure and accessible education tool, but we need more research on the feasibility of such education tools.

Blended Treatments

To use ICBT together with therapist-delivered CBT, sometimes referred to as blended treatment, is another potential avenue for ICBT programs and this needs further study in the future as many traditional therapists see remote treatments as being best suited as an adjunct to treatment, rather than a standalone treatment (Sinclair et al. 2013). ICBT could, for instance, be used to increase exposure frequency between live sessions or be used as a psychoeducational tool, which then frees up the clinicians time to implement exposure tasks with the patient or frees up the clinicians time making it possible for the clinician to see more clients.

In summary, ICBT for OCD has grown substantially over the past 5 years and results demonstrate that ICBT is an acceptable, efficacious, and cost-effective treatment. Despite the progress made in recent years, there are several important areas that require future research and will help clinicians and policy makers to understand the role of ICBT in optimal service provision for OCD.

References

Abramowitz JS, Taylor S, McKay D (2009) Obsessive-compulsive disorder. Lancet 374(9688): 491–499. doi:10.1016/S0140-6736(09)60240-3

American Psychiatric Association (2013) Diagnostic and statistical manual of mental disorders, 5th edn. American Psychiatric Association, Washington, DC

Andersson E, Enander J, Andrén P, Hedman E, Ljótsson B, Hursti T, Rück C (2012) Internet-based cognitive behaviour therapy for obsessive-compulsive disorder: a randomized controlled trial. Psychol Med 42(10):2193–2203. doi:10.1017/S0033291712000244

Andersson E, Hedman E, Ljótsson B, Wikström M, Elveling E, Lindefors N, Rück C (2015) Cost-effectiveness of internet-based cognitive behavior therapy for obsessive-compulsive disorder: results from a randomized controlled trial. J Obsessive-Compulsive Relat Disord 4:47–53

Andersson E, Ljótsson B, Hedman E, Kaldo V, Paxling B, Andersson G, Rück C (2011) Internet-based cognitive behavior therapy for obsessive compulsive disorder: a pilot study. BMC Psychiatry 11:125. doi:10.1186/1471-244X-11-125

Andersson E, Steneby S, Karlsson K, Ljótsson B, Hedman E, Enander J, Rück C (2014) Long-term efficacy of Internet-based cognitive behavior therapy for obsessive-compulsive disorder with or without booster: a randomized controlled trial. Psychol Med 44:2877–2887

Andersson G (2009) Using the Internet to provide cognitive behaviour therapy. Behav Res Ther 47(3):175–180. doi:10.1016/j.brat.2009.01.010

Andrews G, Davies M, Titov N (2011) Effectiveness randomized controlled trial of face to face versus Internet cognitive behaviour therapy for social phobia. Aust N Z J Psychiatry 45(4): 337–340. doi:10.3109/00048674.2010.538840

Anholt GE, Aderka IM, Van Balkom AJLM, Smit JH, Schruers K, Van Der Wee NJA, Van Oppen P (2014) Age of onset in obsessive-compulsive disorder: admixture analysis with a large sample. Psychol Med 44(1):185–194. doi:10.1017/S0033291713000470

Australian Bureau of Statistics (2007) National survey of mental health and wellbeing: summary of results (Cat. no. 4326.0). Canberra

Baer L, Minichiello WE (2008) Reasons for inadequate utilization of cognitive-behavioral therapy for obsessive-compulsive disorder. J Clin Psychiatry 69(4):676

Belloch A, Valle G, Morillo C, Carrió C, Cabedo E (2009) To seek advice or not to seek advice about the problem: the help-seeking dilemma for obsessive-compulsive disorder. Soc Psychiatry Psychiatr Epidemiol 44(4):257–264. doi:10.1007/s00127-008-0423-0

Blanco C, Olfson M, Stein DJ, Simpson HB, Gameroff MJ, Narrow WH (2006) Treatment of obsessive-compulsive disorder by U.S. psychiatrists. J Clin Psychiatry 67(6):946–951

Burton R (1989) The anatomy of melancholy. Clarendon, Oxford

Calvocoressi L, Libman D, Vegso SJ, McDougle CJ, Price LH (1998) Global functioning of inpatients with obsessive-compulsive disorder, schizophrenia, and major depression. Psychiatr Serv 49(3):379–381

Coles ME, Cook LM, Blake TR (2007) Assessing obsessive compulsive symptoms and cognitions on the internet: evidence for the comparability of paper and internet administration. Behav Res Ther 45(9):2232–2240. doi:10.1016/j.brat.2006.12.009

De Boer MJ, Versteegen GJ, Vermeulen KM, Sanderman R, Struys MMRF (2014) A randomized controlled trial of an Internet-based cognitive-behavioural intervention for non-specific chronic pain: an effectiveness and cost-effectiveness study. Eur J Pain. doi:10.1002/ejp.509

Diefenbach GJ, Wootton BM, Bragdon LB, Moshier, SJ, Tolin DF (2015) Treatment outcome and predictors of internet guided self help for obsessive compulsive disorder. Behavior Therapy. doi:10.1016/j.beth.2015.06.001

DuPont RL, Rice DP, Shiraki S, Rowland CR (1995) Economic costs of obsessive-compulsive disorder. Med Interface 8(4):102–109

Enander J, Andersson E, Kaldo V, Lindefors N, Andersson G, Rück C (2012) Internet administration of the Dimensional Obsessive-Compulsive Scale: a psychometric evaluation. J Obsessive-Compulsive Relat Disord 1(4):325–330, http://dx.doi.org/10.1016/j.jocrd.2012.07.008

Ferwerda M, Van Beugen S, Van Burik A, Van Middendorp H, De Jong EMGJ, Van De Kerkhof PCM, Evers AWM (2013) What patients think about E-health: patients' perspective on internet-based cognitive behavioral treatment for patients with rheumatoid arthritis and psoriasis. Clin Rheumatol 32(6):869–873. doi:10.1007/s10067-013-2175-9

Foa EB (2010) Cognitive behavioral therapy of obsessive-compulsive disorder. Dialogues Clin Neurosci 12(2):199–207

Frost RO, Steketee G, Tolin DF (2011) Comorbidity in hoarding disorder. Depress Anxiety 28(10):876–884. doi:10.1002/da.20861

Goodwin R, Koenen KC, Hellman F, Guardino M, Struening E (2002) Helpseeking and access to mental health treatment for obsessive-compulsive disorder. Acta Psychiatr Scand 106(2):143–149. doi:10.1034/j.1600-0447.2002.01221.x

Greist JH, Marks IM, Baer L, Kobak KA, Wenzel KW, Hirsch MJ, Clary CM (2002) Behavior therapy for obsessive-compulsive disorder guided by a computer or by a clinician compared with relaxation as a control. J Clin Psychiatry 63(2):138–145

Grover S, Dutt A (2011) Perceived burden and quality of life of caregivers in obsessive-compulsive disorder. Psychiatry Clin Neurosci 65(5):416–422. doi:10.1111/j.1440-1819.2011.02240.x

Herbst N, Voderholzer U, Thiel N, Schaub R, Knaevelsrud C, Stracke S, Kulz AK (2014) No talking, just writing! Efficacy of an Internet-based cognitive behavioral therapy with exposure and response prevention in obsessive compulsive disorder. Psychother Psychosom 83(3):165–175. doi:10.1159/000357570

Kenwright M, Marks I, Graham C, Franses A, Mataix-Cols D (2005) Brief scheduled phone support from a clinician to enhance computer-aided self-help for obsessive-compulsive disorder: randomized controlled trial. J Clin Psychol 61(12):1499–1508. doi:10.1002/jclp.20204

Kessler RC, Petukhova M, Sampson NA, Zaslavsky AM, Wittchen HU (2012) Twelve-month and lifetime prevalence and lifetime morbid risk of anxiety and mood disorders in the United States. Int J Methods Psychiatr Res 21(3):169–184. doi:10.1002/mpr.1359

Kohn R, Saxena S, Levav I, Saraceno B (2004) The treatment gap in mental health care. Bull World Health Organ 82(11):858–866

Ljotsson B, Hedman E, Andersson E, Hesser H, Lindfors P, Hursti T, Andersson G (2011) Internet-delivered exposure-based treatment vs. stress management for irritable bowel syndrome: a randomized trial. Am J Gastroenterol 106(8):1481–1491. doi:10.1038/ajg.2011.139

Ljotsson B, Hesser H, Andersson E, Lackner JM, El Alaoui S, Falk L, Hedman E (2014) Provoking symptoms to relieve symptoms: a randomized controlled dismantling study of exposure therapy in irritable bowel syndrome. Behav Res Ther 55:27–39. doi:10.1016/j.brat.2014.01.007

Ly KH, Truschel A, Jarl L, Magnusson S, Windahl T, Johansson R, Andersson G (2014) Behavioural activation versus mindfulness-based guided self-help treatment administered through a smartphone application: a randomised controlled trial. BMJ Open 4(1):e003440. doi:10.1136/bmjopen-2013-003440

Marques L, LeBlanc NJ, Wegarden HM, Timpano KR, Jenike M, Wilhelm S (2010) Barriers to treatment and service utilization in an internet sample of individuals with obsessive-compulsive symptoms. Depress Anxiety 27(5):470–475. doi:10.1002/da.20694

Mataix-Cols D, Boman M, Monzani B, Rück C, Serlachius E, Längström N, Lichtenstein P (2013) Population-based, multigenerational family clustering study of obsessive-compulsive disorder. JAMA Psychiatry 70(7):709–717. doi:10.1001/jamapsychiatry.2013.3

Mataix-Cols D, Pertusa A, Leckman JF (2007) Issues for DSM-V: how should obsessive-compulsive and related disorders be classified? Am J Psychiatry 164(9):1313–1314. doi:10.1176/appi.ajp.2007.07040568

Meyer V (1966) Modification of expectations in cases with obsessional rituals. Behav Res Ther 4(1–2):273–280

Monzani B, Rijsdijk F, Harris J, Mataix-Cols D (2014) The structure of genetic and environmental risk factors for dimensional representations of DSM-5 obsessive-compulsive spectrum disorders. JAMA Psychiatry 71(2):182–189. doi:10.1001/jamapsychiatry.2013.3524

Ruscio AM, Stein DJ, Chiu WT, Kessler RC (2010) The epidemiology of obsessive-compulsive disorder in the National Comorbidity Survey Replication. Mol Psychiatry 15(1):53–63. doi:10.1038/mp.2008.94

Sinclair C, Holloway K, Am GR, Auret K (2013) Online mental health resources in rural australia: clinician perceptions of acceptability. J Med Internet Res 15(9):e193. doi:10.2196/jmir.2772

Stengler-Wenzke K, Kroll M, Riedel-Heller S, Matschinger H, Angermeyer MC (2007) Quality of life in obsessive-compulsive disorder: The different impact of obsessions and compulsions. Psychopathology 40(5):282–289. doi:10.1159/000104744

Torres AR, Prince MJ, Bebbington PE, Bhugra DK, Brugha TS, Farrell M, Singleton N (2007) Treatment seeking by individuals with obsessive-compulsive disorder from the british psychiatric morbidity survey of 2000. Psychiatr Serv 58(7):977–982, 58/7/977 [pii]. doi:10.1176/appi.ps.58.7.977

van Oppen P, van Balkom AJ, Smit JH, Schuurmans J, van Dyck R, Emmelkamp PM (2010) Does the therapy manual or the therapist matter most in treatment of obsessive-compulsive disorder? A randomized controlled trial of exposure with response or ritual prevention in 118 patients. J Clin Psychiatry 71(9):1158–1167. doi:10.4088/JCP.08m04990blu

Wagner B, Horn AB, Maercker A (2014) Internet-based versus face-to-face cognitive-behavioral intervention for depression: a randomized controlled non-inferiority trial. J Affect Disord 152–154(1):113–121. doi:10.1016/j.jad.2013.06.032

Waller G (2009) Evidence-based treatment and therapist drift. Behav Res Ther 47(2):119–127. doi:10.1016/j.brat.2008.10.018

Williams MT, Farris SG, Turkheimer E, Pinto A, Ozanick K, Franklin ME, Foa EB (2011) Myth of the pure obsessional type in obsessive-compulsive disorder. Depress Anxiety 28(6): 495–500. doi:10.1002/da.20820

Wootton BM, Dear BF, Johnston L, Terides MD, Titov N (2013) Remote treatment of obsessive-compulsive disorder: a randomized controlled trial. J Obsessive-Compulsive Relat Disord 2(4):375–384. doi:10.1016/j.jocrd.2013.07.002

Wootton BM, Dear BF, Johnston L, Terides MD, Titov N (2014) Self-guided internet administered treatment for obsessive-compulsive disorder: results from two open trials. J Obsessive-Compulsive Relat Disord 3(2):102–108. doi:10.1016/j.jocrd.2014.03.001

Wootton BM, Dear BF, Terides MD, Johnston L, Titov N (2015) Self-guided internet-delivered cognitive behavior therapy (ICBT) for obsessive-compulsive disorder: 12 month follow up. Internet Interv 2(3):243–247

Wootton BM, Titov N, Dear BF, Spence J, Andrews G, Johnston L, Solley K (2011a) An Internet administered treatment program for obsessive-compulsive disorder: a feasibility study. J Anxiety Disord 25(8):1102–1107. doi:10.1016/j.janxdis.2011.07.009

Wootton BM, Titov N, Dear BF, Spence J, Kemp A (2011b) The acceptability of internet-based treatment and characteristics of an adult sample with obsessive compulsive disorder: an internet survey. PLoS One 6(6):e20548. doi:10.1371/journal.pone.0020548

Online Structured Writing Therapy for Post-traumatic Stress Disorder and Complicated Grief

7

Jeroen Ruwaard and Alfred Lange

Abstract

Post-traumatic stress disorder (PTSD) and complicated grief are related disorders for which well-described and effective cognitive-behavioural therapeutic procedures exist that are firmly rooted in theoretical work. As a result, several research groups have been able to successfully translate these procedures into e-mental health applications for the prevention, detection and treatment of the disorders. This chapter reviews online structured writing therapy (oSWT), a standardised therapist-guided Internet-based cognitive-behavioural treatment (ICBT) for post-traumatic stress disorder and complicated grief, which can be fully delivered online, without face-to-face contact between the patient and therapist. This protocol integrates three principal elements of trauma-focused therapy: (1) exposure through self-confrontation, (2) cognitive reappraisal and (3) strengthening of social support. A unique characteristic of oSWT is that it implements these three elements through writing assignments. In the past two decades, oSWT has been validated in a series of controlled studies and in routine clinical practice, with positive results. This chapter reviews these efficacy and effectiveness trials, elaborates on the details of the therapeutic procedures of the treatment protocol and identifies future research themes.

J. Ruwaard (✉)
Department of Clinical, Neuro, and Developmental Psychology, Vrije Universiteit Amsterdam, Amsterdam, The Netherlands
e-mail: j.j.ruwaard@vu.nl

A. Lange
Department of Clinical Psychology, Universiteit van Amsterdam, Amsterdam, The Netherlands
e-mail: a.lange@uva.nl

© Springer International Publishing Switzerland 2016

N. Lindefors, G. Andersson (eds.), *Guided Internet-Based Treatments in Psychiatry*, DOI 10.1007/978-3-319-06083-5_7

Abbreviations

BSI	Brief symptom inventory
DASS	Depression anxiety stress scale
ICBT	Internet-based cognitive behaviour therapy
IES	Impact of event scale
LIWC	Linguistic inquiry and word count
oSWT	Online structured writing therapy
PTSD	Post-traumatic stress disorder
SWT	Structured writing therapy
WAI	Working alliance inventory
WLC	Waiting-list/delayed treatment condition

Introduction

Post-traumatic stress disorder (PTSD) and complicated grief are related disorders that are perhaps best conceptualised in a dimensional spectrum of trauma-related stress disorders (Moreau and Zisook 2002). In both, a significant life event can be identified as the source of symptoms that include persistent, vivid and anxiety-provoking intrusive recollections, active but unsuccessful avoidance of internal and external event-related stimuli, negative cognitions and mood and heightened arousal and reactivity. Hence, the disorders can be treated with similar therapeutic techniques. Well-described and effective cognitive-behavioural therapeutic procedures exist that are firmly rooted in theoretical work (see, e.g. Brewin and Holmes 2003). Principal therapeutic elements include in vivo and in vitro exposure (Foa and Kozak 1986; Thompson 2009), cognitive interventions targeting the negative appraisal of the event and its sequelae (Ehlers and Clark 2000) and the activation of positive social support (Brewin et al. 2000). As will be shown in this chapter, evidence strongly suggests that these elements can be effectively delivered over the Internet, without face-to-face contact between the patient and the therapist, in the form of standardised online structured writing therapy (oSWT).

In the past two decades, the effects of online structured writing in the treatment of trauma-related symptoms have been studied extensively. The substantial evidence base warrants a focused review. It should be noted, though, that online structured writing presents just one possible strategy to deliver Internet-based CBT (ICBT) to people with trauma-related symptoms. Several research groups have successfully explored the use of the Internet, not only for treatment but also the prevention and detection of PTSD and related disorders (e.g. Hirai and Clum 2005; Ivarsson et al. 2014; Klein et al. 2010; Litz et al. 2007; Mouthaan et al. 2013; Ruggiero et al. 2006; Spence et al. 2013; Steinmetz et al. 2012; Van Voorhees et al. 2012; Wang et al. 2013). We will discuss these initiatives only in the context of oSWT. Extensive discussions of these different approaches can be found in several recent reviews (Amstadter et al. 2009; Andersson 2010; Benight et al. 2008; Brunet et al. 2010; Cuijpers et al. 2009). Likewise, we will not discuss developments in virtual reality exposure therapy (VRET, see, e.g. Motraghi et al. 2014; Nelson 2013), which, due to technological advancements, can be expected to enter the online realm soon.

In what follows, we will provide details of the therapeutic procedure of oSWT (section "The three phases of oSWT"), an overview of the available efficacy and effectiveness trials in which the protocol was tested (section "The efficacy and effectiveness of oSWT") and a summary of outcome prediction research (section "Predictors of outcome of oSWT"). The chapter closes with a description of related work (section "Related empirical work") and a general discussion (section "Discussion"). We start with a brief historical account of the therapeutic application of structured writing in face-to-face settings.

The Origins of Online Structured Writing Therapy

Around 1980, a group of Dutch psychiatrists and psychologists developed 'directive therapy', an eclectic mix of CBT and Ericksonian therapy, characterised by pragmatism, problem solving, positive labelling, the application of homework and a focus on enhancing self-esteem and client motivation (Haley 1973; Lange and Van der Hart 1983; Van der Velden 1977 1980, 1989). Its members were among the first to report case studies of the strategic application of structured writing in the treatment of traumatised patients (Lange 1994). Patients were instructed to write essays about the trauma or to write letters to the source of the trauma/grief. Patients wrote these essays at home. Face-to-face sessions were used for psycho-education, for detailed instructions and for discussion of the content of essays and of the impact of writing. At that time, strict protocols defining the frequency or number of writing sessions did not yet exist.

In the late 1980s/early 1990s, James Pennebaker and colleagues started to provide experimental support for the positive health effects of structured writing (Pennebaker 1993; Pennebaker and Susman 1988). In their so-called expressive writing paradigm, they asked participants to write either about a traumatic event or a neutral topic. Writing sessions were brief (15–30 min), repeated (over a period of 3–5 consecutive days) and did not include feedback. Compared to neutral writing, expressive writing was shown to be associated with (long-term) decreases in health problems. Pennebaker initially explained this effect by a psychosomatic inhibition theory, in which disclosure is assumed to free patients from the energy-depleting stress-inducing inhibition of trauma-related feelings and thoughts. In later publications, cognitive changes and prolonged exposure were considered to be contributing factors as well (Lepore and Smyth 2002; Sloan and Marx 2004).

Meanwhile, Alfred Lange, a founding member of the directive therapy group, had started experimental work on structured writing at the University of Amsterdam. Through a series of experimental studies, he and his team developed a standardised protocol for the use of structured writing assignments in the treatment of PTSD and complicated grief (Lange et al. 2002; Schoutrop et al. 2002). In contrast to the

Pennebaker approach, the protocol of Lange and colleagues included longer writing sessions (45 min), focused instructions to implement different therapeutic processes and face-to-face instruction and feedback sessions. When the *World Wide Web* opened up for consumers, around 1995, this protocol provided a natural paradigm for online treatment. The researchers hypothesised that instructions and feedback could be effectively delivered online, without face-to-face contact. To study this, they implemented the protocol in a website that allowed patients and therapists to interact over the Internet through text. Next, they invited psychology students, who had reported highly elevated scores on self-report measures of post-traumatic symptomatology, to follow online treatment through this website (Lange et al. 2000a). Results of this first pilot study were surprisingly positive. After treatment, 19 of the 20 treated students reported strong, reliable and clinically significant reductions in core symptoms of post-traumatic stress, as indicated by the avoidance and intrusion subscales of the Impact of Event Scale (IES; Joseph 2000; Sundin and Horowitz 2003). This heralded the birth of oSWT.

The Three Phases of oSWT

Online structured writing therapy comprises 5 weeks of therapist-guided Internet-based CBT. The treatment consists of three phases, in which writing instructions are varied to implement imaginary exposure, cognitive reappraisal and closure/social sharing. Each week, patients write two essays, which they share with their therapist through a secure website (e-mail is not used because of privacy concerns). Therapists provide written feedback and instructions on this website within one working day (a total of seven times over the course of treatment).

Phase I: Imaginary Exposure

The first module implements imaginary exposure through actualisation of the traumatic event. The module starts with a psycho-educational text on trauma symptoms, the rationale of self-exposure and structured writing. Next, patients receive general writing instructions to engage in four scheduled 45-min writing sessions in the next 2 weeks. The patients are asked to produce detailed, first-person, present-tense narratives of the traumatic event, in which attention is paid to the most painful accompanying thoughts, fears and sensory experiences. They are instructed to write freely, without worrying about chronology, style, grammar, spelling, repetition or the use of proper language.

Phase II: Cognitive Reappraisal

The second module starts with a psycho-educational text about the principles of cognitive restructuring. Next, the patients are requested to write an encouraging letter to a hypothetical friend, who suffers from a traumatic event similar to what has happened to the patient. This change of perspective is used to facilitate the development of benign interpretations, enhanced self-esteem and reduced guilt. Patients are encouraged to acknowledge and reflect on the friend's feelings of guilt and shame, to challenge dysfunctional automatic thinking and behaviour patterns and to correct unrealistic assumptions.

Phase III: Closure/Social Sharing

In the third module, patients use two writing sessions to produce a coherent, dignified account of the traumatic event, in which they reflect on the event and its sequelae, on the therapeutic learning process and on future relapse prevention. In contrast to phase I, proper chronology, style, grammar, form and language are now important. Patients address the letter either to someone who was involved in the traumatic event (e.g. the perpetrator, the deceased child), to a significant other (e.g. a partner, a friend) or to themselves. Ritualistic disclosure of the end product (e.g. posting the letter) provides further opportunities to enhance self-esteem and emotional strength and helps to take leave of the previous episode that was coloured by the traumas.

Box 7.1: Case Description

Mrs H., a 47-year-old train driver, applies for treatment with a referral from her company doctor, in relation to a series of sick leave periods, marital problems and a recent safety incident in which she ignored a red traffic sign.

During the intake, Mrs H. links current symptoms to a traumatic experience that happened 2 years ago, in which a young man committed suicide by jumping under her train. Recurrent nightmares of this event and chronic hyperarousal further indicate PTSD. Mrs H. and the diagnostician agree to focus treatment on the suicide experience through writing therapy.

In phase I of treatment, Mrs H.'s writings appear to display adequate self-confrontation to painful aspects of the suicide experience. Unlike other patients, who sometimes provide only fragmentary descriptions of the traumatic event, Mrs H. sends a clear narrative of her experience in the first writing exercise. In the next three exercises, Mrs H. repeatedly zooms in on specific vivid images and emotions.

In phase II, Mrs H. finds it difficult to formulate supportive advice to an imaginary friend. She addresses the friend, but also the victim, her husband and herself. Two themes emerge. First, she allows herself to express some anger towards the victim and the incident support team, which arrived fairly late on the scene. Second, she introduces the loss of a close family member, who died some months before the suicide incident. Given the impact of this loss on her husband, Mrs H. did not want to burden him with the horrible details of the suicide. Consequently, she never shared her experience with him. As a result, she writes, her husband couldn't understand her short-temperedness and mood swings, which she considers one of the primary reasons for their current marital problems.

In line with the outcome of phase II, Mrs H. uses the last phase (III) of treatment to write a letter to her husband. In this letter, she explains to him why she never spoke about the suicide and how she now regrets this decision. She describes the images that have been haunting her for the past year and explains how these may have led to her short-temperedness and mood swings. She thanks her husband for urging her to seek help and ends the letter with a firm confirmation of her commitment to their relationship.

The case of Mrs H. illustrates how sequences of traumatic events may increase the vulnerability to PTSD. The case also illustrates the importance of social support in PTSD trajectories. By declaring the suicide a taboo subject, Mrs H. deprived herself from cognitive and emotional processing of the traumatic experience and from the positive support of her husband. Phase III in the online guided writing treatment enhances the chance of increases in social support, especially if the final letter is addressed to and shared with a significant other. It would certainly be an option to encourage Mrs H. to end treatment by sharing the letter with her husband.

The Efficacy and Effectiveness of oSWT

The efficacy and effectiveness of the online structured writing protocol for PTSD and complicated grief has been examined in 11 studies (see Table 7.1). This section provides a summary of these studies, supplementing a recent meta-analysis of Van Emmerik et al. (2013).

Pilot Feasibility Trial

As discussed in section "The origins of online structured writing therapy", the first trial of online SWT was an uncontrolled pilot feasibility study (Lange et al. 2000a, b). This study included 24 students with highly elevated symptoms of PTSD, of which 20 completed all online measurements. Pre-post reductions in trauma-related symptoms were found to be large, significant and stable up to 6 weeks after treatment (IES avoidance, $d=.81$[1]; intrusion, $d=1.0$; $P<.001$). Similar effects were observed with regard

[1] In this uncontrolled study, d was calculated as the standardized mean pre-post within-group change score, using the pretest standard deviation as the standardizer. Note that these effect sizes cannot be directly compared to the between-group effect sizes of the comparative studies (which represent the standardized *difference* between the pre-post change scores in the experimental groups).

Table 7.1 Characteristics of the clinical trials of online structured writing therapy

Study ID	Country	Participants	Type	*N*	Exp. groups	Follow-up
Lange 2000	NL	Traumatised students	Pilot	20	oSWT	6 weeks
Lange 2001	NL	Traumatised students	RCT	30	oSWT vs. WLC	18 months
Lange 2003	NL	Traumatised adults; community sample	RCT	101	oSWT vs. WLC	18 months
Wagner 2006	DE	Bereaved adults with complicated grief; community sample	RCT	56	oSWT vs. WLC	18 months
Knaevelsrud 2007	DE	Traumatised adults; community sample	RCT	96	oSWT vs. WLC	18 months
De Haas 2010	NL	Adolescent victims of sexual abuse (14–18 years); community sample	Pilot	8	oSWT	Post-test
Lange 2010	NL	Adolescent victims of sexual abuse (14–24 years); community sample	Baseline control	24	oSWT vs. attention placebo	1 year
Ruwaard 2012	NL	Traumatised adults; referred patients	Routine practice	478	oSWT	6 weeks
Wagner 2012	DE	Arab community sample	Pilot	15	oSWT	Post-test
Kersting 2013	DE	Women who experienced perinatal loss; community sample	RCT	228	oSWT vs. WLC	1 year
Knaevelsrud 2015	DE	Arab community sample	RCT	159	oSWT vs. WLC	3 months

Note: *Abbreviations*: *oSWT* online structured writing therapy, *WLC* waiting-list/delayed treatment control condition

to general psychopathology (anxiety, depression, somatisation and sleeping problems, as measured by the Symptom Check List; SCL, Arrindell and Ettema 2003).

Student Sample RCT

To assess the controlled effects of online treatment, Lange et al. (2001) conducted a small ($N=30$) randomised controlled trial, again in a student population. After online screening, participants were randomly allocated to online SWT ($n=15$) or to a waiting-list/delayed treatment control condition (WLC; $n=15$). At pretest, post-test and 6-week follow-up, patients completed the IES and self-report measures of general psychopathology. Dropout was 13 % (2/15) and study attrition at post-test was 17 % (5/30). A completers analysis showed that oSWT was efficacious with regard to trauma-related symptoms (intrusions, $P<.01$, $d=1.1$; avoidance, $P<.03$, $d=.7$) and general psychopathology, in particular depressive symptoms ($d=1.0$) and somatisation ($d=1.1$). At post-test, 86 and 82 % of the treated patients showed clinically significant improvement with regard to avoidance and intrusion, against 23 and 56 % of the control group. Follow-up measurements showed that improvements had sustained. This RCT strengthened the findings of the pilot study (Lange et al. 2000a) and yielded considerably stronger effect sizes in comparison to the RCTs in which structured writing assignments were delivered face to face (i.e. Schoutrop et al. 2002). The researchers attributed this to the appealing treatment format, the larger number of writing assignments, the transparency of treatment, the preciseness of instructions and the opportunity for the therapists to discuss or reflect on their feedback.

Community Sample RCT

This second RCT aimed to replicate the first controlled trial in a large ($N=184$) adult, non-student Dutch community sample (Lange et al. 2003a, b). Participants were allocated to online treatment ($n=122$) or WLC ($n=62$). Outcomes included trauma-related measures (IES) and measures of general psychopathology (anxiety, depression, somatisation and sleeping problems). Dropout rate was 36 % (44/122). Analyses of completers data ($N=101$; control condition, $n=32$; treatment, $n=69$) confirmed the efficacy of online CBT. At post-test, the control group reported non-significant changes on every outcome measure. In contrast, treated participants reported strong reductions in the severity of trauma-related symptoms and general psychopathology. Between-group differences were significant ($P<.002$) and large (IES: intrusion, $d=1.3$; avoidance, $d=1.4$). In terms of reliable and clinically relevant change (i.e. recovery; Jacobson and Truax 1991), differences between treated and untreated participants were significant (control group, 8 %; oSWT, 50 %; $P<.007$). Follow-up measurements, which were administered up to 18 months after treatment, again showed that treatment gains were stable on the long term.

Adolescent Victims of Sexual Abuse Controlled Trial

In 2007, alarmed by an extremely low percentage of sexually abused adolescent seeking help, a Dutch expert centre on sexuality initiated an adaptation of the online writing protocol to reach out to this group. Therapist feedback and psycho-education were extended, and an extra writing assignment module was added to address the impact of the sexual abuse on physical functioning, body image and intimate relationships. An uncontrolled pilot trial of this protocol gave mixed results (De Haas et al. 2009). The study suffered from large pretreatment withdrawal: out of 90 eligible youngsters, only eight (10 %) started treatment. However, outcomes were promising among those who started (within-group effect IES: $d=1.0$). The researchers then conducted a second trial, in which they aimed to reduce pretreatment withdrawal. The second study was a baseline-controlled repeated measures study: effects of treatment on trauma symptoms (IES), depression, invalidation and strength were compared to changes during a pretreatment attention placebo period (Lange and Ruwaard 2010). Pretreatment withdrawal was reduced in this study, but remained high (82/106; 77 %). However, as in the pilot study, among treatment starters ($n=24$), treatment dropout was low ($n=4$), and comparative effect sizes were moderate to large: .5 (IES; *ns*)$<d<$1.5 (invalidation; $P<.01$), with $n=17$ (71 %) reporting reliable and clinically significant improvement after treatment. The researchers noted that pretreatment withdrawal would likely be reduced if participants would be allowed to follow treatment anonymously, but concluded that this would not be feasible given the professional responsibility of the therapist and strict Dutch healthcare laws.

German Replication RCT

Knaevelsrud and Maercker (2007, 2010) randomly assigned 96 German traumatised adult patients to online structured writing ($n=49$) or a waiting-list control condition ($n=47$). Primary outcomes were the revised Impact of Event Scale (IES-R; Joseph 2000), the depression and anxiety subscales of the Brief Symptom Inventory (BSI; Derogatis and Melisaratos 1983) and the ShortForm-12 (SF-12; Ware et al. 1996), a measure of general functioning. These measures were administered at pretest, at post-test and at 3-month and 18-month follow-up. Results corroborated the outcomes of the Dutch trials. At post-test, between-group effect sizes were moderate to large and significant with respect to each outcome measure (intrusion, $d=.9$; avoidance, $d=.5$). In comparison to the waiting list, oSWT increased the probability of recovery from 21 to 74 %. As in the Dutch studies, follow-up assessments revealed that treatment gains were maintained.

Complicated Grief RTC

Wagner et al. (2006, 2007) conducted an RCT to assess the effects of oSWT-PTSD protocol in a German-speaking sample of patients, who suffered from complicated grief. This study included 55 German-speaking participants, who were randomly assigned to immediate treatment ($n=29$) or to WLC ($n=26$). Outcome measures included the IES, the depression and anxiety subscales of the BSI, the failure-to-adapt scale (Langner and Maercker 2005) and the SF-12. Treatment and study adherence were high: 22 participants (85 %) completed treatment, 25 (96 %) completed a 3-month follow-up and 22 (85 %) completed an 18-month follow-up. At post-test, symptom reductions in the treatment group ($1.0<d<1.7$) were significantly larger than those observed in the control group. The between-group effect sizes varied from $d=.6$ to $d=1.3$, and clinically significant change was observed in

81 % (21/26) of the participants in the treatment group, against 33 % (8/25) in the control group. Results represented completer data, although additional intention-to-treat analyses did not change the statistical significance of the results.

Perinatal Loss RCT

In a second RCT examining the suitability of the oSWT protocol in the treatment of complicated grief, Kersting et al. (2013) included 228 participants, who had experienced the loss of an infant through miscarriage or neonatal death ($n = 115$; WLC: $n = 113$). Attrition was similar on both groups (oSWT, 14 %; WLC, 11 %), and missing data were accounted for in intention-to-treat analyses using last-observation-carried-forward imputation. Outcome measures, including the IES and self-report measures of complicated grief, anxiety and depression, revealed significantly higher symptom reductions in the oSWT group in comparison to the WLC (between-group effects fluctuated from $d = .48$ to $d = .88$). Follow-up assessments, up to 12 months after treatment, showed that symptoms further decreased on the long term.

Victims of Terror in the Middle East (Ilajnafsy) RCT

In the Ilajnafsy project, Knaevelsrud and Wagner explore the use of oSWT in providing humanitarian aid to traumatised Arab patients, who live in conflict zones (Knaevelsrud et al. 2007). For this project, the contents of the original treatment protocol were substantially adapted. Instructions and feedback templates were rewritten towards a more pronounced directive therapeutic stance, quotes and metaphors from the Koran were introduced and participants were instructed to address the final writing in phase III only to themselves (to prevent potentially negative consequences). After an uncontrolled $N = 15$ pilot study, which yielded promising results (Wagner et al. 2012b), a randomised waiting-list controlled study was conducted among 159 Arabic-speaking patients from Iraq (Knaevelsrud et al. 2015). Outcomes of this study were similar to those observed in Western samples: effects of oSWT ($n = 79$) compared favourably to those of WLC ($n = 80$), with moderate to large between-group effect-sizes with regard to intrusion, avoidance, depression, anxiety and somatisation ($.6 < d < 1.0$) and large differential recovery rates (oSWT, 62 %; WLC, 2 %). The study included a highly educated sample that may not be representative of the final target group. Nevertheless, these findings demonstrate that, when cultural differences are carefully taken into account, oSWT may be beneficial for non-Western patients in conflict areas.

Routine Practice Outcomes

Controlled efficacy trials reveal the effects of an intervention under ideal conditions, but provide only limited information on its applicability in routine clinical practice.

To explore the generalisability of the oSWT efficacy trials, Ruwaard et al. (2012) analysed electronic health records of 1500 GP-referred patients of a Dutch online mental health clinic. Of those, 478 traumatized patients started oSWT and $n=361$ (76 %) completed the full treatment. Surprisingly, treatment effects were found to be stronger in comparison to the controlled trials, probably because the routine practice patients presented for treatment with more severe symptoms (Ruwaard 2012). Mixed model linear regression analyses of symptom severity assessments revealed large short-term reductions (up to 6 weeks post-treatment) with regard to primary PTSD symptomatology (intrusion, $d=1.6$; avoidance, $d=1.3$) and negative affect ($d=.7$; as measured by the Depression Anxiety Stress Scale; DASS). Patients gave high ratings to their therapists ($M=8.6$ on a 1–10 scale). Although 29 % of the patients ($n=110$) indicated that they had missed face-to-face contact during therapy, 78 % evaluated ICBT as effective, and 89 % would recommend the online treatment to others. Data were collected retrospectively, in a naturalistic setting. Patients and therapists were not affected by the study during treatment, and therapists' adherence to the protocol was less strictly monitored in comparison to the efficacy trials. Hence, these findings provide strong indications for the acceptability, applicability and effectiveness of oSWT in routine clinical practice.

Predictors of Outcome of oSWT

Patient Characteristics

Many of the oSWT trials explored whether variables such as age, gender, education level or cultural background moderate treatment outcome. No evidence was found that the online treatment is more or less effective for specific demographic groups. Only two identifying predictive variables emerged (Lange et al. 2003a). Patients, who had never shared their traumatic events prior to treatment, were found to benefit more from oSWT than those who had. This finding confirms earlier evidence about the negative impact of not sharing traumatic events (Lange et al. 1999). Second, structured writing was found to be more effective with intentional traumatic events (i.e. those inflicted by neglect or intention), in comparison to non-intentional traumatic events (e.g. accidents or natural disasters).

Therapeutic Alliance

In face-to-face CBT, patient ratings of the quality of the working alliance between the therapist and the patient have been found to correlate with treatment outcome (see, e.g. Martin et al. 2000; Norcross and Wampold 2011). Knaevelsrud and Maercker (2006) investigated the association of therapeutic alliance and outcome in online writing therapy, using the Working Alliance Inventory (WAI; Horvath and Greenberg 1989), a self-report measure of agreement on therapeutic tasks and therapeutic goals and on the degree of mutual trust and acceptance. Patients and therapists completed the WAI after phase I and immediately after treatment. Therapists' alliance ratings did not change during treatment. Patients' alliance ratings, however, did increase. Early alliance scores did not predict treatment outcome, although small to moderate inverse correlations were found between post-treatment patients' alliance ratings and psychopathology assessments (i.e. IES-R, BSI; Knaevelsrud and Maercker 2007). In contrast, Wagner et al. (2012a) did find moderate to large correlations between mid-treatment WAI scores and reductions of core PTSD symptomatology of $.28\ (ns) < r < .49\ (P < .01)$ in the context of the oSWT Ilajnafsy RCT. In sum, preliminary evidence currently suggests that online therapy does not preclude the development of an effective therapeutic working alliance. Yet, findings with regard to its relationship with treatment outcome are mixed.

Adherence to Assignment Instructions

Ruwaard (2009) explored the relation between treatment outcome and adherence to writing assignment instructions. He analysed a text corpus comprising 4255 essays written by the 478 traumatised patients that were included in the routine practice study (Ruwaard et al. 2012). He used Pennebaker's Linguistic Inquiry and Word Count (LIWC; Pennebaker et al. 2007), a programme for automated content analysis that calculates the occurrence of different categories of words. LIWC scores clearly mirrored assignment instructions. For example, frequencies of LIWC's 'I' word category strongly decreased from phase I to phase II, while 'You' words inversely increased, in line with the therapeutic instruction to change perspective in phase II. However, these LIWC scores did not convincingly predict treatment outcome as measured by the self-report questionnaires. After Bonferroni corrections for multiple statistical testing, no statistically significant relationships between LIWC scores and treatment outcome remained.

Cognitive Coping

Lemmen and Maas (2001, see Lange et al. 2003) applied conventional content analysis to study the relation between the development of cognitive coping during treatment and treatment outcome. They created contrast groups out of 101 patients, who had completed writing treatment for PTSD: ten patients who had benefitted most and ten patients who had benefitted least. Independent judges, blind to the groups, rated essays 1, 3, 8 and 10 (presented in random order) on several aspects of cognitive coping: insight in the process of overcoming the traumatic events (e.g. showing reflection on dysfunctional automatic thoughts), functional coping by expressing behavioural adaptation (e.g. decrease in avoidance behaviour, showing more assertiveness; Donnelly and Murray 1991) and orientation on the future (e.g. planning positive things, using words such as 'I will'). In both groups, the increase in coping was significant and large ($F_{3,54} = 40.1$, $P < .001$). As expected, essays did not show an increase in coping during phase I. However, essays written in phase II (cognitive reappraisal) and phase III (closure/

social sharing) reflected large increases in coping. Increases in functional coping were larger in the most improved group in comparison with the least improved group, although these differences were not significant ($F_{1,19}=2.2$, $P<.15$). Since the group, that had profited the least, also showed large benefits in coping, variance in outcome was very small. This may explain the non-significant difference between the two groups.

Related Empirical Work

Several empirical studies have provided indirect further support for the application of structured writing assignments in trauma-focused treatment.

Face-to-Face SWT Versus Regular CBT Versus WLC

Van Emmerik et al. (2008) compared face-to-face structured writing therapy (SWT; $n=44$) to regular face-to-face CBT ($n=41$) and WLC ($n=40$) in an RCT that included 125 adults with a confirmed diagnosis of acute stress disorder or PTSD. Structured writing therapy closely followed the structure of the original online structured writing protocol. Writing assignments were provided as homework assignments and were discussed in five to ten face-to-face feedback sessions. There were no statistically significant differences between the two active treatment conditions on any of the outcome measures (CBT vs. SWT, $.03<d<.4$). Both active treatments, however, were superior to WLC ($.3<d<.7$).

Write Junior

Van der Oord et al. (2010) adapted oSWT into a standardised computer-aided treatment for traumatised children and adolescents ('Write Junior'). In this 'blended' treatment, the young patient completes the writing assignments on a computer during face-to-face sessions, with the help of the therapist, to construct a coherent narrative of the traumatic event, in which elements of self-confrontation, reappraisal and social sharing are integrated. For very young children, drawing replaces computer-based writing. In a small uncontrolled pilot trial of this protocol variant ($n=23$; age of participants: $M=12$ years), strong, significant and stable reductions in PTSD symptomatology were found.

Onco-STEP

Seitz et al. (2014) explored the application of a variant of oSWT in the treatment of young adult survivors of paediatric cancer (age, 20–26 years) with elevated symptoms of PTSS and/or anxiety, in a small ($N=28$) uncontrolled study of what they call Onco-STEP. As the original oSWT protocol, Onco-STEP consists of ten therapist-assisted online structured writing exercises. However, the phases of treatment are structured differently. In the first phase – 'Looking back' (five assignments) – patients address the traumatic cancer-related experience through imaginary exposure and cognitive reappraisal. In the second phase, 'Looking forward' (five assignments), patients address dysfunctional fears of disease progression. In a completer analysis ($n=20$), participants reported moderate and significant reductions in symptoms of PTSD, anxiety, fear of disease progression and depression ($.5<d<1.0$). These results suggest that structured online writing may also be suitable to provide online psychological support to cancer survivors.

Writing Assignments in Other ICBT

Structured writing exercises have been applied in several variants in other Internet-based CBT programmes for PTSD. Hirai and colleagues examined unguided online writing. In the first RCT ($N=27$; Hirai and Clum 2005), they assessed the effects of a self-help ICBT programme that combined relaxation training, cognitive restructuring and exposure through writing. Moderate to large between-group effect sizes were found in favour of ICBT in comparison to a waiting-list comparison group, although between-group effects were significant only with regard to depression, state anxiety, avoidance symptoms and frequency of intrusions ($.8<d<1.3$). In a later RCT ($N=104$; Hirai et al. 2012), they found indications that online writing induces better effects when patients are instructed to write not only about facts of the traumatic event but also about related emotions (as in oSWT). Litz et al. (2007) compared therapist-guided online CBT to online supportive counselling in an RCT ($N=45$). Both treatment programmes included repeated writing. In the ICBT group, writing focused on identified traumatic events. In the supportive counselling group, writing focused on daily concerns. With ICBT, the researchers found a sharper decline of PTSD symptoms over time and higher rates of end-state functioning at 6-month follow-up. In contrast, Possemato et al. (2011) did not find significant differences between trauma-focused vs. non-trauma-focused online writing in a small RTC ($N=31$), although this could have resulted from the low power of the study and the fact that patients completed only three writing sessions. Klein et al. (2010) further added to the evidence by demonstrating promising effects of a 10-week therapist-guided ICBT programme (including online writing) in a small uncontrolled trial ($N=22$) that included patients with a primary clinical diagnosis of PTSD. Pre-post-follow-up assessments revealed significant reductions of PTSD severity and related PTSD symptomatology (although changes in general psychopathology ratings were non-significant). This study also suggested that therapist input might be limited in ICBT, since the reported average duration of therapist guidance during treatment was only 194 min (which the authors contrasted to a standard of 12 h in face-to-face CBT for PTSD; Harvey et al. 2003). More recently, these results were replicated and extended through waiting-list controlled trials by Spence et al. (2011) and Ivarsson et al. (2014). In both studies, large and significant effects of therapist-guided ICBT were found with regard to core symptoms of PTSD and symptoms of general psychopathology, in patient samples with confirmed diagnoses of PTSD.

Discussion

Two decades of research strongly suggest that online structured writing therapy provides a feasible treatment alternative in the management of post-traumatic stress disorder and complicated grief. Preliminary findings further suggest that oSWT may also be a useful psychological intervention in the aftermath of life-threatening medical conditions. The treatment is well accepted by patients, efficacious across different cultural contexts, and findings have been shown to transfer well to routine clinical practice.

Future Research Themes

Effects of oSWT are likely to be equivalent to face-to-face CBT, as evidenced by effect sizes within treated groups and a study in which an offline variant of the protocol was compared to regular CBT (Van Emmerik et al. 2008). However, direct evidence for this equivalence is not available, since all randomised controlled trials of the online treatment have been conducted with waiting-list comparison groups. Clear-cut support for the equivalence hypothesis should be sought in an adequately powered equivalence trial, in which margins of clinical insignificance are defined a priori. Such a trial should also include a proper evaluation of the cost-effectiveness of oSWT. Ideally, this trial would then also systematically vary the number of therapist feedback sessions, to assess the cost/benefit ratio of more or less therapist guidance.

Why Does It Work (1): Specific Factors

The effects of oSWT are partly explained by the elegant way in which the protocol integrates three critical elements of trauma-focused treatment: exposure, cognitive reappraisal and social support. OSWT has a strong exposure component. Full treatment comprises over 7 h of active self-confrontation to a rich array of trauma aspects. The treatment phases ensure that the exposure not only focuses on the traumatic event itself but also on the meaning of the trauma and its sequelae. This promotes broad activation of what Foa et al. have called the 'fear network' in memory (Foa and Kozak 1986). Through repeated, controlled and deliberate activation of this network, fear extinction can be expected to occur through habituation. But oSWT also addresses the 'contents' of this network, by focusing on the development of cognitive reappraisal in phase II, which has been shown to be a critical step (Boelen and van den Hout 2008; Ehlers and Clark 2000; Lange et al. 2003b).

Consolidation of these changes to the autobiographical memory is then promoted in phase III, by asking patients to produce and ritualistically share a coherent and dignified written account of the new perspective.

Why Does It Work (2): Common Factors

It has been argued that specific elements of therapy are 'necessary but only active insofar as they are a component of a larger healing context of therapy' (Messer and Wampold 2002). This context is defined by factors that are common to many psychotherapies, such as a productive working alliance, the clarity and acceptability of therapeutic tasks, the expectancy of change (i.e. hope) and a focus on increased mastery and self-esteem (see, e.g. Frank 1973; Laska et al. 2013; Wampold et al. 2010). These common factors can and should be incorporated in a treatment manual. The oSWT protocol reflects this, for example, in its clear structure (which is communicated throughout treatment and automatically enforced), the extensive use of psycho-education to provide a credible rationale and the highly specific writing instructions (facilitating goal consensus). In the standardised feedback templates of the protocol, which therapists can use for guidance, techniques are built in to promote working alliance and client motivation, such as the use of therapeutic compliments and the importance of explicit 'echoing' of words and phrases of the patient. In our experience, these standardised 'common factor implementations' play an important role in the effectiveness of oSWT. Common factors have been largely ignored in e-mental health research. They deserve wider recognition and more explicit targeted research, especially in relation to treatment adherence.

Therapist Guidance

Outcomes of therapist-guided ICBT are generally superior to those of unguided ICBT (Cuijpers et al. 2009). One explanation for this finding is that therapist guidance ensures an appropriate implementation of critical treatment factors. There is no guarantee that patients confront themselves to the most painful aspects of a trauma in a writing assignment, even when instructions are explicit. Therapists can detect the avoidance of trauma aspects that are too fearful and encourage patients to focus on them. Likewise, therapists are important advisors when patients consider sharing the end result of treatment with someone who was involved in the trauma. According to Brewin and Holmes (2003), 'negative social support' is a stronger predictor of chronic PTSD than the lack of social support. Hence, if sharing a letter could result in negative effects, patients should be advised to not take the risk. Therapist guidance also promotes the impact of common factor strategies. Hope, self-esteem and the working alliance are best promoted through credible admiration and respect for specific individual displays of endurance and resilience (or, conversely, by an accepting stance in the case of reported failures; Lange 1985). In addition, therapists can, when necessary, enhance client motivation by adapting standardised instructions and psycho-educational texts to the characteristics of their patients (e.g. a deaf patient should not be instructed to concentrate on what she heard during the traumatic event). Raising the impact of standardised elements by matching them to the personal situation of the patient requires careful consideration, for which oSWT provides time. The interval of one working day between reception of the patient's material and the moment of giving feedback and instructions allows therapists to reflect and make the right choices.

Acknowledgements and Disclosure of Conflict of Interest The authors would like to acknowledge Bart Schrieken of Interapy PLC, for his valuable contributions. At present, both authors have no financial ties to this company.

References

Amstadter AB, Broman-Fulks J, Zinzow H, Ruggiero KJ, Cercone J (2009) Internet-based interventions for traumatic stress-related mental health problems: a review and suggestion for future research. Clin Psychol Rev 29(5):410–420. doi:10.1016/j.cpr.2009.04.001

Andersson G (2010) Guided, internet-delivered cognitive behavioral therapy for posttraumatic stress disorder and other comorbid anxiety disorders. In: Brunet A, Ashbaugh AR, Herbert CF (eds) NATO science for peace and security series – E: human and societal dynamics, vol 72, Internet use in the aftermath of trauma. IOS Press, Amsterdam, pp 243–254, Retrieved from http://ebooks.iospress.nl/publication/25291

Arrindell WA, Ettema JHM (2003) Symptom checklist SCL-90: Handleiding bij een multidimensionele psychopathologie-indicator. Swets Test Publishers; Harcourt Test Publishers, Lisse/Amsterdam

Benight CC, Ruzek JI, Waldrep E (2008) Internet interventions for traumatic stress: a review and theoretically based example. J Trauma Stress 21(6):513–520. doi:10.1002/jts.20371

Boelen PA, van den Hout MA (2008) The role of threatening misinterpretations and avoidance in emotional problems after loss. Behav Cogn Psychother 36(01):71–88. doi:10.1017/S1352465807004079

Brewin CR, Holmes EA (2003) Psychological theories of posttraumatic stress disorder. Clin Psychol Rev 23(3):339–376. doi:10.1016/S0272-7358(03)00033-3

Brewin CR, Andrews B, Valentine JD (2000) Meta-analysis of risk factors for posttraumatic stress disorder in trauma-exposed adults. J Consult Clin Psychol 68(5):748–766. doi:10.1037//0022-006X.68.5.748

Brunet A, Ashbaugh AR, Herbert CF (eds) (2010) NATO science for peace and security series – E: human and societal dynamics, vol 72, Internet use in the aftermath of trauma. IOS Press, Amsterdam

Cuijpers P, Marks IM, Van Straten A, Cavanagh K, Gega L, Andersson G (2009) Computer-aided psychotherapy for anxiety disorders: a meta-analytic review. Cogn Behav Ther 38(2):66–82. doi:10.1080/16506070802694776

De Haas S, Höing M, Schrieken B, Tsagana A, Wijnker C, Michels C, Lange A (2009) Behandeling via het Internet voor jeugdige slachtoffers van seksueel geweld: een pilotstudie [Online treatment of young victims of sexual violence: a pilot study]. Maandblad Geestelijke Volksgezondheid 64(11):981–997

Derogatis LR, Melisaratos N (1983) The Brief Symptom Inventory: an introductory report. Psychol Med 13(3):595–605

Donnelly DA, Murray EJ (1991) Cognitive and emotional changes in written essays and therapy interviews. J Soc Clin Psychol 10(3):334–350. doi:10.1521/jscp.1991.10.3.334

Ehlers A, Clark DM (2000) A cognitive model of posttraumatic stress disorder. Behav Res Ther 38(4):319–345. doi:10.1016/S0005-7967(99)00123-0

Foa EB, Kozak MJ (1986) Emotional processing of fear: exposure to corrective information. Psychol Bull 99(1):20–35. doi:10.1037/0033-2909.99.1.20
Frank JD (1973) Persuasion and healing. John Hopkins University Press, Baltimore
Haley J (1973) Uncommon therapy: the psychiatric techniques of Milton H. Erickson. MD. Norton, New York
Harvey AG, Bryant RA, Tarrier N (2003) Cognitive behaviour therapy for posttraumatic stress disorder. Clin Psychol Rev 23(3):501–522
Hirai M, Clum GA (2005) An Internet-based self-change program for traumatic event related fear, distress, and maladaptive coping. J Trauma Stress 18(6):631–636. doi:10.1002/jts.20071
Hirai M, Skidmore ST, Clum GA, Dolma S (2012) An investigation of the efficacy of online expressive writing for trauma-related psychological distress in Hispanic individuals. Behav Ther 43(4):812–824. doi:10.1016/j.beth.2012.04.006
Horvath AO, Greenberg LS (1989) Development and validation of the Working Alliance Inventory. J Couns Psychol 36(2):223–233. doi:10.1037/0022-0167.36.2.223
Ivarsson D, Blom M, Hesser H, Carlbring P, Enderby P, Nordberg R, Andersson G (2014) Guided internet-delivered cognitive behavior therapy for post-traumatic stress disorder: a randomized controlled trial. Internet Interv 1(1):33–40. doi:10.1016/j.invent.2014.03.002
Jacobson NS, Truax P (1991) Clinical significance: a statistical approach to defining meaningful change in psychotherapy research. J Consult Clin Psychol 59(1):12–19. doi:10.1037/0022-006X.59.1.12
Joseph S (2000) Psychometric evaluation of Horowitz's Impact of Event Scale: a review. J Trauma Stress 13(1):101–113. doi:10.1023/A:1007777032063
Kersting A, Dölemeyer R, Steinig J, Walter F, Kroker K, Baust K, Wagner B (2013) Brief Internet-based intervention reduces posttraumatic stress and prolonged grief in parents after the loss of a child during pregnancy: a randomized controlled trial. Psychother Psychosom 82(6): 372–381. doi:10.1159/000348713
Klein B, Mitchell J, Abbott J, Shandley K, Austin D, Gilson K, Kiropoulos L, Cannard G, Redman T (2010) A therapist-assisted cognitive behavior therapy internet intervention for posttraumatic stress disorder: pre-, post- and 3-month follow-up results from an open trial. J Anxiety Disord 24(6):635–644. doi:10.1016/j.janxdis.2010.04.005
Knaevelsrud C, Maercker A (2006) Does the quality of the working alliance predict treatment outcome in online psychotherapy for traumatized patients? J Med Internet Res 8(4):e31. doi:10.2196/jmir.8.4.e31
Knaevelsrud C, Maercker A (2007) Internet-based treatment for PTSD reduces distress and facilitates the development of a strong therapeutic alliance: a randomized controlled clinical trial. BMC Psychiatry 7:13. doi:10.1186/1471-244X-7-13
Knaevelsrud C, Maercker A (2010) Long-term effects of an internet-based treatment for posttraumatic stress. Cogn Behav Ther 39(1):72–77. doi:10.1080/16506070902999935
Knaevelsrud C, Wagner B, Karl A, Mueller J (2007) New treatment approaches: integrating new media in the treatment of war and torture victims. Torture (Quarterly Journal on Rehabilitation of Torture Victims and Prevention of Torture) 17(2):67–78
Knaevelsrud C, Brand J, Schulz W, Lange A, Ruwaard J, Wagner B (2015) Internet-based psychotherapy for posttraumatic stress disorder in war-traumatized Arab patients: a parallel group randomized controlled trial. J Med Internet Res 17(3):e71. doi:10.2196/jmir.3582
Lange A (1985) Motivating clients in directive family therapy. In: Zeig JK (ed) Ericksonian psychotherapy, vol 2, Clinical applications. Brunner Mazel, New York
Lange A (1994) Writing assignment in the treatment of grief and trauma's from the past. In: Zeig JK (ed) Ericksonian methods. The essence of the story, 1st edn. Brunner/Mazel, Levittown.
Lange A, Ruwaard J (2010) Ethical dilemmas in online research and treatment of sexually abused adolescents. J Med Internet Res 12(5):e58. doi:10.2196/jmir.1455
Lange A, Van der Hart O (1983) Directive family therapy. Brunner/Mazel, New York
Lange A, De Beurs E, Dolan C, Lachnit T, Sjollema S, Hanewald G (1999) Long-term effects of childhood sexual abuse: objective and subjective characteristics of the abuse and psychopathology in later life. J Nerv Ment Dis 187(3):150–158

Lange A, Van de Ven J, Schrieken B, Bredeweg B, Emmelkamp PM (2000a) Internet-mediated, protocol-driven treatment of psychological dysfunction. J Telemed Telecare 6(1):15–21. doi:10.1258/1357633001933880
Lange A, Van de Ven J, Schrieken B, Emmelkamp P, Bredeweg B, Van der Kolk J, Lydsdottir L, Massaro M, Reuvers A (2000b) 'INTERAPY': the effects of a short protocolled treatment of post-traumatic stress and pathological grief through the Internet. Behav Cogn Psychother 28(2):103–120
Lange A, Van de Ven J, Schrieken B, Emmelkamp PM (2001) Interapy, treatment of posttraumatic stress through the Internet: a controlled trial. J Behav Ther Exp Psychiatry 32(2):73–90
Lange A, Schoutrop MJA, Schrieken B, Van de Ven J (2002) Interapy: a model for therapeutic writing through the internet. In: Lepore SJ, Smyth JM (eds) The writing cure. How expressive writing promotes health and emotional well-being, 1st edn. American Psychological Association, Washington, DC, pp 215–238
Lange A, Rietdijk D, Hudcovicova M, Van de Ven J, Schrieken B, Emmelkamp PM (2003a) Interapy: a controlled randomized trial of the standardized treatment of posttraumatic stress through the internet. J Consult Clin Psychol 71(5):901–909. doi:10.1037/0022-006X.71.5.901
Lange A, Van de Ven J, Schrieken B (2003b) Interapy: treatment of post-traumatic stress via the internet. Cogn Behav Ther 32(3):110–124. doi:10.1080/16506070302317
Langner R, Maercker A (2005) Complicated grief as a stress response disorder: evaluating diagnostic criteria in a German sample. J Psychosom Res 58(3):235–242. doi:10.1016/j.jpsychores.2004.09.012
Laska KM, Gurman AS, Wampold BE (2013) Expanding the lens of evidence-based practice in psychotherapy: a common factors perspective. Psychotherapy (Chicago, IL). doi:10.1037/a0034332
Lemmen A, Maas M (2001) Inhoudsanalyse van cognitieve categorieën in gestructureerde schrijfopdrachten via Interapy [Content analysis of structured writing.]. Department of Clinical Psychology
Lepore SJ, Smyth JM (eds) (2002) The writing cure: how expressive writing promotes health and emotional well-being, 1st edn. American Psychological Association, Washington, DC
Litz BT, Engel CC, Bryant RA, Papa A (2007) A randomized, controlled proof-of-concept trial of an Internet-based, therapist-assisted self-management treatment for posttraumatic stress disorder. Am J Psychiatry 164(11):1676–1683. doi:10.1176/appi.ajp.2007.06122057
Martin DJ, Garske JP, Davis MK (2000) Relation of the therapeutic alliance with outcome and other variables: a meta-analytic review. J Consult Clin Psychol 68(3):438–450. doi:10.1037/0022-006X.68.3.438
Messer SB, Wampold BE (2002) Let's face facts: common factors are more potent than specific therapy ingredients. Clin Psychol Sci Pract 9(1):21–25. doi:10.1093/clipsy.9.1.21
Moreau C, Zisook S (2002) Rationale for a posttraumatic stress spectrum disorder. Psychiatr Clin North Am 25(4):775–790
Motraghi TE, Seim RW, Meyer EC, Morissette SB (2014) Virtual reality exposure therapy for the treatment of posttraumatic stress disorder: a methodological review using CONSORT guidelines. J Clin Psychol 70(3):197–208. doi:10.1002/jclp.22051
Mouthaan J, Sijbrandij M, de Vries G-J, Reitsma JB, van de Schoot R, Goslings JC, Luitse JS, Bakker FC, Gersons BP, Olff M (2013) Internet-based early intervention to prevent posttraumatic stress disorder in injury patients: randomized controlled trial. J Med Internet Res 15(8):e165. doi:10.2196/jmir.2460
Nelson RJ (2013) Is virtual reality exposure therapy effective for service members and veterans experiencing combat-related PTSD? Traumatology 19(3):171–178. doi:10.1177/1534765612459891
Norcross JC, Wampold BE (2011) Evidence-based therapy relationships: research conclusions and clinical practices. Psychotherapy (Chicago, IL) 48(1):98–102. doi:10.1037/a0022161
Pennebaker JW (1993) Putting stress into words: health, linguistic, and therapeutic implications. Behav Res Ther 31(6):539–548. doi:10.1016/0005-7967(93)90105-4

Pennebaker JW, Susman JR (1988) Disclosure of traumas and psychosomatic processes. Soc Sci Med 26(3):327–332. doi:10.1016/0277-9536(88)90397-8

Pennebaker JW, Booth RJ, Francis ME (2007) Operator's manual Linguistic Inquiry and Word Count: LIWC2007. LIWC.net, Austin

Possemato K, Ouimette P, Knowlton P (2011) A brief self-guided telehealth intervention for post-traumatic stress disorder in combat veterans: a pilot study. J Telemed Telecare 17(5):245–250. doi:10.1258/jtt.2011.100909

Ruggiero KJ, Resnick HS, Acierno R, Carpenter MJ, Kilpatrick DG, Coffey SF, Carpenter MJ, Ruscio AM, Stephens RS, Kilpatrick DG, Stasiewicz PR, Roffman RA, Bucuvalas M, Galea S (2006) Internet-based intervention for mental health and substance use problems in disaster-affected populations: a pilot feasibility study. Behav Ther 37(2):190–205. doi:10.1016/j.beth.2005.12.001

Ruwaard J (2009) Computerized text analysis in computer-mediated therapy: the Interapy post-traumatic stress corpus (presentation slides): Presented at the Fourth Meeting of the International Society for Research on Internet Interventions; 14–16 October [presentation slides]. Amsterdam. Retrieved from http://www.slideshare.net/jruwaard/text-analysis-of-the-interapy-pts-corpus

Ruwaard J (2012) The efficacy and effectiveness of online CBT. Department of Clinical Psychology, the University of Amsterdam, Amsterdam

Ruwaard J, Lange A, Schrieken B, Dolan CV, Emmelkamp P (2012) The effectiveness of online cognitive behavioral treatment in routine clinical practice. PLoS One 7(7):e40089. doi:10.1371/journal.pone.0040089

Schoutrop MJA, Lange A, Hanewald G, Davidovich U, Salomon H (2002) Structured writing and processing major stressful events: a controlled trial. Psychother Psychosom 71(3):151–157. doi:10.1159/000056282

Seitz DCM, Knaevelsrud C, Duran G, Waadt S, Loos S, Goldbeck L (2014) Efficacy of an internet-based cognitive-behavioral intervention for long-term survivors of pediatric cancer: a pilot study. Supportive Care Cancer (Official Journal of the Multinational Association of Supportive Care in Cancer) 22(8):2075–2083. doi:10.1007/s00520-014-2193-4

Sloan DM, Marx BP (2004) Taking pen to hand: evaluating theories underlying the written disclosure paradigm. Clin Psychol Sci Pract 11(2):121–137. doi:10.1093/clipsy.bph062

Spence J, Titov N, Dear BF, Johnston L, Solley K, Lorian C, Wootton B, Zou J, Schwenke G (2011) Randomized controlled trial of Internet-delivered cognitive behavioral therapy for post-traumatic stress disorder. Depress Anxiety 28(7):541–550. doi:10.1002/da.20835

Spence J, Titov N, Johnston L, Dear BF, Wootton B, Terides M, Zou J (2013) Internet-delivered eye movement desensitization and reprocessing (iEMDR): an open trial. F1000Research 2:79. doi:10.12688/f1000research.2-79.v2

Steinmetz SE, Benight CC, Bishop SL, James LE (2012) My Disaster Recovery: a pilot randomized controlled trial of an Internet intervention. Anxiety Stress Coping 25(5):593–600. doi:10.1080/10615806.2011.604869

Sundin EC, Horowitz MJ (2003) Horowitz's Impact of Event Scale evaluation of 20 years of use. Psychosom Med 65(5):870–876

Thompson RF (2009) Habituation: a history. Neurobiol Learn Mem 92(2):127–134. doi:10.1016/j.nlm.2008.07.011

Van der Oord S, Lucassen S, Van Emmerik AAP, Emmelkamp PMG (2010) Treatment of post-traumatic stress disorder in children using cognitive behavioural writing therapy. Clin Psychol Psychother 17(3):240–249. doi:10.1002/cpp.670

Van der Velden K (ed) (1977, 1980, 1989) Directieve therapie/1,2,3 [Directive Therapy]. Van Loghum Slaterus, Deventer

Van Emmerik AAP, Kamphuis JH, Emmelkamp PMG (2008) Treating acute stress disorder and posttraumatic stress disorder with cognitive behavioral therapy or structured writing therapy: a randomized controlled trial. Psychother Psychosom 77(2):93–100. doi:10.1159/000112886

Van Emmerik AAP, Reijntjes A, Kamphuis JH (2013) Writing therapy for posttraumatic stress: a meta-analysis. Psychother Psychosom 82(2):82–88. doi:10.1159/000343131

Van Voorhees BW, Gollan J, Fogel J (2012) Pilot study of Internet-based early intervention for combat-related mental distress. J Rehabil Res Dev 49(8):1175–1190. doi:10.1682/JRRD.2011.05.0095
Wagner B, Maercker A (2007) A 1.5-year follow-up of an Internet-based intervention for complicated grief. J Trauma Stress 20(4):625–629. doi:10.1002/jts.20230
Wagner B, Knaevelsrud C, Maercker A (2006) Internet-based cognitive-behavioral therapy for complicated grief: a randomized controlled trial. Death Stud 30(5):429–453. doi:10.1080/07481180600614385
Wagner B, Brand J, Schulz W, Knaevelsrud C (2012a) Online working alliance predicts treatment outcome for posttraumatic stress symptoms in Arab war-traumatized patients. Depress Anxiety 29(7):646–651. doi:10.1002/da.21962
Wagner B, Schulz W, Knaevelsrud C (2012b) Efficacy of an Internet-based intervention for posttraumatic stress disorder in Iraq: a pilot study. Psychiatry Res 195(1–2):85–88. doi:10.1016/j.psychres.2011.07.026
Wampold BE, Imel ZE, Laska KM, Benish S, Miller SD, Flückiger C, Del Re AC, Baardseth TP, Budge S (2010) Determining what works in the treatment of PTSD. Clin Psychol Rev 30(8):923–933. doi:10.1016/j.cpr.2010.06.005
Wang Z, Wang J, Maercker A (2013) Chinese My Trauma Recovery, a Web-based intervention for traumatized persons in two parallel samples: randomized controlled trial. J Med Internet Res 15(9):e213. doi:10.2196/jmir.2690
Ware J, Kosinski M, Keller SD (1996) A 12-Item Short-Form Health Survey: construction of scales and preliminary tests of reliability and validity. Med Care 34(3):220–233

ICBT for Insomnia

8

Annemieke van Straten, Kerstin Blom, Jaap Lancee, and Viktor Kaldo

Abstract

Insomnia is a major public health issue. It affects about 10 % of the population and often leads to impairments in emotional and daily functioning as well as to comorbidity with other (mental) disorders. The high prevalence of insomnia and its related burden of disease call for widely available, high-quality, and effective treatments. Insomnia guidelines indicate that cognitive-behavioral treatment (CBT) is preferred above sleep medication. Unfortunately, face-to-face CBT for insomnia is almost unavailable. Offering CBT via the Internet might be a solution.

To date we have identified ten different Internet CBT programs for insomnia which have published data on the effectiveness of the program: nine for adults and one for adolescent patients. Patients' adherence to these programs was high (range 54–91 %) indicating that many patients accept the Internet format. The results from the trials on symptoms of insomnia are also very encouraging. In general it seems that patients fall asleep quicker and are less often awake during the night. As for traditional CBT for insomnia, the total number of hours asleep improves more modestly, but because sleep is less fragmented, patients tend to feel more refreshed and restored and less worried about sleep. Furthermore, there are also indications that online CBT for insomnia is effective in reducing depression severity.

A. van Straten (✉)
Department of Clinical- Developmental and Neuropsychology, Faculty of Behavioural and Movement Sciences & EMGO Institute for Health and Care Research, VU University Amsterdam, Amsterdam, The Netherlands
e-mail: a.van.straten@vu.nl

K. Blom • V. Kaldo
Department of Clinical Neuroscience, Karolinska Institutet, Stockholm, Sweden
e-mail: kerstin.blom@sll.se; Viktor.kaldo@ki.se

J. Lancee
Department of Clinical Psychology, University of Amsterdam, Amsterdam, The Netherlands

© Springer International Publishing Switzerland 2016
N. Lindefors, G. Andersson (eds.), *Guided Internet-Based Treatments in Psychiatry*, DOI 10.1007/978-3-319-06083-5_8

Several important questions still need to be answered: Is human support necessary or is automated support sufficient? Can the same results be obtained in clinical samples with help-seeking patients or are they only valid in population samples? Can insomnia treatment prevent other psychological disorders? What are the (long) term effects on daily functioning? Is Internet CBT also cost-effective?

Despite these questions, we conclude that time has come to implement Internet-based treatments for insomnia. Health-care practitioners are in need of other treatment options than medication and patients seem to be willing to adhere to the Internet-based interventions. Based on the studies which have been performed, we feel confident to say that Internet-based CBT for insomnia improves insomnia.

Insomnia

Diagnosis

Almost every adult occasionally experiences a period of poor sleep in his or her life. Typically, this occurs in periods of stress. We speak of insomnia when the sleep symptoms persist even when the stressful situation is no longer present. Insomnia is generally characterized by difficulties falling asleep, difficulties staying asleep, or by non-restorative sleep. Often people experience a combination of those difficulties. In order to fulfill insomnia diagnosis, this impaired sleep needs to have a negative impact on the daytime functioning.

The fourth edition of the Diagnostic and Statistical Manual for mental disorders (DSM-IV; APA 1994) made a distinction between primary insomnia, in which there is no other identified condition causing the insomnia, and secondary insomnia in which insomnia is believed to be caused by another mental or medical disorder. Since it has been recognized that it is virtually impossible to reliably distinguish primary from secondary insomnia, this distinction has been abandoned in the newest edition of the DSM (DSM-5; APA 2013). The DSM-5 simply identifies an "insomnia disorder." The criteria are summarized in Table 8.1.

The DSM-5 is not the only diagnostic classification system which includes insomnia. Insomnia is also incorporated into the International Classification of Diseases (ICD-10; WHO 1992) and in the International Classification of Sleep Disorders (ICSD-2; AASM 2005). The three diagnostic classification systems share the general criteria for insomnia (difficulty initiating or maintaining sleep or non-restorative sleep leading to impairments in daytime functioning), but they vary in the required severity of the symptoms and a number of additional requirements. The DSM criteria seem to be the most sensitive, leading to the highest prevalence rates (Roth et al. 2011).

Table 8.1 Summary of the DSM5 criteria for insomnia disorder

1. Symptoms
Dissatisfaction with sleep quantity or quality and one (or more) of the following symptoms:
(a) Difficulty initiating sleep
(b) Difficulty maintaining sleep (frequent awakenings or problems returning to sleep after awakening)
(c) Early morning awakening with inability to return to sleep
2. Severity
(a) The sleep difficulty occurs at least 3 nights per week
(b) The sleep difficulty is present for at least 3 months
(c) The sleep disturbance causes clinically significant distress or impairment in functioning
3. The sleep difficulty cannot be (solely) attributed to
(a) Inadequate opportunity for sleep
(b) Another sleep-wake disorder
(c) The physiological effects of a substance (drugs or medication)
(d) Coexisting mental disorders or medical conditions

Prevalence and Consequences

Insomnia is very common. About a third of the people in the general population experiences one or more symptoms of poor sleep. About 10 % reports a full insomnia disorder including daytime consequences (Ohayon 2002). These daytime consequences typically refer to subjectively reported impairments in cognitive and emotional functioning such as fatigue, mood swings, and concentration problems (Kyle et al. 2010). Among other things, these impairments lead to increased healthcare use and decreased work productivity which in turn leads to high societal costs (Daley et al. 2009a). It has been estimated that poor sleepers cost society about ten times more than good sleepers (Daley et al. 2009b). Moreover, insomnia might be considered a long-term condition: about half of all patients suffer from insomnia for at least 3 years (Morin et al. 2009).

Insomnia also often co-occurs with other mental or medical conditions. Depression and anxiety are two common comorbid conditions (Staner 2010; Baglioni et al. 2011), but insomnia is also associated with cancer, hypertension, and cardiovascular diseases (e.g., Meng et al. 2012; Redline and Foody 2011; Savard and Morin 2011).

Current Treatments

The high prevalence of insomnia and its related burden of disease call for widely available, high-quality, and effective treatments. Currently insomnia is most often treated with pharmacotherapy either with benzodiazepines or benzodiazepine receptor agonists (Z-drugs: zolpidem, zopiclone, zaleplon). Several meta-analyses have shown that pharmacotherapy is effective in enhancing sleep in the short run, but it has also been demonstrated that there are negative side effects, especially in the elderly, while long-term consequences risks and benefits are still unknown (Buscemi et al. 2007; Glass et al. 2005).

Various non-pharmacological treatments have been developed as alternatives. These non-pharmacological treatments can be classified as educational (psychoeducation, sleep hygiene), behavioral (relaxation, sleep restriction, stimulus control, paradoxical intention), or cognitive (identifying and challenging dysfunctional thought about sleep; Edinger and Means 2005; Espie 2006; Morin and Espie 2003). Since the 1990s, it has become popular to offer those treatments in (different) combinations. These combinations are referred to as cognitive-behavioral therapy for insomnia (CBTI). See Table 8.2 for an overview of the core components. Next to those core components, the treatment might include relaxation exercises, paradoxical intention (in which the patient is instructed to stay awake during the night), mindfulness exercises, or problem-solving strategies.

Table 8.2 Core components of CBTI

Component	Description
Sleep education	Information about what instigates sleep, the function of sleep, the normal range of hours of sleep for different age groups, and information about sleep disorders and insomnia
Sleep hygiene	Information about everyday behavior and habits that might promote, or interfere, with good sleep. This usually includes information about lifestyle (e.g., food, caffeine, alcohol, stress) and bedroom (e.g., temperature, light, mattress)
Stimulus control	Patients are taught to associate their bed with sleep again (instead of lying awake). This includes to go to bed and get out of bed at the same time each day, to use the bed for sleep and sex only but not for other activities such as reading or watching television, and to get out of bed in case of lying awake for more than 15 or 30 min. The fixed hours for going to bed and getting up in the morning helps the circadian rhythm to stabilize and facilitate a more pronounced difference between sleep and wakefulness
Sleep restriction	Patients restrict their time in bed. The rationale is that patients sleep fewer hours and become more tired than usual. As a consequence, they have less difficulty falling and staying asleep. Sleep restriction can also be viewed and explained as exposure therapy – exposure to the fear of being very tired during the day
	Usually the number of hours in bed is restricted to the average numbers of hours a patient actually slept in the week prior to starting the sleep restriction. In case the patient actually sleeps for 80–90 % of those limited number of hours, for a prespecified number of days, the sleep window is extended by 15 or 30 min. This continues until the desired number of hours is reached
Cognitive reappraisal	Patients are taught to identify and challenge their misconceptions about sleep (i.e., "I need 8 h of sleep to perform well during the next day"). It might also be aimed at identifying and challenging other thoughts that keep the patient awake at night and thus providing a more general form of cognitive therapy

Unfortunately, not many patients receive CBTI. One reason is that less than half of all the insomnia patients seek help (Morin et al. 2006a). People with insomnia usually believe that medication is the only existing treatment option. They may be reluctant to take sleep medication and therefore reluctant to seek help. A second reason is that CBT for insomnia is not widely available. Moreover, GPs seldom refer to available psychological services for insomnia even when they do exist (Everitt et al. 2014). Offering CBT through the Internet may help overcome these issues.

ICBT Programs for Insomnia

As early as in 1979, it was recognized that insomnia treatment might also be delivered in self-help formats (Alperson and Biglan 1979). During the following 30 years, several self-help programs have been developed in different formats such as books, videos, and audiotapes (e.g., Morin et al. 2005; Riedel et al. 1995). This means that patients receive materials in which the different components of cognitive-behavioral therapy are explained. They are stimulated to practice the established CBTI techniques themselves or with brief therapist support.

The first study on Internet-delivered self-help for insomnia appeared in 2004 (Ström et al. 2004). To date we identified ten different programs which have published data on the effectiveness of the program: nine for adult patients with insomnia (Blom et al. 2015a; Espie et al. 2012; Kaldo et al. 2015a; Lancee et al. 2012; Ritterband et al. 2009; Ström et al. 2004; Suzuki et al. 2008; Van Straten et al. 2014; Vincent and Lewycky 2009) and one for adolescent patients (De Bruin et al. 2014).

The ten programs all include the core CBTI components as described in Table 8.2, and some include additional components, e.g., audio files for relaxation and stress management techniques. Even though the content of the programs is not that different, the way the treatments are presented does vary quite a lot. The treatment by Suzuki offers all the CBT elements, but patients can choose which of those they want to try out (at least three). The treatment of De Bruin is offered during fixed weekly online consultations. The treatments by Blom and Kaldo have both fixed and optional elements, with flexible and active online therapist support. The remaining treatments are fixed structured programs which the patients can work through at their own pace. Some of the programs are mostly text based (e.g., Blom, De Bruin, Lancee, Ström, Kaldo, Van Straten), while others make more use of audiovisual clips (e.g., Vincent) or use an array of different elements to make the intervention more attractive. Examples of these elements are quizzes, games, animations, and a virtual therapist (e.g., Espie, Ritterband). The rationale behind a more interactive design, next to offering patients a more pleasurable experience, is to promote better understanding of the information. It is also suggested that it will retain patients in the intervention.

The interventions also vary in the way patients are supported. This varied from no support at all (Lancee, Vincent) to automated support (Espie, Ritterband, Ström, Suzuki) and weekly personal feedback from a coach or therapist (Blom, De Bruin,

Van Straten, Kaldo). Support is aimed at helping patients through the program and exercises (i.e., providing optimal sleep windows) and to encourage patients to continue. The automated support was personalized and based on bed times and sleep estimates provided by patients in their sleep diary.

Case Description

Farah is a 34-year-old woman with insomnia disorder. Her sleeping problems started when her child, now 3 years old, was a baby and needed feeding several times per night. When the baby grew older and started sleeping through most nights, Farah kept waking up three to four times per night and had trouble going back to sleep. After her parental leave, Farah went back to her job as a manager at a construction company. The work entails long hours and a high level of stress. Farah started having trouble falling asleep, in addition to her frequent nighttime awakenings. She found it hard to relax in the evening. She often checked her email late in the evening to get a head start on next day's work. Her mind was constantly active solving problems, thinking about work and planning their everyday life, making her mentally aroused when trying to sleep. She started worrying a lot about not sleeping and the ramifications of that for her health and performance at work and as a parent. The worrying made it even harder to fall asleep – a catch 22! She was too tired to meet friends and exercise, something she used to do regularly prior to her sleeping problems. Farah has started using sleep medication in order to fall asleep. Her general practitioner (GP) has told her not to use it too frequently, for fear of habituation, and she takes them two or three times per week when she is desperate to sleep. They help her go to sleep, but she still wakes up during the night. It is not a satisfactory solution.

Farah talks to her GP about her issues, and the GP deems online treatment to be suitable for her. He refers her to a mental health service which offers online CBT for insomnia. After filling out an online sleep diary for 1 week, her treatment starts.

Farah logs on to the treatment Internet site and is greeted by a welcome message from her personal online psychologist. The treatment is divided into several chapters, which she can access sequentially, after completing the previous chapter. The treatment consists of educational text to read about insomnia and CBT for insomnia, questions to answer at the end of each chapter on theory and how it applies to her situation, assignments on how to work through the CBT interventions, work sheets to fill out, and a sleep diary that is to be filled out daily throughout treatment.

When Farah has finished a chapter, her writings and answers are automatically sent to her psychologist. The psychologist logs on to the site and looks into Farah's sleep diary and her writings. The psychologist then gets back to her with advice, answers to questions, and encouragement. Farah is expected to complete on average one chapter per week and can send messages to her psychologist whenever she wants. After a couple of weeks' treatment, Farah gets a cold, and at the same time her workload increases dramatically due to a colleague's sick leave. As a result she stops focusing on the ICBT and forgets to log on to the site. When Farah hasn't been heard from for 1 week, her psychologist sends an online message, asking her how she is doing and motivating her to continue with the treatment. After that, Farah is back on track and continues with the next chapter. She will need another two text messages to remind her in the coming weeks, but she always responds quickly and makes it though the treatment chapters on time.

The treatment focuses on behavioral changes such as sleep restriction, stimulus control, and evening routines. Farah struggles with sleep restriction, since it means she has to stay awake until one in the morning the first week and get up at 6 o'clock. The most difficult part is staying awake in the early evening after putting her child to bed. After online consultation with the psychologist, she decides to start a new evening routine and she asks her husband to support her to stick to the routine. It means that she takes a walk after putting her child to bed, that she and her husband watch some television together, and that she takes a bath before going to bed. Quite soon after she starts adhering to the sleep restriction schedule, she notices that she wakes up less often which encourages her further to stick to the routine. The treatment also encompasses cognitive reappraisal, stress management, and how to cope with, and prevent, sleepiness and fatigue. For example, Farah is encouraged to talk to her manager about reducing her workload, and she takes up running again. She also starts meeting her friends every now and then, even if she feels tired. At the end of the treatment, she makes a plan for the future – how to continue with interventions and look for warning signs of relapse.

When Farah has worked through the complete treatment, her insomnia severity has dropped from severe to mild. At the start it took her around 40 min to fall asleep after going to bed, but this decreased to only 10 min. She also wakes up less frequently and worries less about her sleep problems. Even though her actual sleep time has not increased by much, she feels that her sleep quality is much better and daytime fatigue is much less. She doesn't use any sleep medication anymore. She believes her sleep time will increase a bit more when she continues with her sleep restriction schedule for a few more weeks after the treatment.

ICBT for Insomnia: Does It Work?

Relevant Insomnia Outcomes

One of the challenges in insomnia research is that there is no generally accepted primary outcome measure. First, some researchers prefer to obtain objective sleep data (e.g., polysomnography or actigraphy), while others prefer subjective sleep data (sleep diary). Even though objective and subjective data are correlated, they usually lead to different results. Second, sleep is usually expressed in a number of different estimates: sleep onset latency (SOL) which is the number of minutes it takes to fall asleep after switching of the light, number of awakenings (NWAK) during the night, time being awake after sleep onset (WASO), the total sleep time (TST), and the sleep efficiency (SE) which is the percentage of time sleeping while being in bed. Third, some researchers prefer to ask patients directly about their insomnia severity and their sleep quality instead of using sleep diaries. Two often used instruments are the Pittsburgh Sleep Quality Index (PSQI; Buysse et al. 1989) and the Insomnia Severity Index (ISI; Morin et al. 2011; Thorndike et al. 2011). They are validated and offer cutoffs to identify patients with clinically significant symptoms of insomnia. In summary, all the different variables measure different aspects of sleep. Sleep improvements are therefore usually expressed not in one but in a number of different estimates.

Face-to-Face CBT

Several excellent (systematic) reviews have been written on face-to-face CBTI and have concluded that CBTI is effective, has longer-lasting effects than medication, and should be the preferred treatment for insomnia (Montgomery and Dennis 2004; Morin et al. 2006b; Murtagh and Greenwood 1995). This means that people usually fall asleep quicker and are less often awake during the night even though their total number of hours asleep generally only improve modestly. However, since sleep is less fragmented, patients tend to report large improvements on insomnia severity and sleep quality.

Internet-Based CBT

Three meta-analyses have been performed on self-help interventions for insomnia. The first included all self-help formats (e.g., books, audio) and encompassed only one study on an Internet intervention (Van Straten and Cuijpers 2009). This meta-analysis was updated in 2015 (Yan-Yee Ho et al. 2015). The third one specifically focused on the effectiveness of computerized CBT for insomnia (Cheng and Dizon 2012). Six Internet programs were identified in these meta-analyses. The overall conclusion was that Internet-based self-help is effective in improving sleep with moderate effect sizes.

After the publication of the meta-analyses, effectiveness data was published on four new Internet CBT programs (Blom et al. 2015b; De Bruin et al. 2014; Van Straten et al. 2014; Kaldo et al. 2015b). This means that there are currently ten Internet programs for insomnia: nine for adults and one for adolescents. Seven of the ten studies demonstrating effectiveness used a wait-list or treatment-as-usual comparison group, one used a placebo control group (Kaldo et al. 2015a), while two studies compared their online treatment to a face-to-face group therapy (Blom et al. 2015a; De Bruin et al. 2014). Table 8.3 provides a summary of the data of the ten trials.

All trials recruited their patients in the general population. They put advertisements for their studies on relevant websites, in newspapers, etc. Four of the nine trials were small (less than 50 patients), five were moderately large (around 100 patients), and one was very large (more than 400 patients). All trials were aimed at insomnia, but they used different criteria to identify this. Suzuki used no definition

Table 8.3 Summary of effectiveness of the ten identified online CBT programs for insomnia

									Posttest between group effect sizes (Cohen's *d*)[d]				
Author	Country	Insomnia definition	Intervention	Control	Support	Weeks	N	Full adherence	SOL	TST	SE	WASO	NWAK
Studies comparing the Internet treatment against wait-list or treatment-as-usual													
Ström et al. (2004)	Sweden	≥30 min awake, ≥3 nights a week, ≥3 months + daytime problem	Core CBT	WL	Automated + max 2 e-mails	5	109	80 %	0.34	0.01	0.20	−0.04	0.24
Suzuki et al. (2008)	Japan	A desire to improve sleep	Sleep education + sleep hygiene. Then patients can choose from other CBT components	WL	Automated personalized messages	2	43	–	0.33	0.09	0.23	–	–
Ritterband et al. (2009)	USA	Sleep difficulties for ≥3 nights a week, ≥6 months + daytime problem	Core CBT	WL	Automated	6	45	91 %[c]	0.99	0.41	1.23	0.94	0.71

(continued)

Table 8.3 (continued)

									Posttest between group effect sizes (Cohen's *d*)[d]				
Author	Country	Insomnia definition	Intervention	Control	Support	Weeks	N	Full adherence	SOL	TST	SE	WASO	NWAK
Vincent and Lewycky (2009)	Canada	≥30 min awake, ≥4 nights a week, ≥6 months + daytime problem	Core CBT + relaxation	WL	None	5	118	68 %	0.50	0.24	0.23	0.13	0.68
Espie et al. (2012)	Scotland	Sleep difficulties for ≥3 nights a week, ≥3 months + daytime problem	Core CBT + imagery + articulatory suppression + mindfulness + social community of users	TAU[a]	Virtual therapist. Automated support tailored on severity and improvements over time	6	109	78 %	0.45	0.00	0.95	1.03	–
Lancee et al. (2012)	Netherlands	Sleep efficiency <85 % + SLEEP50 score >19	Core CBT + paradoxical intention + relaxation	WL[b]	None	4	418	54 %	0.38	0.34	0.60	0.54	0.08
van Straten et al. (2014)	Netherlands	≥30 min awake, ≥3 nights a week, ≥3 months	Core CBT + relaxation	WL	Weekly online by personal coach	6	118	73 %	0.04	0.57	0.95	–	0.54

Studies comparing the Internet treatment against another active or placebo treatment													
de Bruin et al. (2014)	Netherlands	Sleep difficulties for ≥3 nights a week, ≥1 month	Core CBT + booster session (2 months). Access to lessons on fixed day/time	Group therapy	Automated feedback + weekly online by personal coach	6	26	85 %	0.64[e]	0.08	0.67	0.03	–
Blom et al. (2015a)	Sweden	Sleep difficulties for ≥1 month + daytime problems + ISI >10	Core CBT + mindfulness	Group therapy	Weekly online by personal therapist	8	48	71 %	−0.20[f]	−0.21	−0.07	–	–
Kaldo et al. (2015a)	Sweden	Insomnia diagnosis[g] + ISI >10	Core CBT + stress and fatigue management	Placebo treatment	Weekly online by personal therapist	8	148	82 %[h]	0.35	0.03	0.59	–	–

[a]This study also included a third group (placebo)
[b]This study also included a third group (bibliotherapy)
[c]% that opened the lesson, not clear if they actually performed exercises
[d]Effect sizes calculated based on reported posttest means and standard deviations (derived from standard errors in some studies)
[e]Based on sleep diary and not on actigraphy data, data used on nights before; nonschool days, positive results indicates that Internet treatments performs better than group treatment
[f]Negative results indicate better performance of group therapy/individual face-to-face therapy
[g]According to the American Academy of Sleep Medicine
[h]82 % finished lessons on core components stimulus control + sleep restriction

at all but included everyone who was willing to participate. Lancee used a specific sleep estimate (sleep efficiency <85 %) as well as a cutoff score on a questionnaire. The remaining trials used sleep difficulties (>30 min awake during the night or subjectively defined), frequency of those difficulties (more than three or four nights in a week), and duration of those difficulties (more than 1, 3, or 6 months), and many also used daytime consequences as an inclusion criterion. Five trials excluded patients with (major) depression. All but one study used data from sleep diaries to report their main outcomes.

One very positive result of these studies on Internet interventions for insomnia is that a large proportion of the people who were offered an Internet intervention actually carried out all lessons or at the very least opened every lesson or carried out the core components (sleep restriction and stimulus control). This is even more remarkable since many studies did not provide any feedback, or provided only automated feedback, and because we know that Internet interventions for depression or anxiety require some form of support in order to engage patients to increase adherence and outcomes. We are aware of two studies that specifically examined the additional therapeutic effect of support in (Internet) self-help therapies for insomnia. Those two studies concluded that providing some support, which might be as small as 5 min of support per week per patient, actually did improve both adherence and sleep outcomes (Lancee et al. 2013; Jernelöv et al. 2012). People who received professional support were more engaged in the key therapeutic techniques (Kaldo et al. 2015b). We conclude that even though in insomnia automated feedback might work better than in other disorders, we need more research to solve the issue of the optimal amount and type of support.

Another important finding is that the effect sizes vary for the different sleep estimates. In other words, it is apparently possible to improve one symptom of insomnia (e.g., SOL) without necessarily improving other symptoms (e.g., WASO). Which symptoms improve and which do not (or less) vary for the different trials. In general, based on sleep diary data, it seems that sleep efficiency yields the highest effect sizes. This is understandable since the interventions aim to promote getting out of bed when not sleeping which inflates the sleep efficiency (% of time sleeping while being in bed). The variable least likely to change is the total sleeping time. This is in line with the results on face-to-face treatments for insomnia: the total sleep time does not necessarily increase, but sleep is less fragmented which leads to feeling more rested and restored.

The effect sizes for the sleep efficiency in the superiority trials, the trials which compare the Internet intervention to a wait-list group or a placebo condition, varied: three reported small effect sizes of around 0.20 (Ström, Suzuki, Vincent), two reported a moderate effect sizes of 0.60 (Lancee, Kaldo), and the remaining three reported (very) large effect sizes (Espie, Ritterband, Van Straten). However, based on the data from these superiority trials, it is not possible to determine which of the Internet interventions work best. After all, the studies do not only vary with respect to the intervention itself but also to a lot of other study characteristics (e.g., different inclusion criteria and hence different study populations, different care-as-usual and hence differences with respect to the control groups, difference in quality of the trials, etc.). Overall, the results do, however, demonstrate that Internet interventions are effective in improving sleep. The effects for sleep efficiency are the largest, but they are also considerable for sleep onset latency (SOL) and for wake after sleep onset (WASO).

Two studies compared the Internet intervention to a face-to-face group therapy. One examined adolescents (De Bruin). In this study, the Internet treatment yielded slightly higher effect sizes than the group therapy. However, because of the small number of youngsters included (2*13), these results were not statistically significant. The other study examined adult patients (Blom). This trial showed that even though the within-effect sizes for the group therapy were slightly better than those for Internet treatment, the results of the Internet treatment were non-inferior to the group treatment. It must be noted that Lancee and coauthors performed a second study next to their first wait-list effectiveness study. In this second study, they compared a guided Internet intervention ($n=30$) to face-to-face individual therapy ($n=30$; Lancee et al. 2015). Both groups showed large effect size compared to a wait-list control group. However, the face-to-face group showed significant larger improvements in sleep efficiency ($d=0.72$), but not on total sleep time, than the online group.

ICBT Insomnia and Depression

The co-occurrence of insomnia and depression is extremely common (Taylor et al. 2005). In the past insomnia was usually seen as a symptom of depression, but more recently it has been demonstrated that insomnia often precedes the onset of depression (Riemann and Voderholzer 2003). A meta-analysis showed that people with insomnia have a twofold risk of becoming depressed (Baglioni and Riemann 2012). If insomnia predicts the onset of depression, does this mean that treatment of insomnia can postpone or prevent depression? The answer to this question is still not known, but on the positive side we can say that there are two trials underway (Gosling et al. 2014). Once people have both disorders, treatment is usually aimed at the depression only. The sleep problems are expected to subside along with other depression symptoms. However, people often have residual sleep problems after successful treatment for depression, and there are indications that this predicts relapses of depressive episodes (Carney et al. 2007). Thus, it seems to be better to aim treatment at both disorders. Recently, a study was performed in which patients with both depression and insomnia were randomized to receive either an online treatment for depression or an online treatment for insomnia (Blom et al. 2015b). As expected, this study demonstrated that the insomnia treatment was more effective in reducing insomnia severity. More surprising, however, is that depression outcomes were similar for both treatments. Insomnia trials including depression outcomes do consistently show that depressive symptoms diminish after insomnia treatment. All this indicates that Internet CBT for insomnia might not only be useful to improve sleep but also to treat depression. These interesting findings should be further explored. A remaining question is whether online treatment for insomnia is equally effective on sleep for people with or without depressive symptoms. A recent study of online CBT showed that people with depression benefit from the intervention when support was added, while people without depression did not need the support to improve their sleep (Lancee et al. 2014).

ICBT for Insomnia: Does It Reduce Costs?

Most commonly people with insomnia receive no treatment at all or they receive sleep medication. This means that treatment-as-usual is rather inexpensive if only taking the cost of medications in consideration. However, besides the costs for physicians prescribing sleeping pills, it also means that the patients' sleeping problems most likely are not solved and costs in the longer run due to decreased work and domestic productivity and increased health-care consumptions probably remain high. The costs associated with Internet treatment are strongly dependent on the cost of the development, support, and administration of stable and safe technical platforms as well as the amount of human support that is provided. As has been shown, there are currently several interventions available without human support which yield good effects. Programs without support could be made available to larger groups of patients which is beneficial from a public health perspective. Because these automated interventions are inexpensive, we can also assume that they are cost-effective. Cost-effectiveness of guided Internet treatment for other disorders has been demonstrated (e.g., Hedman et al. 2011). However, as far as we are aware, there are no studies available yet for insomnia which looks into (long term) consequences on sleep, (work) performance, and associated costs. In other words, the cost-effectiveness of online interventions for insomnia, with or without support, is not established yet.

Discussion and Future Challenges

Overall, the results of Internet interventions of insomnia based on CBT are very promising. In comparison to wait-list groups, patients report less insomnia symptoms, and their sleep efficiency improves a lot which indicates that sleep is less fragmented. Therefore, patients feel more refreshed in the morning and experience a higher sleep quality. The effectiveness of online interventions for insomnia is very much in line with the effects of online interventions for other mental disorders such as depression and anxiety (e.g., Arnberg et al. 2014; Richard and Richardson 2012). Therefore, we conclude that the addition of online CBT to the insomnia treatment arsenal is worthwhile.

One of the next challenges is to establish whether online treatment is as effective as face-to-face treatment. For other disorders, there have been a number of studies that compared these two delivery formats. For depression it has been demonstrated that online treatment is as effective as face-to-face treatment (Andersson et al. 2014;

Cuijpers et al. 2010). Only a limited number of such studies have been published for insomnia though. Two studies described in this chapter (Blom and De Bruin) that compared online treatment to group therapy showed that the group therapy did not outperform the online treatment. The third study (Lancee) however, which compared online treatment with individual face-to-face treatment, demonstrated significantly larger effects for the face-to-face treatments. It must be noted that the sample sizes in these three studies were all quite small. Clearly, we need more studies before firm conclusions can be drawn on the comparison between online and face-to-face treatment. However, regardless of the outcome, online treatment remains an interesting option since it is effective and requires less therapist input than the traditional face-to-face formats.

All the studies on Internet interventions on insomnia that have been performed until now included patients from the general population. No studies have been performed yet among populations recruited from regular care, e.g., seeking help from their general practitioner. Since patients seeking help in regular care might be different from the primarily media-recruited participants in the trials, we need studies to ascertain that the same effects could be obtained. It must be noted that there is one bibliotherapy study for insomnia in the GP setting which demonstrated positive effects (Katofsky et al. 2012). Furthermore, the need for easy accessible CBT interventions for insomnia in GP practice has been demonstrated more than once (Everitt et al. 2014).

One of the most problematic features of insomnia is its consequences for daytime functioning. People often feel very tired during the day, are more easily irritated, are less able to concentrate, are more forgetful, etc. Hence, they often experience limitations in their family roles and work. Unfortunately, the studies on Internet interventions typically do not include daytime functioning in their outcomes. Therefore, we do not know to what extent people are able to fulfill their roles again after treatment. We strongly suggest including measures of daytime functioning in all future trials.

Another important feature of insomnia is its co-occurrence with other mental disorders, most notably depression. We do not know yet if it is possible to prevent the onset of depression by treating insomnia, but empirical data to answer this question is on its way. What has been shown is that insomnia treatments are able to reduce depressive symptoms. Moreover, there are even indications that insomnia treatments are equally effective in treating depression as depression treatments (Blom et al. 2015b) for patients with both diagnoses. Since depression is one of the leading causes of disability worldwide, further research into the association between insomnia (treatment) and depression is warranted, especially since (online) insomnia treatments seem to be very acceptable to patients resulting in high adherence rates.

Insomnia also often occurs in the course of other (chronic) somatic diseases. Cancer, especially breast cancer, is an example of a condition in which insomnia is very prevalent (Garland et al. 2014). We are aware of one study examining self-help CBT through video and book for breast cancer survivors with insomnia (Savard et al. 2011) and one examining Internet-based CBT for cancer survivors in general

(Ritterband et al. 2012). Both studies showed promising results. This might indicate that CBT for insomnia is an effective treatment regardless of other somatic health problems. This is in line with the depression literature in which it also has been shown that psychological treatments are effective regardless of other health conditions (Van Straten et al. 2010).

We conclude that time has come to implement Internet-based treatments for insomnia in routine practice. Health-care practitioners are in need of other treatment options than medication, and patients seem to be willing to adhere to the Internet-based interventions. Based on the studies which have been performed, we feel confident to say that Internet-based CBT for insomnia improves sleep. To what extent they are able to improve (long term) daily performance and other (mental) health problems are questions which need to be answered soon.

References

Alperson J, Biglan A (1979) Self-administered treatment of sleep onset insomnia and the importance of age. Behav Ther 10:347e56

American Academy of Sleep Medicine (2005) The International classification of sleep disorders, 2nd edn (ICSD-2). American Academy of Sleep Medicine, Westchester

American Psychiatric Association (1994) Diagnostic and statistical manual of mental disorders (4th ed.) Washington

American Psychiatric Association (2013) Diagnostic and statistical manual of mental disorders, 5th edn. American Psychiatric Publishing, Arlington

Andersson G, Cuijpers P, Carlbring P, Riper H, Hedman E (2014) Guided Internet-based vs. face-to-face cognitive behavior therapy for psychiatric and somatic disorders: a systematic review and meta-analysis. World Psychiatry 13(3):288–295

Arnberg FK, Linton SJ, Hultcrantz M, Heintz E, Jonsson U (2014) Internet-delivered psychological treatments for mood and anxiety disorders: a systematic review of their efficacy, safety, and cost-effectiveness. PlosOne 9(5):e98118

Baglioni C, Riemann D (2012) Is chronic insomnia a precursor to major depression? Epidemiological and biological findings. Curr Psychiatry Rep 14:511–518

Baglioni C, Feige B, Spielhalder K, Nissen C, Voderholzer U, Lombardo C, Riemann D (2011) Insomnia as a predictor of depression: a meta-analytic evaluation of longitudinal epidemiological studies. J Affect Disord 135(1–3):10–19

Blom K, Tarkian Tillgren H, Wiklund T, Danlycke E, Forssén M, Söderström A, Johansson R, Hesser H, Jernelöv S, Lindefors N, Andersson G, Kaldo V (2015a) Internet-vs. group-delivered cognitive behavior therapy for insomnia: a randomized controlled non-inferiority trial. Behav Res Ther 70:47–55

Blom K, Jernelöv S, Kraepelien M, Bergdahl MO, Jungmarker K, Ankartjärn L, Kindefors N, Kaldo V (2015b) Internet treatment addressing either insomnia or depression, for patients with both diagnoses: a randomized trial. SLEEP 38(2):267–277

Buscemi N, Vandermeer B, Friesen C, Bialy L, Tubman M, Ospina M, Klassen TP, Witmans M (2007) The efficacy and safety of drug treatments for chronic insomnia in adults: a meta-analysis of RCTs. J Gen Intern Med 22:1335e50

Buysse DJ, Reynolds CF, Monk TH, Berman SR, Kupfer DJ (1989) The Pittsburgh sleep quality index: a new instrument for psychiatric practice and research. Psychiatry Res 28:193–213

Carney CE, Segal ZV, Edinger JD, Krystal AD (2007) A comparison of rates of residual insomnia symptoms following pharmacotherapy or cognitive-behavioral therapy for major depressive disorder. J Clin Psychiatry 68(2):254–260

Cheng SK, Dizon J (2012) Computerised cognitive behavioural therapy for insomnia: a systematic review and meta-analysis. Psychother Psychosom 81:206–216

Cuijpers P, Donker T, van Straten A, Li J, Andersson G (2010) Is guided self-help as effective as face-to-face psychotherapy for depression and anxiety disorders? A systematic review and meta-analysis of comparative outcome studies. Psychol Med 40(12):1943–1957

Daley M, Morin CM, Le Blanc M, Grégoir JP, Savard J (2009a) The economic burden of insomnia: direct and indirect costs for individuals with insomnia syndrome, insomnia symptoms, and good sleepers. SLEEP 32:55–64

Daley M, Morin CM, Leblanc M, Grégoir JP, Savard J, Baillargeon L (2009b) Insomnia and its relationship to health-care utilization, work absenteeism, productivity and accidents. Sleep Med 10:427–438

de Bruin EJ, Oort FJ, Bögels SM, Meijer AM (2014) Efficacy of internet and group-administered cognitive behavioral therapy for insomnia in adolescents: a pilot study. Behav Sleep Med 12(3):235–254

Edinger JD, Means MK (2005) Cognitive-behavioral therapy for primary insomnia. Clin Psychol Rev 25:539–558

Espie C (2006) Overcoming insomnia and sleep problems: a self-help guide using cognitive behavioral techniques. Robinson, London

Espie CA, Kyle SD, Williams C, Ong JC, Douglas NJ, Hames P, Brown JSL (2012) A randomized, placebo-controlled trial of online cognitive behavioral therapy for chronic insomnia disorder delivered via an automated media-rich web application. SLEEP 35(6):769–781

Everitt H, McDermott L, Leydon G, Yules H, Baldwin D, Little P (2014) GPs' management strategies for patients with insomnia: a survey and qualitative interview study. Br J Gen Pract. doi:10.3399/bjgp14X677176

Garland SN, Johnson JA, Savard J, Gehrman P, Perlis M, Carlson L, Campbell T (2014) Sleeping well with cancer: a systematic review of cognitive behavioral therapy for insomnia in cancer patients. Neuropsychiatr Dis Treat 10:1113–1124

Glass J, Lanctôt K, Herrmann N, Sproule BA, Busto UE (2005) Sedative hypnotics in older people with insomnia: meta-analysis of risks and benefits. Br Med J 331:1169

Gosling JA, Glozier N, Griffiths K, Ritterband L, Thorndike F, Mackinnon A, Bennet A, Bennet K, Christensen H (2014) The GoodNight study – online CBT for insomnia for the indicated prevention of depression: study protocol for a randomised controlled trial. Trials 15:56

Hedman E, Andersson E, Ljótsson B, Andersson G, Rück C, Lindefors N (2011) Cost-effectiveness of Internet-based cognitive behavior therapy vs. cognitive behavioral group therapy for social anxiety disorder: results from a randomized controlled trial. Behav Res Ther 49(11):729–736

Jernelöv S, Lekander M, Blom K, Rydh S, Ljótsson B, Axelsson J, Kaldo V (2012) Efficacy of a behavioral self-help treatment with or without therapist guidance for co-morbid and primary insomnia – a randomized controlled trial. BMC Psychiatry 12:5

Kaldo V, Jernelöv S, Blom K, Ljótsson B, Brodin M, Jörgensen M, Kraepelin M, Rück C, Lindefors N (2015a) Guided internet cognitive behavioral therapy for insomnia compared to a control treatment – a randomized trial. Behav Res Ther 71:90–100

Kaldo V, Ramnerö J, Jernelöv S (2015b) Involving clients in treatment methods – a neglected interaction in the therapeutic relationship. J Consult Clin Psychol 7. doi:10.1037/ccp0000039

Katofsky I, Backhaus J, Junghanss K, Rumpf HJ, Hüppe M, von Eitzen U, Hohagen F (2012) Effectiveness of a cognitive behavioral self-help program for patients with primary insomnia in general practice – a pilot study. Sleep Med 13(5):463–468

Kyle SD, Espie CA, Morgan K (2010) Quality of life and daytime functioning in insomnia. Behav Sleep Med 8:123–140

Lancee J, van den Bout J, van Straten A, Spoormaker VI (2012) Internet-delivered or mailed self-help treatment for insomnia? A randomized waiting-list controlled trial. Behav Res Ther 50:22–29

Lancee J, van den Bout J, Sorbi MJ, van Straten A (2013) Motivational support provided via email improves the effectiveness of internet-delivered self-help treatment for insomnia: a randomized trial. Behav Res Ther 51(12):797–805

Lancee J, Sorbi MJ, Eisma MC, van Straten A, van den Bout J (2014) The effect of support on internet-delivered treatment for insomnia: does baseline depression severity matter? Behav Ther 45(4):507–516

Lancee J, Van Straten A, Morina N, Kaldo V, Kamphuis JH (2015) Guided online or face-to-face cognitive behavioral treatment for insomnia? A randomized wait-list controlled trial. Sleep [Epub ahead of print]

Meng L, Zheng Y, Hui R (2012) The relationship of sleep duration and insomnia to risk of hypertension incidence: a meta-analysis of prospective cohort studies. Hypertens Res 36:985–995

Montgomery P, Dennis J (2004) A systematic review of non-pharmacological therapies for sleep problems in later life. Sleep Med Rev 8(1):47–62

Morin CM, Espie C (2003) Insomnia: a clinical guide to assessment and treatment. Kluwer Academic/Plenum Publishers, New York

Morin CM, Beaulieu-Bonneau S, Leblanc M, Savard J (2005) Self-help treatment for insomnia: a randomized controlled trial. SLEEP 28:1319–1327

Morin CM, Leblanc M, Daley M, Gregoire JP, Merette C (2006a) Epidemiology of insomnia: prevalence, self-help treatments, consultations, and determinants of help-seeking behaviors. Sleep Med 7:123e30

Morin CM, Bootzin RR, Buysse DJ, Edinger JD, Espie CA, Lichstein KL (2006b) Psychological and behavioral treatment of insomnia: update of the recent evidence (1998–2004). SLEEP 29(11):1398–1414

Morin CM, Bélanger L, Leblanc M, Ivers H, Savard J, Espie CA, Mérette C, Baillargeon L, Grégoire JP (2009) The natural history of insomnia. A population-based 3-year longitudinal study. Arch Intern Med 169:447–453

Morin CM, Belleville G, Bélanger L, Ivers H (2011) The insomnia severity index: psychometric indicators to detect insomnia cases and evaluate treatment response. SLEEP 34(5):601–608

Murtagh DRR, Greenwood KM (1995) Identifying effective psychological treatments for insomnia: a meta-analysis. J Consult Clin Psychol 63(1):79–89

Ohayon MM (2002) Epidemiology of insomnia: what we know and what we still need to learn. Sleep Med Rev 6:97–111

Redline S, Foody JA (2011) Sleep disturbances. Time to join the top 10 potentially modifiable cardiovascular risk factors? Circulation 124:2049–2051

Richards D, Richardson T (2012) Computer-based psychological treatments for depression: a systematic review and meta-analysis. Clin Psychol Rev 32:329–342

Riedel BW, Lichstein KL, Dwyer WO (1995) Sleep compression and sleep education for older insomniacs: self-help versus therapist guidance. Psychol Aging 10:54–63

Riemann D, Voderholzer U (2003) Primary insomnia: a risk factor to develop depression? J Affect Disord 76(1–3):255–259

Ritterband LM, Thorndike FP, Gonder-Frederick LA, Magee JC, Bailey ET, Saylor DK, Morin CM (2009) Efficacy of an internet-based behavioral intervention for adults with insomnia. Arch Gen Psychiatry 66(7):692–698

Ritterband LM, Bailey ET, Thorndike FP, Lord HR, Farrel-Carnahan L, Baum LD (2012) Initial evaluation of an internet intervention to improve the sleep of cancer survivors with insomnia. Psychooncology 21(7):695–705

Roth T, Coulouvrat C, Hajak G, Lakoma MD, Sampson NA, Shahly V, Shillington AC, Stephenson JJ, Walsh JJ, Kessler RC (2011) Prevalence and perceived health associated with insomnia based on DSM-IV-TR; international statistical classification of diseases and related health problems, tenth revision; and research diagnostic criteria/international classification of sleep disorders, second edition criteria: results from the America Insomnia Survey. Biol Psychiatry 69:592–600

Savard J, Morin CM (2011) Insomnia in the context of cancer: a review of a neglected problem. J Clin Oncol 19:895–908

Savard J, Villa J, Simard S, Ivers H, Morin CM (2011) Feasibility of a self-help treatment for insomnia comorbid with cancer. Psychooncology 20(9):1013–1019

Staner L (2010) Comorbidity of insomnia and depression. Sleep Med Rev 14:35–46
Ström L, Pettersson R, Andersson G (2004) Internet-based treatment for insomnia: a controlled evaluation. J Consult Clin Psychol 72(1):113–120
Suzuki E, Tsuchiya M, Hirokawa K, Taniguchi T, Mitsuhashi T, Kawamai N (2008) Evaluation of an Internet-based self-help program for better quality of sleep among Japanese workers: a randomized controlled trial. J Occup Health 50:387–399
Taylor DJ, Lichstein KL, Durrence HH, Reidel BW, Bush AJ (2005) Epidemiology of insomnia, depression, and anxiety. SLEEP 28(11):1457–1464
Thorndike FP, Ritterband LM, Saylor DK, Magee JC, Gonder-Frederick LA, Morin CM (2011) Validation of the insomnia severity index as a web-based measure. Behav Sleep Med 9(4):216–223
van Straten A, Cuijpers P (2009) Self-help therapy for insomnia: a meta-analysis. Sleep Med Rev 13:61e71
van Straten A, Geraedts A, Verdonck-De Leeuw I, Andersson G, Cuijpers P (2010) Psychological treatment of depressive symptoms in patients with medical disorders: a meta-analysis. J Psychosom Res 69(1):23–32
van Straten A, Emmelkamp J, de Wit J, Lancee J, Andersson G, van Someren EJ, Cuijpers P (2014) Guided Internet-delivered cognitive behavioural treatment for insomnia: a randomized trial. Psychol Med 44(7):1521–1532
Vincent N, Lewycky S (2009) Logging on for better sleep: RCT of the effectiveness of online treatment for insomnia. SLEEP 32(6):807–815
World Health Organization (1992) The ICD-10 classification of mental and behavioural disorders: clinical descriptions and diagnostic guidelines. World Health Organization, Geneva
Yan-Yee Ho F, Chung K, Yeung W, Ng TH, Kwan K, Yung K, Cheng SK (2015) Self-help cognitive-behavioral therapy for insomnia: a meta-analysis of randomized controlled trials. Sleep Med Rev 19:17–28

9 ICBT for Severe Health Anxiety

Erik Hedman, Brjánn Ljótsson, and Nils Lindefors

Abstract

Severe health anxiety is characterised by a persistent and exaggerated fear of serious illness, based on misinterpretations of bodily symptoms. It is a common condition, especially in medical settings, and associated with functional disability. The disorder exhibits features similar to obsessive-compulsive disorder, panic disorder and generalised anxiety disorder and can be conceptualised as an anxiety disorder.

ICBT for severe health anxiety is a treatment based on systematic exposure and response prevention integrating mindfulness components to facilitate an accepting stance towards thoughts and feelings. The treatment has been found to be highly effective in two large-scale randomised controlled trials and yields improvements above and beyond that of taking part of an active and credible psychological treatment. The treatment seems to be working for most clients and is suitable for those with high levels of health anxiety. The treatment is highly cost-effective and the cost of treatment is offset by net societal economic gains in a short time frame. The research area is however new and there are many important future research questions yet to be answered.

Definition and Epidemiology

Hypochondriasis according to DSM-IV is characterised by a persistent and exaggerated fear of serious illness, based on misinterpretations of bodily symptoms (American Psychiatric Association 2000). Due to the pejorative connotations of the term hypochondriasis and the fact that there is growing evidence indicating that

E. Hedman (✉) • B. Ljótsson • N. Lindefors
Department of Clinical Neuroscience, Karolinska Institutet, Solna, Sweden
e-mail: kire.hedman@ki.se; brjann.ljotsson@ki.se; nils.lindefors@ki.se

© Springer International Publishing Switzerland 2016

N. Lindefors, G. Andersson (eds.), *Guided Internet-Based Treatments in Psychiatry*, DOI 10.1007/978-3-319-06083-5_9

the disorder is best conceptualised as an anxiety disorder (Olatunji et al. 2009), the term severe health anxiety has been proposed and is used synonymously with hypochondriasis throughout this chapter. Severe health anxiety shares behavioural and cognitive features with obsessive-compulsive disorder (e.g. repetitive checking and avoidance behaviours), panic disorder (e.g. misinterpretation of bodily symptoms, safety behaviours) as well as generalised anxiety disorder (e.g. excessive worry, intolerance of uncertainty) and could to some extent be viewed as a blend of these disorders but with a main focus on health-related fear. In DSM-5, hypochondriasis has been replaced by the disorders somatic symptom disorder (SSD) and illness anxiety disorder (IAD) (American Psychiatric Association 2013). These two disorders differ in the sense that the former requires somatic symptoms to be present and the major cause of concern whereas the latter diagnosis does not require somatic symptoms to be the source of the fear. IAD thus capture, for example, individuals highly worried about developing cancer but who do not have distinct bodily sensations that are thought of as evidence of cancer. According to DSM-5, SSD is thought to be most similar to hypochondriasis (American Psychiatric Association 2013), but as both SSD and IAD are new diagnostic entities, there is very limited research on these disorders in every aspect including epidemiological estimates and burden of disease, and—not least—to the authors' knowledge, there is yet no published study on treatment of SSD or IAD. Disorder data in the present chapter therefore generally refer to findings from the literature on severe health anxiety.

Severe health anxiety is fairly common in the general population with prevalence estimates ranging from 1 to 4 % (e.g. Faravelli et al. 1997; Sunderland et al. 2013). In medical settings, the estimated prevalence is however much higher with evidence suggesting that up to 25 % of patients may have significant levels of health anxiety (Tyrer et al. 2011). The disorder is associated with functional disability and increased use of medical resources and is chronic over a 5-year period for a majority of affected individuals if untreated (Barsky et al. 1998, 2001). This means that severe health anxiety causes suffering for many individuals and is also a costly and challenging disorder from a health-care provider and societal perspective. As with most anxiety disorders, the aetiology remains unclear to a large extent, but studies have shown that risk factors include having recently experienced stressful live events and somatic illness (Craig et al. 1993; Barsky et al. 1994). Gender seems to be of little importance as severe health anxiety is evenly distributed among men and women (Bleichhardt and Hiller 2007). As for factors maintaining the disorders, there is more knowledge and largely supporting a cognitive behavioural model. A study by Salkovskis and Warwick clearly showed that reassurance behaviours, such as asking a GP about a symptom, are factors contributing to the maintenance of severe health anxiety (Salkovskis and Warwick 1986). Evidence from treatment studies using exposure therapy also suggests that avoidance behaviours can play a crucial role for the chronicity of severe health anxiety (Furer and Walker 2005).

Treatment of Severe Health Anxiety

Severe health anxiety was considered difficult to treat until the 1990s, but today, there is a solid body of evidence showing that it can be effectively treated with cognitive behaviour therapy (CBT) (Olatunji et al. 2014). The term CBT comprises several somewhat different therapies such as exposure-based therapy, cognitive therapy and applied relaxation. Exposure-based therapy is thought to lead to extinction of health anxiety symptoms through repeated contact with stimuli that trigger the symptoms (e.g. Furer and Walker 2005; Craske et al. 2008), such as to fully experience bodily sensations while refraining from seeking medical reassurance (Visser and Bouman 2001; Seivewright et al. 2008). Cognitive therapy, on the other hand, lacks systematic exposure but often includes behavioural experiments topographically similar to exposure but with a specific aim to test beliefs about illness (Clark et al. 1998; Sorensen et al. 2011). One randomised controlled trial (RCT) has shown that exposure-based therapy can be superiorly an active psychological treatment and at least two RCTs have demonstrated that cognitive therapy can be more effective than active psychological treatments (Clark et al. 1998; Sorensen et al. 2011; Hedman et al. 2014).

Internet-Based Treatment

To the authors' knowledge, there is currently only one research group that has developed and tested the efficacy of ICBT for severe health anxiety (Hedman et al. 2011), namely, our own. Our treatment is based on a model emphasising the role of negatively reinforced avoidance and safety behaviours as maintaining factors of health anxiety (Furer and Walker 2005; Furer et al. 2007). The components of the 12 modules of the treatment are outlined in Table 9.1. The main intervention of the treatment is systematic exposure to health anxiety-related situations or events in combination with response prevention. An example of this could be to be to trigger feared bodily sensations through physical exercise (exposure) while refraining from checking that the pulse is normal (response prevention). Other examples include watching episodes of television shows such as ER or Dr House, where the main theme is a disease that the client fears. Of course, one important aspect in the latter examples is that the client is instructed not to seek reassurance from his or her general practitioner or others if the TV shows would trigger worry about bodily sensations. As suggested by Furer, Walker and Stein (Furer et al. 2007), the treatment also contains specific exercises designed to expose the patients to thoughts about illness where an often effective one is to let the patient write an illness story containing all the feared consequences of being ill, such as experiencing muscular deterioration in ALS or going through painful cancer treatment. As the treatment relies on systematic exposure, all exercises relating to exposure is repeated several times and in different contexts and the client is instructed to monitor thoughts and emotions during exercises.

Table 9.1 Overview of the contents of Internet-based treatment for severe health anxiety

Module	Exposure-based CBT	Main homework assignments
1	Introduction to CBT and mindfulness exercise	Mindfulness training, health anxiety behaviour diary
2	Presentation of the CBT model, continued mindfulness training	Mindfulness training, completion of idiosyncratic health anxiety model, health anxiety behaviour diary
3	Cognitive processes, continued mindfulness training	Work relating to cognitive processes, mindfulness training, health anxiety behaviour diary
4	Interoceptive exposure, continued mindfulness training	Exposure exercises
5	Response prevention, continued mindfulness training	Exposure exercises
6	Exposure to health anxiety-provoking stimuli	Exposure exercises
7	Exposure to illness thoughts	Exposure exercises
8	Continued exposure and response prevention	Exposure exercises
9	Continued exposure and response prevention	Exposure exercises
10	Continued exposure and response prevention	Exposure exercises
11	A summary of the treatment	Exposure exercises, writing a summary of the treatment focusing on most helpful interventions
12	Maintaining gains and relapse prevention	Exposure exercises, writing a plan on how to continue improving and how to prevent and handle relapse

Starting in the early phase of treatment, mindfulness training is used as a means to enhance exposure. This means that mindfulness is not used as a stand-alone intervention but as a way to increase the probability that clients conduct often highly anxiety-provoking exposure exercises and that they will not use distraction as a means to cope with worrying sensations. The treatment therefore differs from the mindfulness-based cognitive therapy of McManus and co-workers (McManus et al. 2012) where mindfulness is used as the main intervention of the treatment. In our treatment, the training in mindfulness comprises daily exercises in directing attention to different stimuli including the body while observing thoughts and emotions without trying to change them. During later stages of the treatment when exposure is introduced, the client is encouraged to use skills in mindfulness to increase tolerance for aversive internal reactions. Although it is not exactly clear how mindfulness achieves it effects, it has been suggested that it could facilitate extinction learning during exposure through increasing awareness of multiple conditioned triggers of anxiety (Treanor 2011). The general stance that clients are encouraged to accept aversive thoughts and feelings when conducting exposure and using mindfulness means that the treatment to some extent uses elements of third-wave CBT but within an exposure-extinction paradigm. As described in Table 9.1, the treatment, besides exposure and mindfulness training, also entails psychoeducation about CBT and severe health anxiety, and relapse prevention.

When it comes to the treatment structure, it is similar to the many of the Swedish ICBT treatments for other disorders in the sense that it to a large extent is built upon extensive self-help texts with relatively few advanced technical features. Integrated in the treatment platform where the client accesses the treatment are also worksheets, a system for symptom assessment and a secure messaging function. The contact between the therapist and client is almost exclusively in form of text messages and therapists generally spend about 10 min weekly per patient making it a minimal therapist contact treatment.

Studies on Internet-Based CBT for Severe Health Anxiety

Efficacy and Long-Term Outcomes

The protocol underlying the so far only published Internet-based treatment for severe health anxiety was first tested in an open clinical trial using a conventional face-to-face delivery format and was found to be effective in reducing health anxiety, as well as general anxiety and depressive symptoms (Hedman et al. 2010). Thereafter, the treatment was adopted for being delivered as an Internet-based treatment and has of today been tested in two randomised controlled trials for clients with severe health anxiety. In the first trial ($N=81$), the treatment was compared to a basic attention control condition that did not receive active treatment (Hedman et al. 2011). The results showed that ICBT yielded large effects on the primary outcome of health anxiety (Health Anxiety Inventory; HAI) with a between-group d of 1.62 at post-treatment. The treatment also produced large within-group improvements on the same measure (pre to post $d=1.94$; pre to 6-month follow-up $d=2.09$) and on measures of general anxiety, depressive symptoms and anxiety sensitivity (pre to post d range=0.90–1.19). At 6-month follow-up, 80 % of participants who had received ICBT no longer met diagnostic criteria for severe health anxiety (Hedman et al. 2011).

One main limitation of this trial was that the control group did not receive active treatment. In a subsequent trial ($N=158$), we therefore pitted the treatment against behavioural stress management comprising mainly applied relaxation and interventions aimed at reducing stress (Hedman et al. 2014). This was considered a tough test not least because applied relaxation has been found to be effective in the treatment for both panic disorder and generalised anxiety disorder. Assessments of treatment credibility and working alliance showed that the two treatments were equal in these regards. In line with prediction, exposure-based ICBT was found to yield significantly larger improvements on the primary outcome compared to behavioural stress management. Within-group improvements in ICBT were large on the primary outcome HAI (pre to post $d=1.78$), but as participants receiving behavioural stress management also made substantial improvements, the between-group effect size at post-treatment was clearly smaller than in the previous RCT (*d*=0.26). The findings can be viewed as important as they show that systematic exposure causes improvements above and beyond those that can be achieved through taking part of a credible and active psychological treatment entailing systematic behaviour change (Hedman et al. 2014).

As for long-term effects, a recently published study showed that ICBT for severe health anxiety can lead to improvements that are sustained for at least one year post-treatment (Hedman et al. 2013a). The effect size (pre to 1-year follow-up) on the primary outcome HAI was *d*=1.95 which is largely the same as the pre to post *d* of 1.94. The same stability of improvements was found on measures of general anxiety, depressive symptoms and anxiety sensitivity (Hedman et al. 2013a). It thus seems as ICBT for severe health anxiety can lead to large improvements that are long-term enduring.

Predictors and Mediators

Although ICBT is effective, not all clients respond sufficiently to treatment and it is therefore of importance to investigate predictors of improvement, which could facilitate the clinician in making treatment decisions. In a predictor study, based on the first RCT described above, we found that more health anxiety at baseline predicted more anxiety at 6-month follow-up but also larger improvements thus indicating that ICBT is a suitable treatment also for clients with more severe symptoms (Hedman et al. 2013b). Depressive symptoms were however found to be a negative predictor in the sense that more depressive symptoms at baseline predicted less improvement of health anxiety. This means that it could be clinically important that clients with comorbid depression are carefully monitored during the treatment so that signs of nonresponding could be dealt with early and additional treatment options discussed (e.g. structured therapist support via telephone). Interesting findings of the study were also that demographic characteristics and computer skills seemed to be largely unrelated to outcome meaning that ICBT suits equally well for old and young, men and women and highly computer skilled or not. When it comes to therapy process-related variables, the only one having a significant impact on outcome was treatment adherence operationalised as number of completed modules (Hedman et al. 2013b). In line with predictor research from other domains, this indicates that it is important that the client actually engages in the exposure exercises throughout the treatment.

When it comes to mediators, only one study has so far been published on ICBT for severe health anxiety (Hedman et al. 2013c). In that study, we investigated putative mechanisms and found that intolerance of uncertainty, reduced attention to bodily symptoms and reduced perceived risk of disease mediated subsequent improvement in health anxiety. The findings support a cognitive behavioural model of severe health anxiety and are interesting as they show that a treatment highly focused on exposure and response prevention produces significant effect on these largely cognitive mediators, which in turn are related to outcome. An interesting venue for future research in this domain is to investigate the potential role of reduced avoidance as a mechanism of change.

Case Description

Cathy, 39, has always been more anxious than others, but in the last few years, especially since her uncle died in cancer, her worry regarding her health has become close to impossible to handle. She fears two things more than anything else—cancer and ALS. Since at least a year, Cathy easily gets caught up in different bodily sensations that could be a sign of either of these two terrible diseases. Lately, her worry has become a really big problem as it is on her mind nearly all the time. When worried, she finds it difficult to concentrate at work and it has also become a large problem in the relationship with her husband Steve as she often wants to talk about her potential symptoms and get reassurance. Sometimes, she needs to call Steve at work several times a day to be fully convinced that she is not sick. From different health sites on the Internet, she has learned that feelings of dizziness and feeling weak might be early symptoms of ALS, which has led to two things. First, she is constantly scanning her body for these potential disease symptoms, and she does it so much that it has practically become an automatic behaviour that she does not initiate deliberately. Second, when she discovers a worrying sensation, such as a feeling that she is a bit unsteady, she instantly looks it up on Google. Although she at this stage is not overly worried, it almost always ends up with her being extremely fearful as the following occurs: she performs searches on her present symptom and the feared diseases, e.g. "dizziness AND ALS". Starting with relatively credible health-care sites, she finds that dizziness indeed might be a symptom of ALS, although dizziness also is common for other reasons. Cathy gets a little bit more worried and scrutinises the entire list of symptoms common in ALS patients and finds that headache and having and trouble remembering things could also be part of the early symptom presentation. Now, Cathy starts getting really worried as she has had headache almost every day the past week and she sometimes feels that she forgets thing a bit too often at work. So, she now knows that she has at least three of potential symptoms and continues googling about ALS and becomes almost terrified when she finds blogs written by people with ALS who document their lives. Reading about the certain deterioration and losing control of one's body is just too much. Cathy is at this time point convinced that she actually has ALS and starts crying and reaches for the telephone to schedule an appointment with her GP. To her great luck, she gets the opportunity to talk to her GP directly on the phone and he convinces her that her bodily sensations are perfectly normal and no signs of ALS. Cathy feels very relieved and for a while almost a bit shameful for jumping to conclusions so rapidly. A few hours later, she however comes to think of a case she heard where the doctor said everything was alright but where it turned out that the patient had a severe form of cancer. As Cathy's doctor didn't even perform any kind of examination but just talked to her on the phone, how could he really know that it is not ALS? And the worry is back…

Fortunately, Cathy finds out that there is effective ICBT that might be of help for her health anxiety and she seeks help. In treatment, she is trained to conduct mindfulness exercises where she actively directs attention to her body but instead of reacting with reassurance seeking behaviours she observes her thoughts and emotions without trying to control them. This is rather difficult but gets even more so when the exposure and response prevention start. She is encouraged to actively confront situations that might trigger her anxiety, such as reading obituaries or doing heavy work-out exercises at the gym and at the same time refraining from not doing anything to control the anxiety but rather to use mindfulness as a way to fully experience symptoms of anxiety. One of the treatment parts that Cathy fears the most but also gains most from is to write a disease story where she writes a story of everything bad that could happen would she develop ALS. She writes about becoming weak, how she cannot take care of herself, how Steve is forced to put her in a nursing home and how she eventually loses the ability to speak and how people she loves cries at her bed without her being able to talk to them. Cathy pictures how this would be and finds it really painful, but after a while, she realises that even if it actually would be horrible to get alS, she doesn't have to fear the thought of it. After 12 weeks of treatment, Cathy is still more worried about her health than most people but she is no longer so afraid of her bodily sensations and what is especially important is that she knows that she through her actions can let health anxiety play a much smaller role in her life than before.

Cost-Effectiveness

The cost-effectiveness of ICBT for severe health anxiety has been investigated in a prospective so-called "piggyback" study of the first RCT described above where ICBT was compared to a basic control condition that did not receive active treatment (Hedman et al. 2013a). A societal perspective was used, which means that both direct costs, e.g. costs for medical utilisation, and indirect costs, e.g. unemployment costs, were taken into account. The results of the study showed that the incremental cost-effectiveness ratio was £1244 in favour of ICBT, which meant that each case of remission from severe health anxiety caused by ICBT generated a total net societal saving of £1244 (Hedman et al. 2013a). These findings are encouraging as they indicate that there is no conflict between resources and treatment-generated improvement as society makes a net gain for each successfully treated case. As a majority of patients achieve remission from severe health anxiety, this means that even if society were willing to pay £0 for a case of remission, it would still be cost-effective to provide ICBT for clients with severe health anxiety. Of note is that one aspect that makes ICBT rather favourable on cost-effectiveness analyses is that the therapist time required is as little as about 10 min weekly per patient, making it possible for a therapist to have up to 80 clients in treatment at the same time.

Clinical Implementation and Dissemination

This is a rather short paragraph as, to the authors' knowledge, ICBT for severe health anxiety is not yet offered anywhere else but in clinical trials. Within a short time frame, the treatment will be implemented at the Internet Psychiatry Clinic in Stockholm, Sweden, and offered for all citizens of Stockholm County as part of regular psychiatric care.

Discussion and Future Challenges

As ICBT for severe health anxiety is a rather new field of research, there are many areas that are yet to be explored. First of all, there are only two RCTs of ICBT for severe health anxiety, and both have been performed by the same research group. Thus, more studies by independent research groups are needed to confirm the efficacy of the treatment. Furthermore, ICBT for severe health anxiety should be directly compared to face-to-face treatment in an RCT. In other clinical disorders, such as social anxiety disorder and panic disorder, results from RCTs suggest that therapist-guided ICBT can in fact be at least as effective as face-to-face treatment (Andersson et al. 2014). One important aspect of that kind of comparison is also that it enables investigation of potential moderators of outcome, i.e. if there are treatment specific predictors. Such information could be of high value when making treatment recommendations and could also potentially lead to larger overall proportions of treatment responders as each client would be recommended the treatment he or she most likely would improve from. Data from studies of other anxiety disorders suggest that although many predictors seem to be common to both kinds of delivery formats, there is some indication that comorbid psychiatric symptoms may play a larger role in ICBT than in face-to-face CBT (Hedman et al. 2012). Other venue for future research is to investigate whether ICBT for severe health anxiety can be provided with maintained effect sizes in other contexts and for other populations. To date, all clients have been recruited and treated in Sweden and it is therefore important to see if effects are as high when offered to clients in other countries and in other health-care systems than the Swedish. Last but not least, as noted above, there is no research at all when it comes to effectiveness and dissemination of ICBT for health anxiety. Investigating the treatment when provided in a regular psychiatric or primary care context is essential as it cannot be taken for granted that the treatment works equally well when delivered in routine health care. However, judging from effectiveness evidence on other common psychiatric disorders, there is a very good chance that the large effect sizes can be maintained in regular health-care settings (Andersson and Hedman 2013).

References

American Psychiatric Association (2000) Diagnostic criteria from dsm-iv-tr. American Psychiatric Association, Washington, DC

American Psychiatric Association (2013) Diagnostic and statistical manual of mental disorders, 5th edn. American Psychiatric Publishing, Arlington

Andersson G, Hedman E (2013) Effectiveness of guided internet-delivered cognitive behaviour therapy in regular clinical settings. Verhaltenstherapie 23:140–148

Andersson G, Cuijpers P, Carlbring P, Riper H, Hedman E (2014) Internet-based vs. Face-to-face cognitive behaviour therapy for psychiatric and somatic disorders: a systematic review and meta-analysis. World Psychiatry 13:288–295

Barsky AJ, Wool C, Barnett MC, Cleary PD (1994) Histories of childhood trauma in adult hypochondriacal patients. Am J Psychiatry 151:397–401

Barsky AJ, Fama JM, Bailey ED, Ahern DK (1998) A prospective 4- to 5-year study of dsm-iii-r hypochondriasis. Arch Gen Psychiatry 55:737–744

Barsky AJ, Ettner SL, Horsky J, Bates DW (2001) Resource utilization of patients with hypochondriacal health anxiety and somatization. Med Care 39:705–715

Bleichhardt G, Hiller W (2007) Hypochondriasis and health anxiety in the German population. Br J Health Psychol 12:511–523

Clark DM, Salkovskis PM, Hackmann A, Wells A, Fennell M, Ludgate J, Ahmad S, Richards HC, Gelder M (1998) Two psychological treatments for hypochondriasis. A randomised controlled trial. Br J Psychiatry 173:218–225

Craig TK, Boardman AP, Mills K, Daly-Jones O, Drake H (1993) The south London somatisation study. I: longitudinal course and the influence of early life experiences. Br J Psychiatry 163:579–588

Craske MG, Kircanski K, Zelikowsky M, Mystkowski J, Chowdhury N, Baker A (2008) Optimizing inhibitory learning during exposure therapy. Behav Res Ther 46:5–27

Faravelli C, Salvatori S, Galassi F, Aiazzi L, Drei C, Cabras P (1997) Epidemiology of somatoform disorders: a community survey in florence. Soc Psychiatry Psychiatr Epidemiol 32:24–29

Furer P, Walker JR (2005) Treatment of hypochondriasis with exposure. J Contemp Psychother 35:251–267

Furer P, Walker JR, Stein MB (2007) Treating health anxiety and fear of death: a practitioner's guide. Springer, New York

Hedman E, Ljótsson B, Andersson E, Rück C, Andersson G, Lindefors N (2010) Effectiveness and cost offset analysis of group CBT for hypochondriasis delivered in a psychiatric setting – an open trial. Cogn Behav Ther 39(4):239–250

Hedman E, Andersson G, Andersson E, Ljotsson B, Ruck C, Asmundson GJ, Lindefors N (2011) Internet-based cognitive-behavioural therapy for severe health anxiety: randomised controlled trial. Br J Psychiatry 198:230–236

Hedman E, Andersson E, Ljótsson B, Andersson G, Andersson E, Schalling M, Lindefors N, Ruck C (2012) Clinical and genetic outcome determinants of internet- and group-based cognitive behavior therapy for social anxiety disorder. Acta Psychiatr Scand 126:126–136

Hedman E, Andersson E, Lindefors N, Andersson G, Ruck C, Ljotsson B (2013a) Cost-effectiveness and long-term effectiveness of internet-based cognitive behaviour therapy for severe health anxiety. Psychol Med 43:363–374

Hedman E, Lindefors N, Andersson G, Andersson E, Lekander M, Ruck C, Ljotsson B (2013b) Predictors of outcome in internet-based cognitive behavior therapy for severe health anxiety. Behav Res Ther 51:711–717

Hedman E, Andersson E, Andersson G, Lindefors N, Lekander M, Ruck C, Ljotsson B (2013c) Mediators in internet-based cognitive behavior therapy for severe health anxiety. PLoS One 8:e77752

Hedman E, Axelsson E, Görling A, Ritzman C, Ronnheden M, El Alaoui S, Andersson E, Lekander M, Ljótsson B (2014) Internet-delivered exposure-based cognitive-behavioural therapy and behavioural stress management for severe health anxiety: randomised controlled trial. Br J Psychiatry 205(4):307–314

McManus F, Surawy C, Muse K, Vazquez-Montes M, Williams JM (2012) A randomized clinical trial of mindfulness-based cognitive therapy versus unrestricted services for health anxiety (hypochondriasis). J Consult Clin Psychol 80:817–828

Olatunji BO, Deacon BJ, Abramowitz JS (2009) Is hypochondriasis an anxiety disorder? Br J Psychiatry 194:481–482

Olatunji BO, Kauffman BY, Meltzer S, Davis ML, Smits JA, Powers MB (2014) Cognitive-behavioral therapy for hypochondriasis/health anxiety: a meta-analysis of treatment outcome and moderators. Behav Res Ther 58:65–74

Salkovskis PM, Warwick HM (1986) Morbid preoccupations, health anxiety and reassurance: a cognitive-behavioural approach to hypochondriasis. Behav Res Ther 24:597–602

Seivewright H, Green J, Salkovskis P, Barrett B, Nur U, Tyrer P (2008) Cognitive-behavioural therapy for health anxiety in a genitourinary medicine clinic: randomised controlled trial. Br J Psychiatry 193:332–337

Sorensen P, Birket-Smith M, Wattar U, Buemann I, Salkovskis P (2011) A randomized clinical trial of cognitive behavioural therapy versus short-term psychodynamic psychotherapy versus no intervention for patients with hypochondriasis. Psychol Med 41:431–441

Sunderland M, Newby JM, Andrews G (2013) Health anxiety in australia: prevalence, comorbidity, disability and service use. Br J Psychiatry 202:56–61

Treanor M (2011) The potential impact of mindfulness on exposure and extinction learning in anxiety disorders. Clin Psychol Rev 31:617–625

Tyrer P, Cooper S, Crawford M, Dupont S, Green J, Murphy D, Salkovskis P, Smith G, Wang D, Bhogal S, Keeling M, Loebenberg G, Seivewright R, Walker G, Cooper F, Evered R, Kings S, Kramo K, McNulty A, Nagar J, Reid S, Sanatinia R, Sinclair J, Trevor D, Watson C, Tyrer H (2011) Prevalence of health anxiety problems in medical clinics. J Psychosom Res 71:392–394

Visser S, Bouman TK (2001) The treatment of hypochondriasis: exposure plus response prevention vs cognitive therapy. Behav Res Ther 39:423–442

ICBT for Eating Disorders

10

Alexandra Keyes and Ulrike Schmidt

Abstract

Eating disorders (EDs) are severe and disabling conditions that are difficult to treat. A specific form of cognitive-behavioural therapy focused on the ED is recognised as the gold standard in treatment of bulimia nervosa (BN) and binge eating disorder (BED); however access to this type of treatment is limited in many countries. Online self-help ICBT interventions are therefore an effective way to bridge this gap as part of a stepped care approach to treating EDs. Research shows that ICBT programmes are effective at reducing ED psychopathology and bulimic symptoms and improving quality of life compared to other forms of self-help intervention (bibliotherapy/CD-ROM) and wait list control. In addition ICBT programmes are most effective when delivered with specialist therapist guidance. Despite the support for ICBT programmes for ED, treatment adherence remains an issue and dropout rates can be considerable. Research suggests that treatment adherence is lower in BN patients who are younger and show more dietary restraint and lower BMI at baseline. Furthermore, evidence for the cost-effectiveness of ICBT programmes is as yet limited. Future research is therefore needed to address these issues in order to maximise the effectiveness of, adherence to and scalability of ICBT programmes for EDs.

A. Keyes, MSc, BSc
Section of Eating Disorders (PO59), Psychological Medicine, Institute of Psychiatry,
De Crespigny Park, London SE5 8AF, UK
e-mail: alexandra.keyes@kcl.ac.uk

U. Schmidt, MD, PhD, FRCPsych (✉)
Section of Eating Disorders (PO59), Institute of Psychiatry,
De Crespigny Park, London SE5 8AF, UK
e-mail: ulrike.schmidt@kcl.ac.uk

© Springer International Publishing Switzerland 2016

N. Lindefors, G. Andersson (eds.), *Guided Internet-Based Treatments in Psychiatry*, DOI 10.1007/978-3-319-06083-5_10

Clinical Features, Epidemiology, Treatments and Outcome of Eating Disorders (ED)

Eating disorders (ED) are severe and disabling conditions that can be categorised into three main diagnoses: anorexia nervosa, bulimia nervosa and binge eating disorder (Smink et al. 2013).

Anorexia nervosa (AN) is characterised by distorted body image and extreme dieting that leads to severe weight loss and a pathological fear of weight gain (Smink et al. 2013). AN has an average prevalence rate of 0.3 % (Kessler et al. 2013) and a lifetime prevalence rate of 0.8 % by age 20 (Stice et al. 2013) and of 0.6–0.9 % in adult women and 0.3 % in men (Hoek and Van Hoeken 2003; Hudson et al. 2007). The typical age of onset peaks at 19–20 years (Stice et al. 2013) and average duration of illness is around 6 years (Simon et al. 2005). AN is a life-threatening illness that has twice the mortality rate of other psychiatric disorders and a suicide rate that is 200 times that of the general population (Yanovski 2003). People with AN experience high levels of disability and physical and psychological co-morbidity (Palmer et al. 2002).

In terms of outcome, a review of German and English studies found that out of 5,590 AN patients, less than one-half recovered on average, whereas one-third improved, and 20 % remained chronically ill (Castellini et al. 2011). Evidence also shows that early detection and treatment (within 3 years of onset) of AN lead to better outcomes (Treasure and Russell 2011). There is clear evidence supporting the use of family-based treatments in adolescents with AN, i.e. those with a recent onset, whereas there is no leading treatment for adults with AN (NICE 2009). Different forms of specialist therapies have all been used in recent clinical trials, prominently including a specific form of enhanced CBT for eating disorders (CBT-E) (Fairburn et al. 2013), specialist supportive clinical management, focal psychodynamic therapy and MANTRA (Maudsley Model of Anorexia Nervosa for Adults) (e.g. Group TCfEPsMHP 2012; Hay et al. 2009; Keski-Rahkonen et al. 2009; Sánchez-Ortiz et al. 2011b) with little difference between them in outcome. A systematic review of treatments for AN showed an advantage for specialist psychotherapy over treatment as usual and a promising study of relapse prevention with CBT (CBT-AN) (Wilson and Zandberg 2012). Further evidence, and RCTs in particular, is needed to evaluate the effectiveness of specific forms of psychotherapy for AN (Bailer et al. 2004).

Bulimia nervosa and binge eating disorder show certain similarities and therefore will be classified together as 'bulimic eating disorders'. *Bulimia nervosa* (BN) is characterised by frequent episodes of binge eating followed by compensatory strategies to avoid weight gain, such as vomiting or laxative abuse (Smink et al. 2013). The lifetime prevalence of BN in adults is approximately 1 % (Hoek and Van Hoeken 2003) [1.5 % in women and 0.5 % in men (Hudson et al. 2007)]. *Binge eating disorder* (*BED*) has recently been recognised as a separate ED diagnosis in the new version of the DSM (Smink et al. 2013). BED is characterised by recurrent episodes of binging with associated feelings of lack of control, guilt, embarrassment or disgust. In BED, episodes of binging are not followed by compensatory strategies to avoid weight gain. The lifetime prevalence for BED is 3 % in adults (Hoek and Van Hoeken 2003) [3.5 % in females compared to 2 % in men (Hudson et al. 2007)]. More recently, population prevalences of bulimic behaviours have been found to have doubled since 1995, reaching 7.2 % for binge eating and 1.5 % for purging in 2005 (Loeb et al. 2000). In both disorders (BN and BED), onset typically occurs during a developmentally sensitive time in adolescence and young adulthood (Palmer et al. 2002). Without effective treatments, both conditions typically run a chronic course and even partial syndromes are associated with poor health outcomes (Thiels et al. 2003). BN and BED are often accompanied by or lead to obesity (Loeb et al. 2000; Traviss et al. 2011; Waller et al. 2012), with their combination growing rapidly and predicted to grow further (Fernández-Aranda et al. 2009; Traviss et al. 2011; Waller et al. 2012). Bulimic disorders are associated with medical complications, severe psychiatric co-morbidity and social disruption (Carrard et al. 2011b; de Zwaan et al. 2002; Delinsky et al. 2006; Hudson et al. 2007). Greater co-morbidity is linked with increased severity of bulimic symptoms, greater obesity, more obesity-related complications and poorer outcomes (Vocks et al. 2010).

National Institute for Health and Care Excellence (NICE) guidelines recommend specially adapted versions of cognitive-behavioural therapy (CBT) for BN and BED (Stefano et al. 2006). Several systematic reviews (Shapiro et al. 2007; Sysko and Walsh 2008; Wilson et al. 2010; Wilson and Zandberg 2012) and a recent trial (Carrard et al. 2011a) suggest that individual or group CBT is superior to waiting list and is at least as effective as other psychological treatments and sometimes superior to credible comparison treatments. With best available forms of CBT, 30–50 % of people with bulimic eating disorders are symptom-free at the end of treatment, with gains maintained at follow-up.

Quality of life is poor in all eating disorders (Braun and Clarke 2006; Murray et al. 2003; Skevington et al. 2004) with significant burden for the individual and their families (Morris 1979; Robins et al. 2001; Trottier et al. 2013a, b). Carers of people with AN often have high levels of distress, including depression and anxiety (Sherer et al. 1982; Woodruff and Cashman 1993). Caregiver distress and difficulty were found to be higher in carers of AN compared to psychosis (Clark et al. 1991). AN carers also reported higher perception of care burden as well as tangible disruptions to their lives result of the nature and demands of their loved one's illness (King et al. 1996). A recent study found that approximately 30 % of a sample of AN carers exhibited clinically significant distress which was associated with high levels of objective burden (Sánchez-Ortiz et al. 2011a).

The total costs of EDs are substantial. In a recent report, the Australian Institute of Health and Welfare (AIHW) supplied costs estimates for EDs. Total annual expenditure came to $80.4 million, with the majority ($57.8 million) being accounted for by hospital admissions for sufferers of AN. Overall, the inpatient cost per person for EDs is estimated at $13, 123. Hospital inpatient costs for AN are more than twice as high as either BN or other EDs (McClay et al. 2013). Sufferers of BN and BED may also be high consumers of medical and social care due to significant associated psychological and medical problems and their chronic nature (Grover et al. 2011; Pretorius et al. 2009, 2010). For example, healthcare utilisation (total service days, outpatient psychotherapy and emergency department visits) is increased in BN/BED patients and is comparable to other psychiatric disorders ((BEAT) BED (2013)). Therefore, the economic burden of bulimic eating disorders (e.g. service utilisation and societal costs including lost productivity) is estimated to be substantial at approximately £1.26 billion in England per year (Dickerson et al. 2011; Vaz et al. 2014).

Existing ICBT Programmes for Eating Disorders

Cognitive-behavioural self-help programmes for eating disorders exist in many formats such as manuals, books, CD-ROMs and online programmes (Treasure and Russell 2011). Internet-based self-help programmes have advantages over other forms of intervention due to higher levels of interactivity, feedback and additional support via e-mail, for example (Treasure and Russell 2011). Given the much stronger evidence base for CBT in bulimic disorders compared to AN, the majority of existing ICBT programmes are aimed at BN and BED populations. Moreover, the clinical needs and high medical risk of AN make it much harder to use distance treatment approaches, leading some authors to suggest that such approaches are contraindicated in AN (Treasure et al. 2010). Despite these concerns, a small number of Internet-based approaches for people with AN and their families have been developed. Existing programmes are outlined below.

ICBT for Anorexia Nervosa

This is a 9-month web-based relapse prevention programme for anorexia nervosa (VIA) designed for use after inpatient treatment (Patton et al. 2008). The content of the programme follows approved manuals, self-help manuals and aftercare manuals for AN and related disorders. The core of VIA is based on CBT strategies such as self-monitoring, stimulus control, operant methods, vicarious learning, exposure treatment and cognitive restructuring of dysfunctional thoughts and core beliefs. These strategies are implemented by supplying information to users and by written and behavioural exercises. Users are also supported by electronic message boards and weekly therapist e-mail support (Patton et al. 2008).

Overcoming Anorexia Online

OAO is an interactive, multimedia online intervention for carers of people with AN (Darby et al. 2009). The intervention uses a CBT and systemic framework and comprises eight modules covering topics such as why people develop and value AN, the implications of this in terms of engagement with treatment, how AN developed in their loved one, helpful communication styles and mealtime support. Workbooks and other materials can be downloaded and users are supported by moderated message boards. The intervention is intended to be used with a low level of guidance (Hay et al. 2008).

Overcoming Bulimia Online

This is an interactive multimedia structured programme that includes eight modules incorporating cognitive-behavioural as well as motivational strategies and psychoeducation. Users receive clinician e-mail support once every 1–2 weeks and the programme takes 3 months to complete at the user's pace (Musiat and Schmidt 2010).

CBT4BN

This is an Internet-based manualised version of CBT in which group intervention is conducted via a therapeutic chat group. The intervention consists of 16 weekly 1.5 hour sessions. Sessions cover the following topics: introduction to CBT, nutrition, challenging automatic thoughts, alternatives to binging and purging, problem-solving and relapse prevention. Study worksheets and self-monitoring exercises via the website are used. Users also receive e-mail support from therapists (Haby et al. 2012).

CD-ROM CBT Intervention for BED

This is a CD-ROM-based CBT programme for the treatment of obesity and unhealthy eating behaviours, covering topics such as nutrition, physical activity, psychoeducation on unhealthy eating, basic concepts of CBT and relapse prevention (Hay 2013). The intervention is based on a similar manual-based intervention 'Cognitive-Behavioural Manual for Healthy Weight Control' (Polnay et al. 2013). The intervention follows a 10-week programme and users receive a weekly phone call for technical support.

Salut BN

This is a structured ICBT programme that includes seven modules consisting of lessons, exercises and examples, incorporating motivation, self-observation, behaviour modification, problem-solving, cognitive restructuring, assertiveness and relapse prevention. Users receive weekly e-mail support from clinicians and the programme lasts between 4 and 7 months (Mehler 2011).

Salut BED

'Salut BED' is a structured ICBT programme for BED that includes eleven modules, which incorporates lessons and exercises covering motivation, self-monitoring, binge triggers, meal plans, strategies to prevent binges, physical activity, problem-solving, assertiveness, automatic thoughts, cognitive restructuring and relapse prevention (Spindler and Milos 2007). Users are required to contact their assigned clinician at least once a week for support. The programme lasts up to 6 months.

Student Bodies+

This is a structured ICBT programme designed for subthreshold EDs (binging, purging and/or restriction). The programme includes eight modules, incorporating cognitive and affective factors (knowledge and attitudes), sociocultural norms and peer norms (thinness ideal, dietary and exercise practices) and behavioural factors (coping, goal setting, food preparation and exercise patterns). Interactive components of the programme include: symptom checklists with individualised feedback, self-monitoring logs and moderated discussion groups. The programme has an 8-week duration (Steiger and Bruce 2007).

Student Bodies 2-BED

This is a semi-structured ICBT programme for BED that incorporates cognitive-behavioural principles, combining psychoeducation and behavioural interventions such as self-monitoring, goal setting, stimulus control and appetite awareness (Sanderson et al. 2011). The programme also introduces emotion regulation skills. Users take part in asynchronous discussion groups and have the option of face-to-face meetings with an assigned mentor. The programme has a 16-week duration.

Guided Self-Help for BN (GSH)

GHS is a structured ICBT programme that includes ten modules incorporating psychoeducation, awareness training, motivation, self-control and self-monitoring, cognitive restructuring, behavioural experiments, body experience, self-esteem and relapse prevention (Hudson et al. 2010). Users receive 25 scheduled clinician feedback 'moments' over approximately 13 hour and the programme lasts 20 weeks.

iBT: Internet-Assisted Cognitive-Behavioural Therapy

This programme is based on a self-help book 'Overcoming Binge Eating' (Mond et al. 2009). The book includes psychoeducation and a structured self-help programme consisting of six modules: self-monitoring, importance of regular eating pattern, alternative activities, problem-solving, dieting and related forms of avoidance and relapse prevention. Users also receive e-mail support for the duration of the online intervention. The programme has a 3-month duration (Hay et al. 2010).

Other Online Interventions

Internet-Based Guided Self-Help for AN (iMANTRA)

This is an Internet-based intervention package for relapse prevention work in people with AN. It is based on an existing manualised cognitive interpersonal outpatient therapy: the Maudsley Model of Treatment for Adults with Anorexia Nervosa (MANTRA) (Pasold et al. 2013). The online intervention is based on this manual and users download workbooks comprising exercises to target four maintaining factors in AN: rigid thinking styles, socio-emotional impairments, pro-anorexia beliefs and relationships with close others. For the duration of the intervention, users also receive individual e-mail support from a trained therapist.

Smart Eating for EDs

This is an Internet-based pure self-help (IB-SH) programme that includes modules covering healthy eating, family education, health assessment and monitoring, motivation enhancement, self-help strategies and psychological health promotion (Pohjolainen et al. 2010). Users receive e-mail support and complete online assessments which also offers feedback. The programme lasts 1 month.

E-Mail Therapy Unguided Self-Directed Writing for BN (USW)

This intervention encourages users to engage in therapeutic writing (Aardoom et al. 2013) with minimal therapist intervention. Users are sent an e-mail and asked to spend some time at least twice a week writing about their difficulties and to send this to trained professionals (Winn et al. 2007).

ICBT Interventions for Eating Disorders: The Evidence

As mentioned above, most available ICBT interventions have been designed for bulimic disorders, although interventions for patients with AN and carers of AN sufferers are now beginning to emerge. As yet, much of the evidence base on ICBT interventions for ED primarily relates to online interventions for BN, BED and EDNOS. Several systematic and narrative reviews have summarised the evidence concerning self-help CBT interventions for these eating disorders and these have included ICBT interventions (Perkins et al. 2004; Treasure and Russell 2011; Winn et al. 2004). Only one systematic review has focused on ICBT interventions for ED specifically (Campbell et al. 2011) (Table 10.1).

Table 10.1 Randomised controlled trials evaluating ICBT for EDs

Study	Population	Conditions	Duration	Effect size Within groups	Between groups
Grover et al. (2011)	Carers of people with AN ($n=64$)	Overcoming Anorexia Online with limited clinician supportive guidance (by e-mail or phone) or usual care	4 months 6-month follow-up	Not reported	Not reported
Fichter et al. (2012)	Participants ($n=258$ females) with AN	ICBT/relapse prevention (RP) TAU	9 months No follow-up	Not reported	Not reported
Hoyle et al. (2013)	Carers of people with AN ($n=37$) Participants ($n=17$) with AN	Overcoming Anorexia Online Guidance (OAO-G) vs no guidance (OAO-NoG)	7 weeks 3-month follow-up	OAO-G: level of expressed emotion (pre to post $d=0.50$, pre to follow-up $d=0.60$), ED impact scale (pre to post $d=0.13$, pre to follow-up $d=0.11$), starvation (pre to post $d=0.37$, pre to follow-up $d=0.57$), bulimic behaviours (pre to post $d=0.07$, pre to follow-up $d=0.39$) OAO-NoG: Level of Expressed Emotion (pre to post $d=0.07$, pre to follow-up $d=0.11$), ED impact scale (pre to post $d=0.34$, pre to follow-up $d=0.49$), starvation (pre to post $d=0.61$, pre to follow-up $d=0.79$), bulimic behaviours (pre to post $d=0.20$, pre to follow-up $d=0.05$)	Not reported
Shapiro et al. (2007)	Participants ($n=66$) with BED	CBT (CD-ROM) CBT (group) WLC	10 weeks 18-week follow-up	Not reported	Not reported

Ljotson et al. (2007)	Participants (n=65 females, n=4 males) with full or subthreshold BN or BED	Internet-based guided self-help (IB-GSH) WLC	3 months 6-month follow-up	Not reported	EDE-Q global (post d=1.15) Objective binge eating episodes (post d=0.68)
Jones et al. (2008)	Participants (n=73 females, n=32 males) with full or subthreshold BED	ICBT WLC	16 weeks 9-month follow-up	Binge eating episodes (pre to post d=−0.93, pre to follow-up d=−0.80)	BMI, all binge eating episodes (follow-up d=0.06)
Robinson and Serfarty (2008)	Participants (n=93 females, n=4 males) with BN, BED or EDNOS	E-mail behavioural therapy Unguided self-directed writing WLC	3 months No follow-up	Not reported	ET vs USW: none USW vs WLC none
Carrard et al. (2011a)	Participants (n=74 females) with full or subthreshold BED	ICBT WLC	6 months 6-month follow-up	EDE-Q global (pre to post d=−1.19), objective binge eating episodes (pre to post d=−0.95)	EDE-Q global (post d=0.3), objective binge eating episodes (post d=0.45)
Sánchez-Ortiz et al. (2011a, b)	Participants (n=76 females) with BN or EDNOS	ICBT WLC	3 months 3-month follow-up	EDE global (pre to post d=−1.29, pre to follow-up d=−1.75), objective binge eating episodes (pre to post d=−0.80, pre- to follow-up d=−1.07), self-induced vomiting (pre to post d=−0.49, pre to follow-up d=−0.76), purging episodes (pre to post d=−0.60, pre to follow-up d=−0.87)	EDE global (post d=1.2, follow-up d=0.99), objective binge eating episodes (post d=0.40)
Jacobi et al. (2012)	Participants (n=126 females) with subthreshold ED	ICBT WLC	8 weeks 6-month follow-up	Not reported	EDE-Q global (follow-up d=0.50), binge episodes (follow-up d=0.43), purging episodes (follow-up d=0.33)

(continued)

Table 10.1 (continued)

Study	Population	Conditions	Duration	Effect size Within groups	Between groups
Ruwaard et al. (2012)	Participants ($n=104$ females, $n=1$ male) with full or subthreshold ED	ICBT Unguided self-help (USH, book-based) WLC	20 weeks 1-year follow-up	EDE-Q global (pre to post $d=-1.22$, pre to follow-up $d=-1.17$), binge eating (pre to post $d=-1.04$, pre to follow-up $d=-0.96$), purging (pre to post $d=-0.75$, pre to follow-up $d=-0.66$)	ICBT vs WLC: EDE-Q global (post $d=0.51$), binge eating (post $d=0.44$), purging (post $d=0.45$) ICBT vs USH: EDE-Q global (post $d=0.37$), binge eating (post $d=0.72$), purging (post $d=0.53$) USH vs WLC: none
Wagner et al. (2013)	Participants ($n=155$ females) with BN purging type or EDNOS with binge eating or purging	ICBT Guided bibliotherapy (BIB-GSH)	4–7 months 7- and 18-month follow-up	Objective binge eating (pre to post $d=-0.24$, pre to follow-up 7 $d=-0.32$, follow-up 18 $d=-0.49$) Purging episodes (pre to post $d=-0.33$, pre to follow-up 7 $d=-0.36$, follow-up 18 $d=-0.53$), laxative misuse (pre to follow-up 18 $d=-0.18$), excessive exercise (pre to follow-up 18 $d=-0.38$), fasting (pre to post $d=-0.40$, pre to follow-up 7 $d=-0.41$, follow-up 18 $d=-0.61$	None

Reviewed trials differ in the populations studied (adults, adolescents, BN or BED and full or partial syndromes); the care settings involved (primary, secondary or tertiary); the availability, intensity and duration of guidance provided; the type of guidance offered (face-to-face, phone or e-mail); and the expertise and training of self-help guides. Nonetheless, evidence suggests that Internet-based self-help CBT interventions are clearly superior to waiting list control in reducing ED psychopathology and frequency of binge eating and purging and in improving ED-related quality of life (Campbell et al. 2011). Self-help ICBT treatments were also found to be more effective for individuals with less co-morbid psychopathology, binge eating as opposed to restrictive problems and individuals with binge eating disorder as opposed to bulimia nervosa (Campbell et al. 2011). This is further supported by the fact that BED patients were found to complete self-help programmes more often than BN patients and to benefit more as a result (Winn et al. 2004). Furthermore, online interventions reduce the risk of therapeutic drift, given their reliance on written and online materials.

ICBT programmes for eating disorders differ in terms of the level of guidance offered to users. Some programmes include regular e-mail or phone guidance, whereas others are unguided forms of intervention whereby the users complete sessions themselves at their own pace. Research shows that Internet-based self-help programmes that are delivered with guidance are as effective as the 'gold-standard' therapist-aided individual CBT in reducing or stopping bulimic symptoms with gains maintained over follow-up (Winn et al. 2004). Specifically, abstinence from binging was observed in more patients receiving guided forms of ICBT compared to unguided programmes. Guided programmes are also associated with better ED outcomes in terms of reductions in weight and shape concern, restraint and frequency of binge episodes (Winn et al. 2004). Furthermore, it was found that inclusion of face-to-face assessment and support from therapists enhanced study compliance, with higher levels of adherence predicting better ED outcomes (Campbell et al. 2011). Across studies, the study dropout rate is 16 % for Internet interventions, which is lower than self-help delivery in other forms such as CD-ROM (30 %) or bibliotherapy (29 %) (Winn et al. 2004). Another systematic review of self-help ICBT interventions found that study dropout rates ranged from 5.3 to 76.8 % (Campbell et al. 2011).

Case Description

Case History

The Problem

Holly is a 21-year-old university student with a 9-month history of bulimia nervosa. She typically eats little during the day (no breakfast, a salad for lunch and for dinner) but binges and vomits most evenings and often all day at the weekend.

Background
Both Holly's maternal grandparents were obese, and as long as Holly could remember, her mother had struggled with her weight and had been on diets. Holly was plump as a child, and when she reached puberty, her mother tried to impress on her that she had inherited the family's tendency to obesity and therefore needed to watch what she ate. Her younger brother would at times call her 'fat legs'. Throughout her teens Holly was very sensitive about her weight and appearance and disliked her legs and tummy.

When Holly started university studies, she made new friends who accepted her for who she was and for a period her weight and appearance seemed to matter less. She also had a nice boyfriend a couple of years older than her who she got on very well with. However, when he finished university studies (2 years ahead of her), he decided to take up the offer of a job in New Zealand and said to her that because of the distance involved they should now finish their relationship. Holly felt very hurt and rejected and began to dwell on what was wrong with her and that perhaps he had 'ditched' her because she was 'too fat'. She went on a strict diet and enrolled in daily exercise classes. Six 6 months later she had lost so much weight that her periods became irregular and her best friend said she looked scrawny. Holly was now living on salad and water and not much else. Having always been a good student, she found it much harder to concentrate, plagued as she was by thoughts about food and weight. She disliked her legs and tummy more than ever. She did much less well in her second year exams than expected and was very disappointed. One night Holly got very drunk and then went on a big food binge. 'I no longer had the will power to control myself constantly', Holly said. After this, regular binges set in and soon after she began to make herself sick after each binge to compensate. Binges became more frequent and more prolongued. Her weight rapidly increased, beyond her previous highest weight. Holly felt desperately out of control and consulted her general practitioner.

Assessment and Treatment
Holly was referred to a specialist eating disorder unit where she was seen for an initial assessment and given the diagnosis of bulimia nervosa. She was found to be anaemic and to have somewhat lowered potassium levels, as a result of her alternating food restriction, binging and purging. The eating disorders specialist explained to her that CBT was the treatment of choice for bulimia and that she had the option of either attending a CBT group or to work through the programme Overcoming Bulimia Online supported by e-mail by one of the unit's therapists. As the date and time of the CBT group clashed with Holly's university commitments, she decided to give the online treatment a go. She liked the idea of being able to start therapy immediately rather than having to wait for treatment. She also liked the idea that she could do things to help herself to overcome her problem. She was given log-in details and straightforward instructions on how best to use

the online programme. For example, she learnt that it would be best if she set aside a particular time each week to work through an online module and to 'talk' to her e-mail therapist. Within a couple of days after her assessment, she was contacted by her e-mail support therapist who sent her a friendly welcome e-mail and who informed Holly that he would check in with her once or twice a week to enquire about her progress, answer any questions and support her use of the programme. Holly immediately started working through the first online module which gave her basic information about her bulimia. Although she had felt that she knew a lot about bulimia, she discovered a number of additional thought-provoking facts about it, e.g. the many negative effects this could have on her body and how dieting and purging maintains binge eating. She liked the clear and simple format of the programme and enjoyed the many interactive exercises. She found the case formulation (the vicious cycle of bulimia) particularly instructive. She realised that her bulimia was triggered by both her extreme undereating/dieting during the day and by stress/boredom, e.g. at weekends when she had little structure in her day and therefore felt even more tempted to binge than usual. After she had completed her own personalised case formulation online, she began to make changes to her daily diet, supported and encouraged in this endeavour by her e-mail therapist. Holly worked through all eight sessions of the programme. She learnt to self-monitor her food intake and reflect on her progress. She gradually returned to three balanced meals and also added regular snacks to her diet, to avoid letting herself get so hungry that a binge became likely. To her surprise, although she had predicted that her weight would skyrocket if she did allow herself to eat more regularly, her weight stabilised and over time even dropped a little. Her food cravings and binges waned. Working through the later modules, Holly learnt to problem solve and to think about how to cope with times when she felt particularly vulnerable and prone to binging. This involved finding more structure at weekends and during holidays and also identifying events that made her feel stressed, anxious or low and therefore tempted to soothe herself with a binge. Holly also learnt from the programme to identify unhelpful (e.g. catastrophic or distorted) cognitions that 'tripped her up' and to reframe these in an alternative less negative way. By the end of the 8-week programme, Holly's bulimic episodes had significantly reduced to one or two binges a week only. She felt a lot more in control of her life and able to contemplate a future where she would be free of all bulimic episodes. She stayed in e-mail contact with her therapist for another couple of months using the skills she had learnt in the programme and reflecting on situations that she had handled particularly well or that had been particularly difficult. Although her therapist only checked in with her a couple of times a week, Holly felt very supported and encouraged by his e-mails and by the end of the follow-up period was symptom-free.

Cost-Effectiveness

Access to evidence-based psychological interventions is key to achieving better outcomes in mental health treatment (Poulsen et al. 2013). However, the cost of delivering individual therapy is high for both patients and healthcare services. There is a need therefore to develop cost-effective alternatives to face-to-face psychological therapy (Stuhldreher et al. 2012). Given the technological advances seen in recent years, the translation of psychological interventions such as CBT into online self-help programmes represents a relatively cheap and easily disseminable solution.

ICBT programmes are brief and focal interventions and are therefore cost-effective in terms of a scalable implementation of evidence-based therapy (Perkins et al. 2004). Studies of the cost-effectiveness of guided self-help (CBTgsh) for EDs have shown encouraging results. For example, one study showed that a stepped care approach using CBTgsh for BN as the first step, followed by fluoxetine and therapist-delivered CBT if needed, resulted in substantially lower cost per effectively treated patient than immediate therapist-delivered CBT augmented with medication if needed (Crow et al. 2013). In addition, mean cost of CBTgsh treatment including supervision was significantly lower than for family therapy in adolescents with BN (Darby et al. 2009). It was also estimated that CBTgsh in addition to TAU resulted in significantly more binge-free days and a lower societal cost in terms of reduced TAU service use at 12-month follow-up in participants with symptoms of binge eating (Crow et al. 2013).

Evidence investigating the cost-effectiveness of online CBT programmes for EDs is currently lacking. On the face of it, ICBT programmes may be considered as less costly alternatives relative to face-to-face therapy. Even with guidance, these programmes require fewer guidance/support sessions than individual CBT therapy and e-mail guidance takes less therapist time per contact, suggesting that the direct costs of these interventions are low. Moreover, online interventions may also be less costly for patients in terms of travel cost and time spent traveling. However, the cost of developing and maintaining online intervention programmes also needs to be considered and is not insignificant. Large-scale randomised controlled trials with integrated health economic analyses are needed to compare the cost-effectiveness of ICBT programmes in comparison to face-to-face CBT and other forms of self-help interventions.

Clinical Implementation and Dissemination

A recent systematic review on self-help interventions in bulimic ED in general suggests that patients with BED, who are older, have a higher BMI and show less dietary restraint, are less likely to drop out of self-help interventions and might benefit substantially more from these than BN patients (Winn et al. 2004). In treating eating disorders, the first step is usually to re-establish a regular pattern of eating. This may present difficulties for patients receiving treatment due to different motivations, fears and concerns regarding changing eating behaviours and the impact this might have on their body weight. For example, BED patients typically hope to lose weight during treatment, despite the fact that weight loss is not the primary focus of CBT interventions for BED. Typically, they show unstructured eating behaviour outside binge eating episodes which requires the application of structure and the normalisation of meals without increasing calories consumed outside of binge episodes (Winn et al. 2004). Conversely, BN is characterised by an intense fear of gaining weight (Striegel-Moore et al. 2005) which may be worsened by changing patterns of dieting, binging and compensatory behaviours. Restriction is common outside of binge episodes and eating is associated with feelings of guilt (Striegel-Moore et al. 2005). BN patients need to increase the amount of calories consumed outside of binge episodes in order to normalise their eating behaviour, and motivation to do this is often low (Economics, Deloitte Access 2012). Self-help interventions should therefore aim to address these fears in the initial stages of treatment, in order to maximise compliance and improve outcome.

Provision of therapist guidance alongside self-help is associated with higher intervention completion rates, higher abstinence from binge eating and greater reduction of dietary restraint in BN patients (Winn et al. 2004). BN patients may therefore need more support and encouragement whilst undertaking self-help programmes (Winn et al. 2004). Guidance from mental health specialists (as opposed to other healthcare workers) is associated with better treatment completion rates and larger effects on key outcomes (Winn et al. 2004); therefore services may need to consider the implications of this in terms of cost and resources. Guides should also be trained sufficiently in how to guide patients through self-help treatment, as well as frequent monitoring of intervention deliverance in order to maximise treatment success (Winn et al. 2004).

Discussion and Future Challenges (Limitations Included)

Summary

Research suggests that online self-help CBT interventions are an effective way of increasing accessibility to evidence-based treatments for BN and BED (Perkins et al. 2004). Studies have shown that online CBT programmes are more effective at reducing ED psychopathology and frequency of bulimic symptoms compared to other forms of self-help (Campbell et al. 2011; Perkins et al. 2004; Winn et al. 2004). Guidance from specialist clinicians is also associated with improved adherence and outcomes in BN patients. Lower dropout rates were observed in BED patients who were older and showed less dietary restraint and higher BMI at baseline (Winn et al. 2004). ICBT programmes can contribute to improving access to effective treatment for patients with BN and BED, especially if features of their delivery are carefully considered (Winn et al. 2004).

Limitations

Evidence supporting online guided self-help is based on a relatively small number of studies (approx. 35). Many existing RCTs are small scale and underpowered (McElroy et al. 2012). Furthermore, adherence to these treatment approaches is currently suboptimal (Winn et al. 2004). Study and intervention dropout rates are lowest in online interventions compared to bibliotherapy or CD-ROM (Winn et al. 2004); however poor user adherence is still a barrier to intervention completion and good outcome. Furthermore, online interventions have the potential to offer materials in varied and engaging formats that are interactive and hold the users' attention and interest (Vocks et al. 2010). However, many existing online self-help packages were developed 10–15 years ago and may be somewhat outdated in terms of content as they do not include state-of-the-art CBT techniques (Stefano et al. 2006). Such programmes may also appear outdated in terms of technological applications and graphics compared to current existing software. Furthermore, therapist guidance appears to have an important impact on adherence to and outcomes from self-help interventions, but regular assistance is costly and practically difficult for services to maintain and may make treatment dissemination more difficult. Lastly, there is a lack of evidence into the cost-effectiveness of ICBT programmes for eating disorders.

Recommendations for Future Research

An important direction for future research is to directly compare different Internet-based treatments for ED and to compare Internet-based treatments to face-to-face treatments for ED (Campbell et al. 2011). Two randomised controlled trials that compare Internet-based CBT with traditional face-to-face CBT are ongoing in participants with BN (Haby et al. 2012) and BED (de Zwaan et al. 2012) (Table 10.2), yet future research is needed to replicate and support these findings.

Future research should also address adherence issues with current ICBT programmes and establish what works for whom and how programmes can be improved to maximise treatment adherence. In order to make direct comparisons between research studies, the lack of standard for reporting adherence or participation needs to be addressed (Winn et al. 2004). This will also allow future studies to determine the degree to which participation depends on intervention or patient characteristics and the level of participation required to achieve a certain outcome (Winn et al. 2004). In order to achieve this, researchers need to distinguish between study and intervention dropout; participants who terminated the intervention should not be excluded from post-intervention assessments and detailed information on 'dosage' used of the programme should be provided (Winn et al. 2004).

Table 10.2 Ongoing trials evaluating ICBT for EDs

Study	Sample	Conditions	Duration	Outcome measures
Bulik et al. (2012)	Participants ($n=180$) with BN	ICBT4BN: online intervention CBTF2F: face to face	20 weeks 3-month, 6-month and 12-month follow-up	ED psychopathology, general psychopathology, body weight, self-efficacy, quality of life
De Zwaan et al. (2012)	Participants ($n=175$) with BED	ICBT (guided self-help) Individual CBT	4 months 6- and 18-month follow-up	Frequency of binge eating episodes, specific ED psychopathology, general psychopathology, body weight, quality of life and self-esteem
Aardoom et al. (2013)	Participants with mild to severe ED symptoms (n not reported)	Featback: Internet-based psychoeducation, monitoring and feedback Featback + weekly support Featback + 3× weekly support WLC	8 weeks 3- and 6-month follow-up	ED psychopathology, quality of life, self-esteem, motivation to change
Jenkins et al. (2014)	Participants (min. $n=52$, $n=17$ per arm) with binge eating episodes	E-mail supported GSH Face-to-face GSH WLC	12 weeks 6-month follow-up	Frequency of objective binge eating episodes, overall eating psychopathology, self-esteem, functional impairment and healthcare usage

Another important gap in the literature is the lack of studies exploring the cost-effectiveness of online self-help programmes for EDs. Future studies should therefore aim to address this, as well as exploring optimal dosage of sessions and therapist guidance in order to establish what optimal guidance is and what is expected of a 'good guide' (Winn et al. 2004).

Conclusion

ICBT programmes are shown to be effective at improving ED psychopathology and reducing frequency of bulimic symptoms in ED patients. Future research is needed to address methodological issues in current studies; to establish cost-effectiveness, optimal levels of dosage and guidance; and to address issues of treatment adherence. Overall, online self-help programmes represent a major advance in bridging the gap for ED treatment in terms of improving access to evidence-based interventions.

References

BEAT (2013) Waiting times equality: survey of 500 eating disorder patients. Available online at http://www.b-eat.co.uk/support-us/campaigning/waiting-times-for-treatment

Aardoom JJ, Dingemans AE, Spinhoven P, Furth EF (2013) Treating eating disorders over the internet: a systematic review and future research directions. Int J Eat Disord 46(6):539–552

Bailer U, de Zwaan M, Leisch F, Strnad A, Lennkh-Wolfsberg C, El-Giamal N, Hornik K, Kasper S (2004) Guided self-help versus cognitive-behavioral group therapy in the treatment of bulimia nervosa. Int J Eat Disord 35:522–537

Braun V, Clarke V (2006) Using thematic analysis in psychology. Qual Res Psychol 3:77–101

Bulik CM, Marcus MD, Zerwas S, Levine MD, Hofmeier S, Trace SE Kordy H (2012) CBT4BN versus CBTF2F: Comparison of online versus face-to-face treatment for bulimia nervosa. Contemporary clinical trials, 33(5):1056–1064

Campbell IC, Mill J, Uher R, Schmidt U (2011) Eating disorders, gene–environment interactions and epigenetics. Neurosci Biobehav Rev 35:784–793

Carrard I, Crépin C, Rouget P, Lam T, Golay A, Van der Linden M (2011a) Randomised controlled trial of a guided self-help treatment on the Internet for binge eating disorder. Behav Res Ther 49:482–491

Carrard I, Fernandez-Aranda F, Lam T, Nevonen L, Liwowsky I, Volkart A, Rouget P, Golay A, Van der Linden M, Norring C (2011b) Evaluation of a guided internet self-treatment programme for bulimia nervosa in several European countries. Eur Eat Disord Rev 19:138–149

Castellini G, Sauro CL, Mannucci E, Ravaldi C, Rotella CM, Faravelli C, Ricca V (2011) Diagnostic crossover and outcome predictors in eating disorders according to DSM-IV and DSM-V proposed criteria: a 6-year follow-up study. Psychosom Med 73:270–279

Clark MM, Abrams DB, Niaura RS, Eaton CA, Rossi JS (1991) Self-efficacy in weight management. J Consult Clin Psychol 59:739

Crow SJ, Agras WS, Fairburn CG, Mitchell JE, Nyman JA (2013) A cost effectiveness analysis of stepped care treatment for bulimia nervosa. Int J Eat Disord 46(4):302–307

Darby A, Hay P, Mond J, Quirk F, Buttner P, Kennedy L (2009) The rising prevalence of comorbid obesity and eating disorder behaviors from 1995 to 2005. Int J Eat Disord 42:104–108

de Zwaan M, Mitchell JE, Howell LM, Monson N, Swan-Kremeier L, Roerig JL, Kolotkin RL, Crosby RD (2002) Two measures of health-related quality of life in morbid obesity. Obes Res 10:1143–1151

de Zwaan M, Herpertz S, Zipfel S, Tuschen-Caffier B, Friederich H-C, Schmidt F, Gefeller O, Mayr A, Lam T, Schade-Brittinger C (2012) INTERBED: internet-based guided self-help for overweight and obese patients with full or subsyndromal binge eating disorder. A multicenter randomized controlled trial. Trials 13:220

Delinsky SS, Latner JD, Wilson GT (2006) Binge eating and weight loss in a self-help behavior modification program. Obesity 14:1244–1249

Dickerson JF, DeBar L, Perrin NA, Lynch F, Wilson GT, Rosselli F, Kraemer HC, Striegel-Moore RH (2011) Health-service use in women with binge eating disorders. Int J Eat Disord 44:524–530

Economics, Deloitte Access (2012) Paying the price: the economic and social impact of eating disorders in Australia. NSW, Australia: The Butterfly Foundation

Fairburn CG, Cooper Z, Doll HA, O'Connor ME, Palmer RL, Dalle Grave R (2013) Enhanced cognitive behaviour therapy for adults with anorexia nervosa: a UK–Italy study. Behav Res Ther 51:R2–R8

Fernández-Aranda F, Núñez A, Martínez C, Krug I, Cappozzo M, Carrard I, Rouget P, Jiménez-Murcia S, Granero R, Penelo E (2009) Internet-based cognitive-behavioral therapy for bulimia nervosa: a controlled study. Cyber Psychol Behav 12:37–41

Fichter, M, Quadflieg N, Nisslmuller K, Lindner S, Osen B, Huber T Wunsch-Leiteritz W (2012) Does internet-based prevention reduce the risk of relapse for anorexia nervosa? Behaviour research and therapy 50(3):180–190

Group TCfEPsMHP (2012) How mental illness loses out in the NHS

Grover M, Naumann U, Mohammad-Dar L, Glennon D, Ringwood S, Eisler I, Williams C, Treasure J, Schmidt U (2011) A randomized controlled trial of an Internet-based cognitive-behavioural skills package for carers of people with anorexia nervosa. Psychol Med 20:1–11
Haby MM, Markwick A, Peeters A, Shaw J, Vos T (2012) Future predictions of body mass index and overweight prevalence in Australia, 2005–2025. Health Promot Int 27:250–260
Hay P (2013) A systematic review of evidence for psychological treatments in eating disorders: 2005–2012. Int J Eat Disord 46:462–469
Hay PJ, Mond J, Buttner P, Darby A (2008) Eating disorder behaviors are increasing: findings from two sequential community surveys in South Australia. PLoS One 3:e1541
Hay P, Bacaltchuk J, Stefano S, Kashyap P (2009) Psychological treatments for bulimia nervosa and binging. Cochrane Database Syst Rev 4:CD000562
Hay P, Buttner P, Mond J, Paxton SJ, Rodgers B, Quirk F, Darby A (2010) Quality of life, course and predictors of outcomes in community women with EDNOS and common eating disorders. Eur Eat Disord Rev 18:281–295
Hoek HW, Van Hoeken D (2003) Review of the prevalence and incidence of eating disorders. Int J Eat Disord 34:383–396
Hoyle D, Slater J, Williams C, Schmidt U, Wade TD (2013) Evaluation of a web-based skills intervention for carers of people with anorexia nervosa: A randomized controlled trial. International Journal of Eating Disorders 46(6):634–638
Hudson JI, Hiripi E, Pope HG Jr, Kessler RC (2007) The prevalence and correlates of eating disorders in the National Comorbidity Survey Replication. Biol Psychiatry 61:348–358
Hudson JI, Lalonde JK, Coit CE, Tsuang MT, McElroy SL, Crow SJ, Bulik CM, Hudson MS, Yanovski JA, Rosenthal NR (2010) Longitudinal study of the diagnosis of components of the metabolic syndrome in individuals with binge-eating disorder. Am J Clin Nutr 91:1568–1573
Jenkins PE, Luck A, Burrows A, Boughton N (2014) Comparison of face-to-face versus email guided self-help for binge eating: study protocol for a randomised controlled trial. Trials, 15(1):181
Jones M, Luce KH, Osborne MI, Taylor K, Cunning D, Doyle AC, Taylor CB (2008) Randomized, controlled trial of an internet-facilitated intervention for reducing binge eating and overweight in adolescents. Pediatrics,121(3):453–462
Keski-Rahkonen A, Hoek H, Linna M, Raevuori A, Sihvola E, Bulik C, Rissanen A, Kaprio J (2009) Incidence and outcomes of bulimia nervosa: a nationwide population-based study. Psychol Med 39:823–831
Kessler RC, Berglund PA, Chiu WT, Deitz AC, Hudson JI, Shahly V, Aguilar-Gaxiola S, Alonso J, Angermeyer MC, Benjet C, Bruffaerts R, de Girolamo G, de Graaf R, Maria Haro J, Kovess-Masfety V, O'Neill S, Posada-Villa J, Sasu C, Scott K, Viana MC, Xavier M (2013) The prevalence and correlates of binge eating disorder in the World Health Organization World Mental Health Surveys. Biol Psychiatry 73:904–914, http://dx.doi.org/10.1016/j.biopsych.2012.11.020
King TK, Clark MM, Pera V (1996) History of sexual abuse and obesity treatment outcome. Addict Behav 21:283–290
Ljotsson B, Lundin C, Mitsell K, Carlbring P, Ramklint M, Ghaderi A (2007) Remote treatment of bulimia nervosa and binge eating disorder: A randomized trial of Internet-assisted cognitive behavioural therapy. Behaviour Research and Therapy, 45(4):649–661
Loeb KL, Wilson GT, Gilbert JS, Labouvie E (2000) Guided and unguided self-help for binge eating. Behav Res Ther 38:259–272
McClay C-A, Waters L, McHale C, Schmidt U, Williams C (2013) Online cognitive behavioral therapy for bulimic type disorders, delivered in the community by a nonclinician: qualitative study. J Med Internet Res 15(3). p. e46
McElroy SL, Guerdjikova AI, Mori N, O'Melia AM (2012) Current pharmacotherapy options for bulimia nervosa and binge eating disorder. Expert Opin Pharmacother 13:2015–2026
Mehler PS (2011) Medical complications of bulimia nervosa and their treatments. Int J Eat Disord 44:95–104

Mond JM, Hay PJ, Rodgers B, Owen C (2009) Comparing the health burden of eating-disordered behavior and overweight in women. J Womens Health 18:1081–1089

Morris R (1979) Conceiving the self. Basic Books, New York

Murray K, Pombo-Carril MG, Bara-Carril N, Grover M, Reid Y, Langham C, Birchall H, Williams C, Treasure J, Schmidt U (2003) Factors determining uptake of a CD-ROM-based CBT self-help treatment for bulimia: patient characteristics and subjective appraisals of self-help treatment. Eur Eat Disord Rev 11:243–260. doi:10.1002/erv.519

Musiat P, Schmidt U (2010) Self-help and stepped care in eating disorders. In: W.S. Agras (Ed.), The Oxford handbook of eaing disorders, Oxford University Press, New York, pp. 386–401

National Institute for Health and Care Excellence (NICE) (2009) Eating disorders: core interventions in the treatment and management of anorexia nervosa, bulimia nervosa and related eating disorders. [CG9] Available online: https://www.nice.org.uk/guidance/cg009

Palmer RL, Birchall H, McGrain L, Sullivan V (2002) Self-help for bulimic disorders: a randomised controlled trial comparing minimal guidance with face-to-face or telephone guidance. Br J Psychiatry 181:230–235

Pasold TL, McCracken A, Ward-Begnoche WL (2013) Binge eating in obese adolescents: emotional and behavioral characteristics and impact on health-related quality of life. Clin Child Psychol Psychiatry 19(2):299–312

Patton GC, Coffey C, Carlin JB, Sanci L, Sawyer S (2008) Prognosis of adolescent partial syndromes of eating disorder. Br J Psychiatry 192:294–299

Perkins S, Winn S, Murray J, Murphy R, Schmidt U (2004) A qualitative study of the experience of caring for a person with bulimia nervosa. Part 1: the emotional impact of caring. Int J Eat Disord 36:256–268

Pohjolainen V, Räsänen P, Roine RP, Sintonen H, Wahlbeck K, Karlsson H (2010) Costutility of treatment of bulimia nervosa. Int J Eat Disord 43:596–602

Polnay A, James V, Hodges L, Murray G, Munro C, Lawrie S (2013) Group therapy for people with bulimia nervosa: systematic review and meta-analysis. Psychol Med 44(11):2241–2254

Poulsen S, Lunn S, Daniel SI, Folke S, Mathiesen BB, Katznelson H, Fairburn CG (2013) A randomized controlled trial of psychoanalytic psychotherapy or cognitive-behavioral therapy for bulimia nervosa. Am J Psychiatry 171:109–116

Pretorius N, Arcelus J, Beecham J, Dawson H, Doherty F, Eisler I, Gallagher C, Gowers S, Isaacs G, Johnson-Sabine E (2009) Cognitive-behavioural therapy for adolescents with bulimic symptomatology: the acceptability and effectiveness of internet-based delivery. Behav Res Ther 47:729–736

Pretorius N, Rowlands L, Ringwood S, Schmidt U (2010) Young people's perceptions of and reasons for accessing a web-based cognitive behavioural intervention for bulimia nervosa. Eur Eat Disord Rev 18:197–206

Robins RW, Hendin HM, Trzesniewski KH (2001) Measuring global self-esteem: construct validation of a single-item measure and the Rosenberg self-esteem scale. Pers Soc Psychol Bull 27:151–161

Robinson P, Serfaty M (2008) Getting better byte by byte: a pilot randomised controlled trial of email therapy for bulimia nervosa and binge eating disorder. European Eating Disorders Review, 16(2):84–93

Sánchez-Ortiz V, House J, Munro C, Treasure J, Startup H, Williams C, Schmidt U (2011a) "A computer isn't gonna judge you": a qualitative study of users' views of an internet-based cognitive behavioural guided self-care treatment package for bulimia nervosa and related disorders. Eat Weight Disord EWD 16:e93

Sánchez-Ortiz V, Munro C, Stahl D, House J, Startup H, Treasure J, Williams C, Schmidt U (2011b) A randomized controlled trial of internet-based cognitive-behavioural therapy for bulimia nervosa or related disorders in a student population. Psychol Med 41:407

Sanderson K, Patton GC, McKercher C, Dwyer T, Venn AJ (2011) Overweight and obesity in childhood and risk of mental disorder: a 20-year cohort study. Aust N Z J Psychiatry 45:384–392

Shapiro JR, Reba-Harrelson L, Dymek-Valentine M, Woolson SL, Hamer RM, Bulik CM (2007) Feasibility and acceptability of CD-ROM-based cognitive-behavioural treatment for binge-eating disorder. European Eating Disorders Review 15(3): 175–184

Sherer M, Maddux JE, Mercandante B, Prentice-Dunn S, Jacobs B, Rogers RW (1982) The self-efficacy scale: construction and validation. Psychol Rep 51:663–671

Simon J, Schmidt U, Pilling S (2005) The health service use and cost of eating disorders. Psychol Med 35:1543–1551

Skevington SM, Lotfy M, O'Connell KA (2004) The World Health Organization's WHOQOL-BREF quality of life assessment: psychometric properties and results of the international field trial. A report from the WHOQOL group. Qual Life Res 13:299–310

Smink FR, van Hoeken D, Hoek HW (2013) Epidemiology, course, and outcome of eating disorders. Curr Opin Psychiatry 26:543–548

Spindler A, Milos G (2007) Links between eating disorder symptom severity and psychiatric comorbidity. Eat Behav 8:364–373

Stefano S, Bacaltchuk J, Blay S, Hay P (2006) Self-help treatments for disorders of recurrent binge eating: a systematic review. Acta Psychiatr Scand 113:452–459

Steiger H, Bruce KR (2007) Phenotypes, endophenotypes, and genotypes in bulimia spectrum eating disorders. Can J Psychiatry Revue Canadienne de psychiatrie 52:220–227

Stice E, Marti CN, Rohde P (2013) Prevalence, incidence, impairment, and course of the proposed DSM-5 eating disorder diagnoses in an 8-year prospective community study of young women. J Abnorm Psychol 122:445

Striegel-Moore RH, Dohm FA, Kraemer HC, Schreiber GB, Crawford PB, Daniels SR (2005) Health services use in women with a history of bulimia nervosa or binge eating disorder. Int J Eat Disord 37:11–18

Stuhldreher N, Konnopka A, Wild B, Herzog W, Zipfel S, Löwe B, König HH (2012) Cost-of-illness studies and cost-effectiveness analyses in eating disorders: a systematic review. Int J Eat Disord 45:476–491

Sysko R, Walsh BT (2008) A critical evaluation of the efficacy of self-help interventions for the treatment of bulimia nervosa and binge-eating disorder. Int J Eat Disord 41:97–112

Thiels C, Schmidt U, Treasure J, Garthe R (2003) Four-year follow-up of guided self-change for bulimia nervosa. Eat Weight Disord EWD 8:212

Traviss GD, Heywood-Everett S, Hill AJ (2011) Guided self-help for disordered eating: a randomised control trial. Behav Res Ther 49:25–31

Treasure J, Russell G (2011) The case for early intervention in anorexia nervosa: theoretical exploration of maintaining factors. Br J Psychiatry 199:5–7

Treasure J, Claudino AM, Zucker N (2010) Eating disorders. Lancet 375:583–593

Trottier K, McFarlane T, Olmsted MF, McCabe R (2013a) The weight influenced self-esteem questionnaire (WISE-Q): factor structure and psychometric properties. Body Image 10(1):112–120

Trottier K, McFarlane T, Olmsted MP (2013b) A test of the weight-based self-evaluation schema in eating disorders: understanding the link between self-esteem, weight-based self-evaluation, and body dissatisfaction. Cogn Therapy Res 37:122–126

Vaz AR, Conceição E, Machado PP (2014) Early response as a predictor of success in guided self-help treatment for bulimic disorders. Eur Eat Disord Rev 22:59–65

Vocks S, Tuschen-Caffier B, Pietrowsky R, Rustenbach SJ, Kersting A, Herpertz S (2010) Meta-analysis of the effectiveness of psychological and pharmacological treatments for binge eating disorder. Int J Eat Disord 43:205–217

Wagner G, Penelo E, Wanner C, Gwinner P, Trofaier ML, Imgart H, Karwautz AF (2013) Internet-delivered cognitive–behavioural therapy v. conventional guided self-help for bulimia nervosa: long-term evaluation of a randomised controlled trial. The British Journal of Psychiatry, 202(2):135–141

Waller G, Stringer H, Meyer C (2012) What cognitive behavioral techniques do therapists report using when delivering cognitive behavioral therapy for the eating disorders? J Consult Clin Psychol 80:171

Wilson GT, Zandberg LJ (2012) Cognitive–behavioral guided self-help for eating disorders: effectiveness and scalability. Clin Psychol Rev 32:343–357

Wilson GT, Wilfley DE, Agras WS, Bryson SW (2010) Psychological treatments of binge eating disorder. Arch Gen Psychiatry 67:94

Winn S, Perkins S, Murray J, Murphy R, Schmidt U (2004) A qualitative study of the experience of caring for a person with bulimia nervosa. Part 2: carers' needs and experiences of services and other support. Int J Eat Disord 36:269–279

Winn S, Perkins S, Walwyn R, Schmidt U, Eisler I, Treasure J, Berelowitz M, Dodge L, Frost S, Jenkins M (2007) Predictors of mental health problems and negative caregiving experiences in carers of adolescents with bulimia nervosa. Int J Eat Disord 40:171–178

Woodruff SL, Cashman JF (1993) Task, domain, and general efficacy: a reexamination of the self-efficacy scale. Psychol Rep 72:423–432

Yanovski SZ (2003) Binge eating disorder and obesity in 2003: could treating an eating disorder have a positive effect on the obesity epidemic? Int J Eat Disord 34:S117–S120. doi:10.1002/eat.10211

Internet-Based Therapies for Child and Adolescent Emotional and Behavioral Problems

11

Susan H. Spence, Sonja March, Sarah Vigerland, and Eva Serlachius

Abstract

This chapter discusses the development and evaluation of Internet-delivered cognitive behavior therapy (ICBT) in the treatment of emotional and behavior disorders in children and adolescents. Although most evaluations of ICBT to date have focused on adults, the literature regarding its use with young people is rapidly expanding. Results thus far have been strongly encouraging, with many studies showing positive outcomes in terms of reduction in symptoms associated with a broad range of psychological disorders and in enhancing emotional well-being and psychosocial functioning. However, the research is still in its early stages and it is difficult to draw firm conclusions regarding the effectiveness of ICBT with young people. The wide variation in the way that ICBT is used also makes it hard to identify the most effective formats for treatment delivery, particularly in terms of level of therapist involvement, parent participation, group online interactivity, and type of Internet material. Despite these reservations, the evidence to date provides a strong case for continued research into the development and evaluation of ICBT approaches with young people in order to determine the most effective approaches. What is clear, however, is that young people find ICBT a very appropriate method of intervention. Nevertheless, one of the big challenges is to find methods of enhancing client engagement, motivation, and compliance with the therapy content.

S.H. Spence (✉)
School of Applied Psychology and Australian Institute for Suicide Research and Prevention, Griffith University, Brisbane, Australia
e-mail: s.spence@griffith.edu.au

S. March
School of Psychology, University of Southern Queensland, Queensland, Australia

S. Vigerland • E. Serlachius
Department of Clinical Neuroscience, Centre for Psychiatric Research and Education, Karolinska Institutet, Stockholm, Sweden

© Springer International Publishing Switzerland 2016
N. Lindefors, G. Andersson (eds.), *Guided Internet-Based Treatments in Psychiatry*, DOI 10.1007/978-3-319-06083-5_11

Introduction

Emotional and behavioral problems among children and adolescents present a significant issue in terms of the distress and interference to young people themselves and to their families. Such problems also generate a major cost to the community in terms of the provision of treatment or the adverse psychosocial impacts if left untreated. Numerous prevalence studies have been conducted in many countries across the world. Exact figures vary according to the study, as the result of variation in definitions and methodology. The results of one of the largest studies to date, based on data from the USA, found estimates of 12-month and 30-day prevalence of 40.3 % and 23.4 %, respectively, for at least one form of mental health problem in 13–17-year-olds (Kessler et al. 2012). Of those who experienced a diagnosed mental health problem over the past 12 months, only around 45 % had received some form of treatment. It would also seem that those with ADHD, conduct disorders, or oppositional defiant disorders are much more likely to have received help than those with anxiety or depression (Costello et al. 2014). The prevalence of mental health problems among younger children is also a cause for concern, although at a lower prevalence rate which gradually increases with age (Merikangas et al. 2010).

It is also clear that mental health issues in young people cannot be assumed to remit automatically without treatment, with many children and adolescents showing strong patterns of repeated episodes and comorbidity (Kessler et al. 2012). There is therefore a very strong case for early intervention in the treatment of emotional and behavioral problems in children and adolescents and ensuring that as many young people as possible have access to effective interventions.

Potential Benefits of Internet-Delivered Cognitive Behavioral Therapy for Young People

Children, adolescents, and their families are entitled to evidence-based mental health care, and access to care should not be influenced by geographical location, socioeconomic conditions, age, gender, sexual orientation, or disability. However, given the high prevalence rates of mental health problems in young people, it is clearly well beyond the capacity of current health services to provide sufficient numbers of trained therapists to treat all children and adolescents who experience emotional and behavioral difficulties. Thus, it is essential that we develop and resource novel and effective ways to make evidence-based psychotherapies available on a broader scale. In addition to the lack of sufficient local clinical services and frequent long waiting lists, there are several other reasons why young people do not receive help, including lack of awareness that a problem exists, embarrassment and worries about the stigma associated with attending a mental health clinic, concerns about confidentiality, lack of knowledge about available services, and financial concerns (Boyd et al. 2007).

Cognitive behavior therapy (CBT) has been found to be effective in treating a wide range of mental health problems in children and adolescents, including depression, anxiety disorders, and conduct disorders (James et al. 2013; McDermott et al. 2010; Scott 2008). Research regarding the impact of CBT for adolescent eating disorders is less well developed, but preliminary findings suggest positive results, albeit with many cases benefiting also from family-based interventions (Gowers 2006). The delivery of structured CBT using the Internet (ICBT) has the potential to increase the availability of treatment for young people. It also requires less therapist time per patient, it eliminates the effects of geographical distances between therapists and patient, and patients do not need to schedule appointments during their day. Indeed, both parents and children have reported the Internet to be an acceptable format for treatment with both the flexibility and anonymity identified as important factors (Stallard et al. 2010). It also has the advantage of emphasizing patients' autonomy in that it allows them to decide when and where to work on their treatment. Also, ICBT teaches skills that the patient can benefit from long after the completion of treatment and the online platform offers the opportunity to repeat the educational content of the treatment when needed and potentially to enhance the self-efficacy of patients.

Additional Advantages for Children, Adolescents, and Their Families

There are additional benefits of ICBT that are likely to be of particular advantage for children, adolescents, and their families. First of all, the Internet is a medium that young people are used to and, many times, is their preferred method of communication. Research suggests that young people already use the Internet as a key mode of communication and find it easier to communicate about thoughts and feelings online than face to face (Livingstone and Bober 2004). Socially anxious adolescents in particular see the Internet as a valuable tool for intimate self-disclosure (Valkenburg and Peter 2007). Similarly, the Internet potentially provides a more comfortable form of communication for individuals with autism spectrum disorder because of the visual anonymity and the more flexible pace of interaction (Benford and Standen 2009).

ICBT also provides particular benefits for parents who are often involved in the treatment and/or transport of their children and who may need to take time away from work to attend sessions. Furthermore, in instances where only one parent is able to come to sessions or if parents live apart and only one parent takes part in the treatment, ICBT could be a way of informing or communicating with the parent that cannot be present at traditional face-to-face sessions.

It is important to note that we are not suggesting that ICBT will replace traditionally delivered CBT conducted by professional therapist. Rather, we propose that ICBT offers an opportunity to treat more patients than could be the case purely with face-to-face delivery of therapy.

A Review of the Literature Evaluating Internet-Based Cognitive Behavior Therapies for Emotional and Behavioral Problems in Children and Adolescents

This chapter will focus specifically upon clinical trials that evaluate the impact of cognitive behavioral interventions that are delivered using the Internet as space precludes from considering the broad range of treatments that use other computer technologies, such as CD-ROMs, videoconferencing, or virtual reality simulations, but we acknowledge their potential in the treatment of child and youth mental health problems. We also note that the Internet is now widely used to provide online education for mental health clinicians and as a source of information for clinicians, parents, and young people about the nature of mental health problems, type of treatments, and availability of therapy. Again, it is beyond the scope of this chapter to discuss these important uses of the Internet. Rather, we will focus this chapter specifically on interventions that make use of the Internet to deliver the majority of treatment components, with either no or minimal direct contact with a therapist.

There are now a substantial number of studies that report the development and evaluation of Internet-delivered psychological therapies for young people, and these relate to almost every conceivable emotional and behavior disorder. As will be noted below however, there are still relatively few randomized controlled trials in this area. The most commonly used approach has been CBT, no doubt due to its high level of suitability for adaptation to Internet delivery given its high level of structure, ease of manualization, and time-limited nature. Approaches have varied in terms of the level of therapist involvement, with most programs including at least some monitoring by and/or feedback from a clinician (Jones et al. 2008; March et al. 2009; Spence et al. 2011; Vigerland et al. 2013). Issues of poor treatment compliance tend to occur when children and/or families participate on a purely self-help basis or with minimal support, such as completing the program in class under teacher supervision (O'Kearney et al. 2009).

ICBT studies have also varied in terms of the level of parent participation. In some instances the interventions have been delivered solely through parents, particularly for problems among young children, such as encopresis (Ritterband et al. 2013) and disruptive behavior (Sanders et al. 2012). In others, participation has been limited to the young person, such as programs for smoking cessation and depression among adolescents (O'Kearney et al. 2009; Patten et al. 2006), or has involved both parents and children, such as in the treatment of child anxiety (March et al. 2009; Spence et al. 2011). Interventions have also varied considerably in length and in the way in which material is delivered in terms of level of interactivity, use of downloadable visual and spoken content, amount of reading material, requirements for homework completion, and so on. These issues need to be taken into account in interpreting the results regarding the effectiveness of online psychotherapies. We are, as yet, a long way from knowing what the ideal format is for delivering ICBT.

ICBT for Disruptive Behavior and Substance Use

Disruptive Behavior Disorders Most of the studies relating to oppositional defiant and conduct disorder have focused on parent training approaches with young children. For example, Sanders and colleagues conducted an interesting trial examining the use of an online version of the Triple P program (Sanders et al. 2012). The study randomly assigned 116 parents of 2–9-year-olds who showed disruptive behavior problems, to either the online program or a control condition that did not receive intervention but allowed parents to have normal access to the Internet. Parenting skills were taught through eight modules, with 43 % of parents completing all modules. Significantly greater improvements in child behavior and parenting style were found for the online program compared to the control condition, with benefits being maintained at 6-month follow-up. A subsequent non-inferiority study demonstrated that the online version of Triple P was not less effective than the more well-researched self-help workbook version of the program (Sanders et al. 2014), with both conditions demonstrating clinical improvements at posttreatment, which were maintained at 6-month follow-up. These results, combined with similar findings reported by Enebrink et al. (2012), suggest that online interventions have a role to play in the treatment of childhood conduct problems. The key challenge will be discovering the best methods of encouraging parents to take up such programs and to engage in their content through to program completion.

Substance Use

A number of Internet programs have been developed for the prevention or reduction of substance use problems, such as tobacco, alcohol, or illicit substance use. For example, Schinke et al. (2011) conducted an RCT examining the effects of a ten-session program, based on family interaction theory, and that aimed to enhance relationship quality between adolescent, African American, or Hispanic girls and their mothers. The results suggested that, in comparison to a no-intervention control condition, girls receiving the program were less depressed and reported higher self-efficacy in their ability to refuse cigarettes, alcohol, and drugs, lower alcohol use, and lower expectations that they would use tobacco, alcohol, or prescription drugs. Further RCTs evaluating this treatment program have shown positive effects in the prevention of substance use among girls aged 10–14 years (Fang et al. 2010), preventing alcohol use among late adolescent urban youth (Schwinn and Schinke 2010), reducing underage drinking among adolescent girls (Schinke et al. 2009a), and preventing substance use among 11–13-year-old girls (Schinke et al. 2009b).

Schwinn et al. (2010) also developed the RealTeen program, an Internet-based, 12-session program incorporating general personal and social skills training, drug use information, and drug refusal skills among adolescent girls. This self-help program incorporates blogs, pen pals, and a private diary, in addition to the skill-building content of the program. At 6-month follow-up, girls in the treatment group reported less marijuana and total substance use compared to the no-intervention control.

Programs such as these have produced some positive results, but their longer-term impact remains to be determined. As with other populations of young people, it is also unclear whether the impact is a direct result of the intervention or reflects a nonspecific treatment effect. Controlled trials with attention-placebo control conditions are warranted.

Eating Disorders and Body Image Problems

Given the relatively high incidence of body image problems and disordered eating, particularly in teenage girls, it is important that interventions are readily accessible to these young people. To date most of the research has focused on adult populations, with a recent literature review suggesting positive effects for ICBT in treating disordered eating symptoms (Aardoom et al. 2013). With adolescents, Heinicke et al. (2007) developed and evaluated an online program for adolescent girls aged 12–18 years who self-identified as having body image or eating problems. The intervention involved six, 90-min weekly small-group, synchronous online discussion sessions, using a chat room and a manual to guide content, facilitated by a therapist. The intervention produced clinically significantly greater short-term improvements in body dissatisfaction, disordered eating, and depression at post-assessment compared to a wait-list control condition, and the benefits were maintained at 6-month follow-up.

Positive benefits were also reported by Jones et al. (2008) for a 16-session Internet-facilitated program, for male and female adolescents, that included psycho-education; interactive components for self-monitoring of diet, exercise, and thoughts; an asynchronous discussion group; and a handbook for parents. Weekly letters focusing on reinforcement, encouragement, and motivational messages were also mailed to participants. Compared to a waitlist group, participants reported greater improvements in their body mass index, binge eating, and weight and shape concerns.

Pretorius et al. (2009) developed and empirically tested a program with 13–20-year-olds who experienced bulimia nervosa or an eating disorder with strong bulimic symptoms. The intervention involved eight, 30–40 min interactive multimedia web-based CBT sessions, accompanied by a workbook, homework, and an anxiety reduction audio session. A message board provided peer support and participants had an online therapist who provided e-mail support and advice. In an uncontrolled effectiveness study, the authors found significant reductions in eating disorder symptoms and service contacts from pretreatment to posttreatment that were maintained at 6-month follow-up. However, the authors noted that the majority of adolescents still had significant symptoms. It was also unclear whether there was any association between the completion of sessions and level of improvement.

Thus, again the results to date are encouraging for this group of young people, but the limited research data to date prevents us from being able to draw firm conclusions about treatment effectiveness.

ICBT for Depression, Anxiety, and Obsessive-Compulsive Disorder

Depression

Several ICBT programs have been evaluated in terms of impact upon depression. Some of these have involved preventative interventions, rather than the treatment of young people with clinical depression. For example, O'Kearney et al. (2006) evaluated the preventative effects of a self-directed ICBT program (MoodGYM) that was initially developed for the treatment of depression in adults. The study involved 78 boys aged 15–16 years who were allocated to either MoodGYM or to standard personal development activities. There were no significant differences in depression change scores between the groups at post intervention or follow-up, but it should be noted that participants were not initially selected on the basis of having high depression scores. There was a very small short-term reduction in the risk of being depressed in the MoodGYM group (based on a composite of depression and attributional style scores) but this effect was not maintained at 12-week follow-up. Subsequently, O'Kearney et al. (2009) allocated 157 girls aged 15 and 16 years to either MoodGYM or their usual curriculum. Although there were no significant differences in depression between conditions at posttreatment, those in MoodGYM showed significantly greater reductions in depression scores at 20-week follow-up than the control group, with girls who demonstrated high depression scores before intervention showing the strongest benefits. It is important to note that only 30 % of participants in the MoodGYM group completed three or more of the five modules and those with initially higher depression scores were less likely to complete the full set of modules. Calear et al. (2009) conducted a larger scale evaluation of MoodGYM allocating 1,477 students from 30 schools to either MoodGYM or waitlist control. Overall, there was no significant difference between conditions in depression scores over time to 6-month follow-up, but analyses showed that for boys, there was a stronger decline in depression scores for those in the MoodGYM group than the control, with no effects for girls. Interestingly, the study showed significant decreases in anxiety associated with participation in MoodGYM. Again, compliance was weak with only 62 % of students completing more than three of the five modules. Clearly, further research with an attention-placebo control condition is warranted to exclude the possibility of changes being due to nonspecific intervention factors.

An intervention called Grip Op Je Dip Online (Master Your Mood: MYM; van der Zanden et al. 2012) that uses an Internet chat room has been developed in the Netherlands. The course comprises CBT modules presented by a mental health professional within the chat room, using text and images, with six sessions of 90 min duration, available at a set time every week, followed by home exercises. A randomized controlled trial assigned 244 young people aged 16–25 years who reported scores above ten on the CES-D to either MYM or a waitlist (van der Zanden et al. 2012). The MYM group showed significantly greater reductions in depression and anxiety and stronger clinical change than the control group at the 12-week assessment. The reductions in symptoms in the MYM condition were maintained at the 24-week assessment. However, only 20 % of the MYM group participated in all sessions, and 20 % of the intent-to-treat MYM sample did not attend any sessions. There was no association between number of sessions attended and outcome, which raises interesting questions about the mechanism of change in generating improvement.

Van Voorhees and colleagues (2005, 2008, 2009) developed the CATCH-IT program for youth aged 14–21 years, as a physician-initiated intervention within primary care contexts. The intervention includes 14 Internet-based sessions based on CBT, interpersonal psychotherapy, behavioral activation, and community resiliency concepts. Eighty-four young people at increased risk for depressive disorders were randomized to primary care physician motivational interview (MI) + Internet program or brief advice (BA) + Internet program. For both groups, depression scores and the percentage of those with clinically significant depression symptoms declined from baseline to 12 weeks, but the condition involving motivational interviewing demonstrated a significantly greater reduction in hopelessness and suicidal ideation (Van Voorhees et al. 2009).

Hoek et al. (2012) published a randomized controlled trial in which 45 12–18-year-olds were allocated to an Internet-based self-help problem-solving therapy or a waitlist control group (WLC). Participants were supported by computer-generated and brief, therapist-formulated e-mails. Results showed overall improvement over time for both groups on depressive and anxiety symptoms, with no significant differences between the groups or between completers and non-completers. Forty-five percent of participants completed three or more lessons and 27 % completed all five.

Although the studies outlined above provide some encouraging results, we are clearly a long way from being able to draw firm conclusions about the impact of ICBT for either the treatment or prevention of depression in young people. Completion rates appear to be an issue, and it is probable the results would be stronger with a higher level of therapist guidance than has been the case to date, with ICBT being used as an adjunct to rather than replacement for direct therapist contact. Indeed, with the use of methods such as Skype, therapist contact can be achieved without the need for clinic attendance and could be provided using very short or fortnightly contacts for example, thereby still achieving reductions in therapist contact times.

Anxiety and Obsessive-Compulsive Disorders Several controlled trials examining the benefits of ICBT with clinically anxious children and adolescents have now been reported. The most widely researched ICBT program with young people to date is the BRAVE-ONLINE Program (hereafter referred to as BRAVE). An initial RCT using BRAVE, reported by Spence et al. (2006b), demonstrated the feasibility of adapting CBT sessions for child anxiety for Internet delivery, with minimal impact upon treatment outcome compared to clinic delivery when half the sessions were presented online. Subsequently, March et al. (2009) published an RCT evaluating the efficacy of BRAVE when delivered fully online in the treatment of children anxiety disorders. Seventy-three children with anxiety disorders (7–12 years) and their parents were randomly assigned to either ICBT (BRAVE) or waitlist (WL). At posttreatment assessment, children in the ICBT condition showed small but significantly greater reductions in anxiety symptoms and increases in functioning than WL participants. These improvements were enhanced during the 6-month follow-up period, with 75 % of ICBT children free of their primary diagnosis, comparable with findings from clinic-based treatment studies in this area. Sixty percent of parents and 33 % of children had completed all sessions at the 12-week assessment point, with families continuing to finish sessions over the following weeks such that, by 6-month follow-up, 72.3 % of parents and 62 % of children had completed all Internet sessions. At follow-up, on average, parents had completed 5.34 out of 6 sessions and children had completed 8.66 out of 10 sessions.

A further RCT from the same research group (Spence et al. 2011) then compared the relative efficacy of Internet versus individual clinic delivery of BRAVE versus a waitlist control, with adolescents with anxiety disorders. One hundred-fifteen adolescents (12–18 years) were randomly assigned to one of the three conditions. Assessment at 12 weeks post baseline showed significantly greater reductions in anxiety diagnoses and anxiety symptoms for both ICBT and CLIN conditions compared with the WL. These improvements were maintained or further enhanced for both conditions, with minimal differences between them, at 6- and 12-month follow-ups. Seventy-eight percent of adolescents of completers in the ICBT group no longer met criteria for the principal anxiety diagnosis at 12-month follow-up compared with 81 % in the CLIN group. The average number of completed sessions was 7.5 out of 10 for adolescents and 4.5 out of 5 for parents, although only 39 % of adolescents and 66 % of parents had completed all of their sessions during the specified treatment period. As in the previous study, families tended not to have finished all therapy sessions at the posttreatment assessment point and continued to complete sessions over the next few weeks. By 12-month follow-up, adolescents in the NET condition had completed an average of 8.20 out of 10 sessions and parents had completed 4.70 out of 5 sessions, with 57 % of adolescents and 79 % of parents completing all treatment sessions.

A frequently asked question about ICBT relates to the impact of lack of face-to-face contact upon the clients' perceptions of their relationship with a therapist. A study reported by Anderson et al. (2012) examined this question within the BRAVE program. Adolescents who completed BRAVE online reported equivalent and positive working alliance scores with respect to the quality of the therapist-client relationship compared to their peers who received face-to-face treatment. This finding was important as there was no face-to-face contact with the therapist in the online delivery and relatively little e-mail or phone contact compared to the clinic delivery. Interestingly, the parents who participated in the online program also reported positive working alliance scores, although they were slightly lower than those of parents who received the clinic format. The results go some way toward reassuring those therapists who are concerned about the impact of online delivery (albeit therapist mediated) upon the therapist-client relationship.

An RCT examining ICBT in the treatment of social anxiety disorder and public speaking fears in adolescents was reported by Tillfors et al. (2011). Nineteen speech-anxious high school students with SAD were randomized to ICBT or to a waitlist control (WL). Significant improvements were found on measures of social anxiety, general anxiety, and depression and effects were maintained at 1-year follow-up. The average number of modules finished during the treatment period was 2.9 (of 9) and none of the students completed all nine sessions.

Vigerland et al. (2013) published the account of an open trial to evaluate ICBT for children with specific phobia. Thirty children (8–12 years) with specific phobia received 6 weeks of ICBT with therapist support. At posttreatment, there were significant and large reductions on diagnosis severity and self-report measures from parents and children showed small to moderate effects on anxiety symptoms. These improvements were enhanced during the 3-month follow-up period, with 50 % of ICBT children free of their primary diagnosis at that point. Eighty percent of participants completed nine or more of the 11 modules.

A recent pilot study by Lenhard et al. (2014) investigated the efficacy of ICBT for adolescents with obsessive-compulsive disorder (OCD). Twenty-one adolescents (13–17) with OCD received 12 weeks of ICBT with therapist support.

Treatment yielded significant improvements on all clinician-, parent-, and most self-administered outcome measures, with a large effect size of $d = 2.29$ (95 % CI 1.5–3.07) on the primary outcome measure. At 6-month follow-up, 71 % were classified as responders and 76 % as being in remission. Participants completed on average 8.29 of the 12 treatment sessions.

Summary regarding ICBT Outcomes with Children and Adolescents

In summary, compared to the large number of published studies that have evaluated ICBT for adults, it is surprising that so few have focused on children and adolescents. Although the research is limited, studies involving a wide range of psychological disorders have generally reported significant improvements in mental health outcomes. However, until we have more, carefully randomized controlled trials, we cannot draw firm conclusions about the impact of ICBT with young people.

Where benefits have been reported, it is not clear whether they can be attributed specifically to the interventions. The lack of attention-placebo control groups in many studies means that it is not possible as yet to demonstrate that any effects are not just due to nonspecific intervention factors. Furthermore, most studies have demonstrated relatively low rates of compliance with ICBT session content; thus where improvements are found, it is uncertain how any changes were brought about. It would be valuable in future studies to determine whether ICBT for young people results in improvements in the skills and knowledge that the interventions aim to teach and whether these improvements in turn mediate the treatment outcome in terms of emotional and behavioral symptoms. Many of these points, however, could equally be applied to clinic-based psychotherapies. A further complicating factor in reviewing the literature regarding ICBT with young people is that studies have differed a good deal in terms of the way in which treatment is delivered, particularly regarding the type and level of input from a therapist, parent participation, the extent of communication between participants with each other (e.g., in chat rooms), and degree of interactivity of the Internet material. Thus, ICBT can mean many things making it difficult to draw conclusions about what works and what doesn't. When the number of studies increases sufficiently, however, it will be feasible to conduct meta-analyses to identify those therapy formats that are associated with the best outcomes.

Meanwhile, it is clear that a consistent factor in the literature is the need to identify ways to increase client engagement and compliance with therapy tasks, to enhance motivation, and to develop methods to reduce early dropout from sessions. Research into the characteristics of those children and families who respond best to ICBT, and those who do not, will also be valuable in enabling us to better target ICBT interventions to those most likely to benefit.

The few studies that have examined this issue have demonstrated inconsistent results. While one study has demonstrated that compliance is not related to treatment outcome (e.g., van der Zanden et al. 2012), others have highlighted more complex relationships. With respect to the BRAVE Program, Anderson et al. (2012) showed that while overall levels of working alliance and treatment compliance did not predict response to the online treatment, these effects were moderated by age. That is, higher working alliance and program compliance predicted better treatment outcome for teenagers (and parents of teenagers), but not for children. Studies examining predictors, mediators, moderators, and mechanisms of change in ICBT interventions are sparse and warrant further attention before firm conclusions can be drawn.

Program Examples

The following section provides examples of two programs that aim to treat anxiety problems in children and adolescents. The aim of this section is to illustrate some of the practical points in the development and implementation of ICBT with young people.

BRAVE-ONLINE

The BRAVE-ONLINE Program is an ICBT program designed for the treatment of anxiety disorders in young people from 7 to 18 years of age (Spence et al. 2005, 2006a). There are age-specific versions for children (7–12 years) and adolescents (13–18 years), with corresponding parent programs. BRAVE is completed online, using a desktop or laptop computer, with more recent versions also allowing access via tablets. The participant receives automated feedback and reinforcement from the program in the form of quizzes, corrective/reinforcement messages, and personalized e-mails. The research studies to date have used a therapist-mediated approach in which the "therapist" monitors the participant's responses and provides brief feedback using an e-mail template system, supplemented by a 15–30 min phone call midway through the program to establish the participant's exposure hierarchy. Aside from the midway exposure phone call (which can also be conducted via e-mail), there is no "real-time" component to BRAVE (e.g., no live forums or live therapist contact). E-mail feedback is sent within 1–3 days following completion of a session, and e-mail questions are responded to on an as-needs basis.

BRAVE has undergone several phases of development, targeted pilot testing, and evaluation and is designed to be developmentally appropriate, engaging, and interactive. In addition to the therapist-mediated version, a self-help version is currently being trialed in Australia (see Dissemination section below).

Program Content The program is comprised of ten sessions for children and adolescents and six sessions for parents (five extended sessions for parents of adolescents). Sessions are completed in order, with a 7-day time delay between sessions to maximize opportunities for skill consolidation and translation. Sessions include information provision, illustration through examples and stories, skill consolidation through engaging activities (completion of worksheets and quizzes), and home practice activities to enhance skill consolidation and generalization. BRAVE utilizes evidence-based techniques including training in detection of physiological signs of anxiety (B stands for body signs), relaxation training (R stands for relax), cognitive strategies such as thought detection, cognitive restructuring and coping statements (A stands for activate helpful thoughts), training in graded exposure and problem solving (V stands for victory over your fears), and training in self- and parent reinforcement (E stands for enjoy and reward yourself). The parent program includes additional parent training strategies to assist the management of children's anxious behaviors (e.g., ignoring fearful behavior) and to assist parents to "coach" their child or adolescent.

The following screenshots in Fig. 11.1 illustrate some of the key concepts from the program, although the actual screens are highly interactive, and many include sound effects, movements, and downloadable materials.

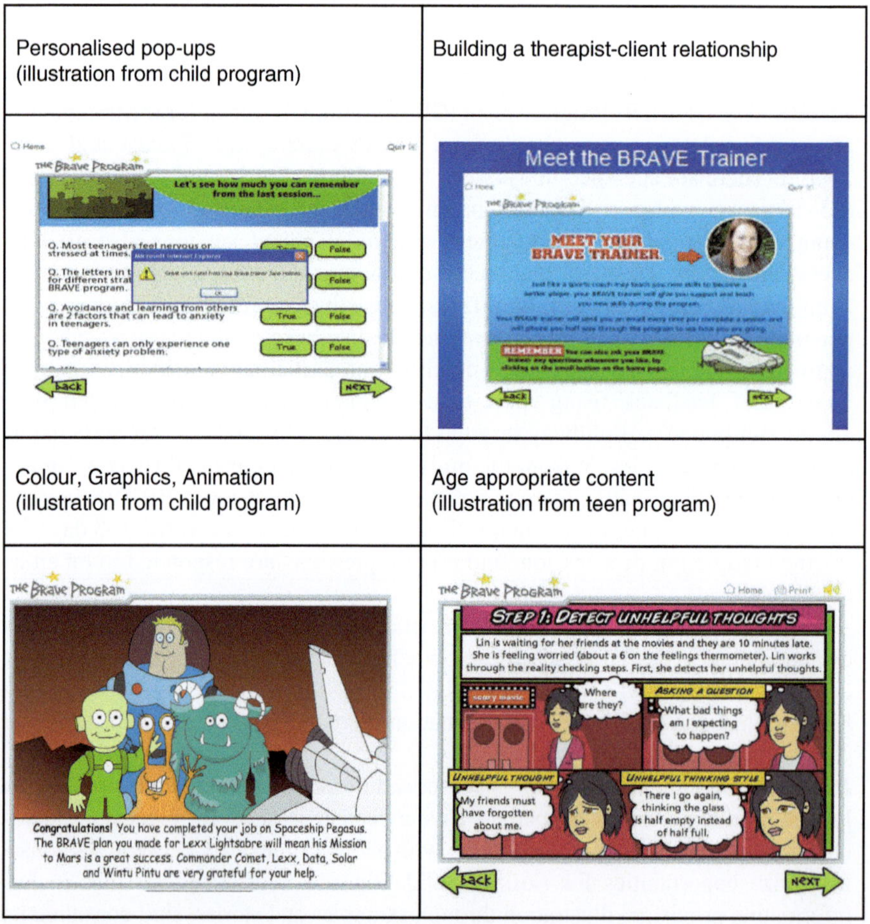
Personalised pop-ups
(illustration from child program)
Building a therapist-client relationship
Let's see how much you can remember from the last session...
Q. Avoidance and learning from others are 2 factors that can lead to anxiety in teenagers.
Q. Teenagers can only experience one type of anxiety problem.
True
False
back
NEXT
Meet the BRAVE Trainer
MEET YOUR BRAVE TRAINER
Colour, Graphics, Animation
(illustration from child program)
Age appropriate content
(illustration from teen program)
THE BRAVE PROGRAM
Congratulations! You have completed your job on Spaceship Pegasus. The BRAVE plan you made for Lexx Lightsabre will mean his Mission to Mars is a great success. Commander Comet, Lexx, Data, Solar and Wintu Pintu are very grateful for your help.
STEP 1: DETECT UNHELPFUL THOUGHTS
Lin is waiting for her friends at the movies and they are 10 minutes late. She is feeling worried (about a 6 on the feelings thermometer). Lin works through the reality checking steps. First, she detects her unhelpful thoughts.
Where are they?
ASKING A QUESTION
What bad things am I expecting to happen?
UNHELPFUL THOUGHT
My friends must have forgotten about me.
UNHELPFUL THINKING STYLE
There I go again, thinking the glass is half empty instead of half full.
Home
Print

Fig. 11.1 Examples of strategies used in BRAVE-ONLINE

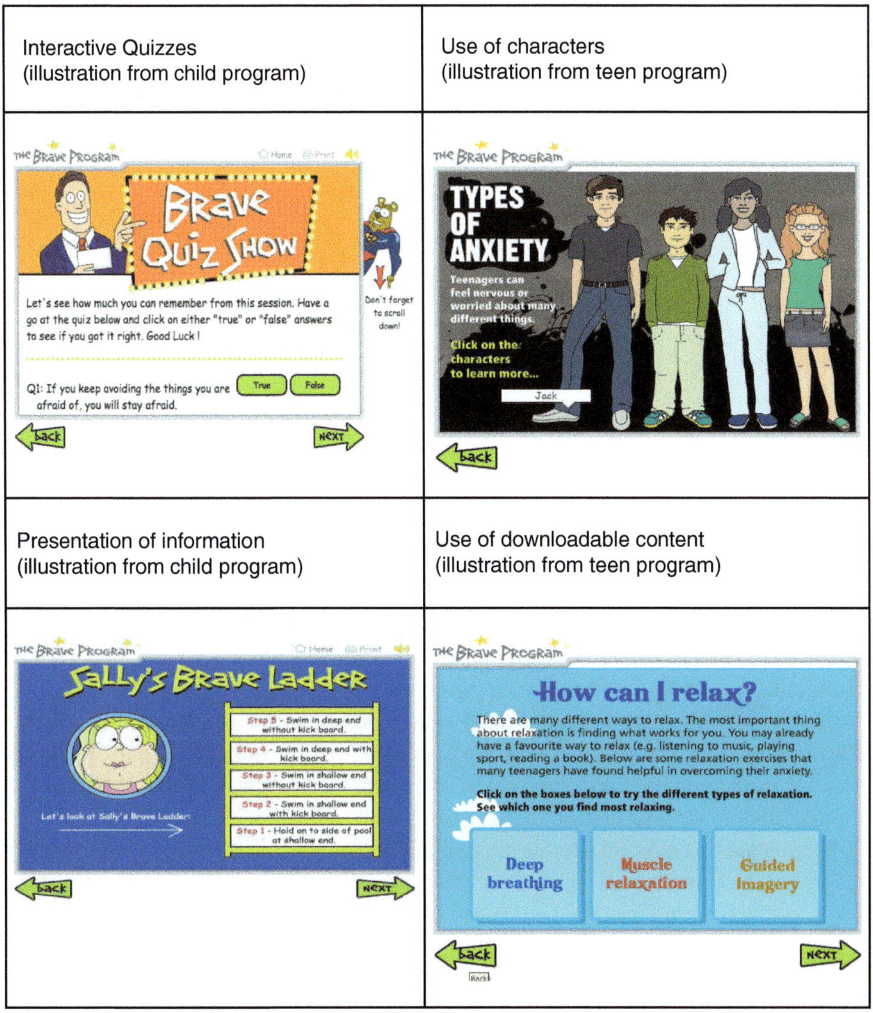
Interactive Quizzes
(illustration from child program)
Use of characters
(illustration from teen program)
The Brave Program
Brave Quiz Show
Let's see how much you can remember from this session. Have a go at the quiz below and click on either "true" or "false" answers to see if you got it right. Good Luck!
Q1: If you keep avoiding the things you are afraid of, you will stay afraid.
True
False
Don't forget to scroll down!
back
Next
The Brave Program
TYPES OF ANXIETY
Teenagers can feel nervous or worried about many different things.
Click on the characters to learn more...
Jack
back
Presentation of information
(illustration from child program)
Use of downloadable content
(illustration from teen program)
The Brave Program
Sally's Brave Ladder
Step 5 - Swim in deep end without kick board.
Step 4 - Swim in deep end with kick board.
Step 3 - Swim in shallow end without kick board.
Step 2 - Swim in shallow end with kick board.
Step 1 - Hold on to side of pool at shallow end.
Let's look at Sally's Brave Ladder
back
Next
The Brave Program
How can I relax?
There are many different ways to relax. The most important thing about relaxation is finding what works for you. You may already have a favourite way to relax (e.g. listening to music, playing sport, reading a book). Below are some relaxation exercises that many teenagers have found helpful in overcoming their anxiety.
Click on the boxes below to try the different types of relaxation. See which one you find most relaxing.
Deep breathing
Muscle relaxation
Guided Imagery
back
Next

Fig. 11.1 (continued)

Client Satisfaction In terms of client satisfaction, evaluations of BRAVE have shown that it is perceived favorably by children, adolescents, and parents, who endorse the online format as an appealing and convenient mode of treatment delivery. The program has now demonstrated efficacy across a number of trials, as outlined above, with rates of improvement similar to face-to-face CBT by follow-up. BRAVE appears to offer a viable, evidence-based alternative for those families unable or unwilling to attend traditional therapy, although it is a time-intensive program that requires some therapist support.

Recent Developments with Brave In addition to the RCTs described above demonstrating the significant benefits of the BRAVE program with children and adolescents, Donovan and March (2014) amended the parent program and evaluated its efficacy in a sample of parents of preschool aged children (3–5 years) with anxiety disorders. Results revealed significant improvements in child anxiety compared to waitlist participants and highlight the potential for variants of the program to be utilized with different age groups. The BRAVE program, as an intervention that takes a transdiagnostic approach to anxiety, is also currently being compared to a newly developed, social phobia-specific version of the program in an RCT with children and adolescents experiencing social anxiety. A UK-based study is also in progress that examines the role of the parent BRAVE program in an adolescent sample. Further, it is being examined in a community effectiveness trial in a New Zealand sample following the Christchurch earthquakes. A self-help version of the program has been developed and is currently being disseminated to Australian young people.

The BarnInternetprojektet (BiP)

(Translated as the Stockholm Child Internet Project) focuses on developing and evaluating ICBT for children with anxiety disorders (Vigerland et al. 2013), ICBT for adolescents with obsessive-compulsive disorder (OCD) (Lenhard et al. 2014) or non-suicidal self-injury (NSSI), and ICBT for children and adolescents with functional gastrointestinal disorder (FGID) (Bonnert et al. 2014).

General Description of the BiP Programs

All BiP programs can be thought of as an interactive e-learning system with therapist support. The aim of the treatment is to teach participants techniques for overcoming their problems and the material is presented in short slides containing a limited amount of information that the participants work through.

Participants have access to the treatment platform for 10–12 weeks. Throughout the treatment, participants have contact with a therapist, mostly through written messages within the platform but also, if needed, over the telephone. Telephone calls are often limited to 1–2 calls and reasons for calling could, for example, be that the participant is lagging behind treatment or need extra support with exposure exercises.

All current BiP interventions typically contain information about the disorder, the rational for treatment, goal setting, foreseeing and managing obstacles, problem solving, planning of exposure exercises, and relapse prevention. The content of the treatments is presented in a varied manner with reading material, films, animations, illustrations, and exercises aimed at consolidating knowledge, practicing new skills, relating personally to the content, or increasing interactivity.

All exercises are saved in an accessible way in the treatment platform so that it is easy for the participants to go back and revise their answers. They also receive comments and feedback from their therapist on all exercises and the technical platform also allows participants to comment on worksheets. Hence, conversations about particularly important worksheets, such as treatment goals or exposure hierarchy, are easily accessible. It is important to note that the communication does not have to be, and seldom is, synchronous. The participants can send written messages to their therapist at any time during treatment. Therapists have the possibility to comment on worksheets or reply to messages at any time but typically log in every weekday. Therapists provide feedback, prompts, and encouragement. All participants have their own assigned therapist throughout the treatment.

Adapting the Program for Different Age Groups There are some differences in the treatment for children (8–12 years), compared to the treatment for adolescents (13–17 years). For children, the parents are highly involved in the treatment and are responsible for conducting the treatment together with the child. Some parts are directed only to parents where they receive information and instructions on how to help their child in the best way. In the parts that are directed to the child and their parents, less written material and more animations are used to explain the concepts of fear, anxiety, exposure, etc.

In the adolescent programs, the parents and adolescents complete separate content and work more independently. Parents access the same psycho-education and rationale for treatment as their adolescents but are also given exercises on how to be supportive of their adolescent during the program without necessarily being directly involved.

<table>
<tr><td>Animated psycho-education about feelings directed at children</td><td>Psycho-education about coping strategies and an audio file with a breathing exercise</td></tr>
<tr><td>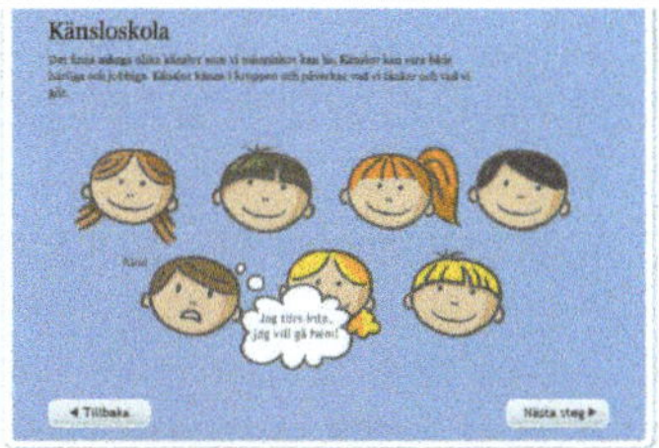
</td><td>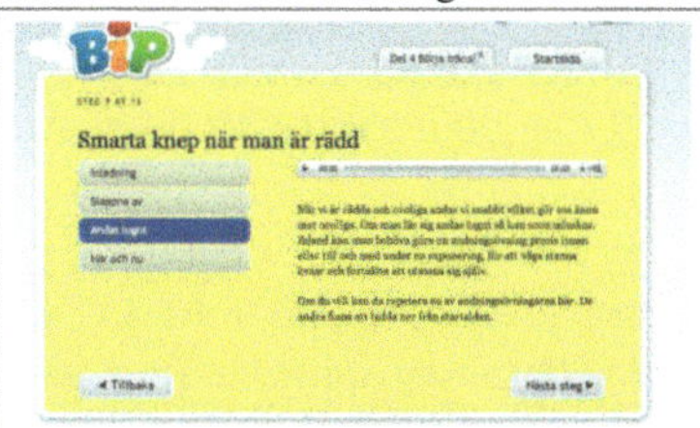
</td></tr>
<tr><td>Whiteboard animation of psycho-education about OCD</td><td>Downloadable material</td></tr>
<tr><td>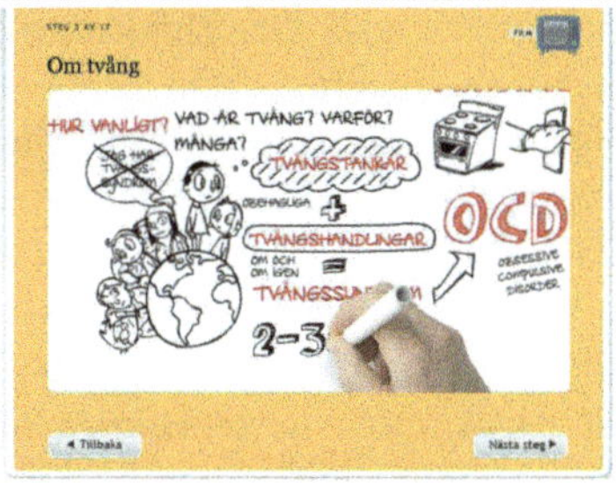
</td><td>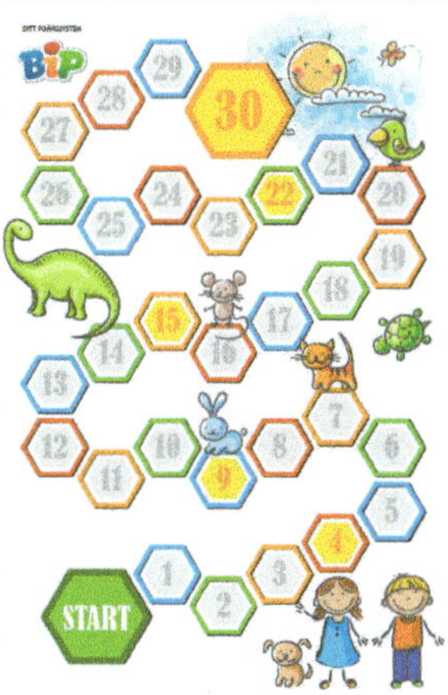
</td></tr>
<tr><td>Goal ladder</td><td>Drag and drop exercise</td></tr>
<tr><td>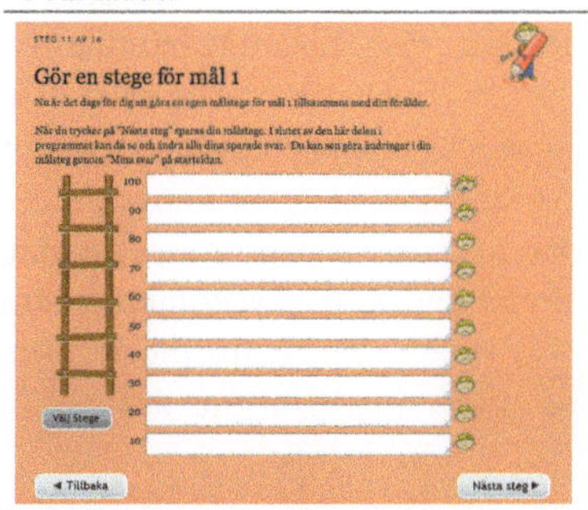
</td><td>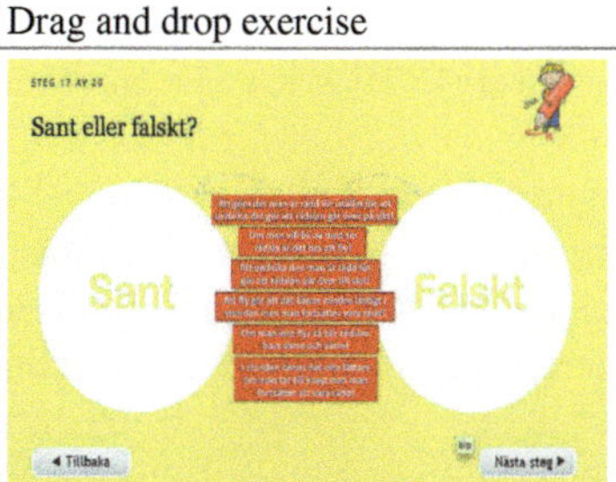
</td></tr>
</table>

Recent and Future Developments with BiP To date, three pilot studies and one RCT have been completed, with three RCTs currently in progress. A smart phone application has recently been developed that is used in conjunction with ICBT to facilitate compliance with homework assignments, as well as for collecting more detailed data on treatment activity and progress.

Discussion

Clinical Issues and Challenges in Implementation of ICBT for Children

There are numerous clinical issues and implementation challenges that have been reported or are potentially of importance for ICBT interventions for children. While families who are motivated, engaged, and compliant and appear to respond well to ICBT, there are some families who fail to respond in the same manner. Similar to ICBT interventions delivered with adults, the loss of face-to-face contact with a therapist in combination with inflexible (manualized) programs is likely to pose a number of clinical challenges for children, parents, and clinicians. First, some families fail to complete all ICBT sessions (or progress much slower than in face-to-face therapy), even with therapist prompting via e-mail or telephone. It seems likely that for some, set appointment times and expectations from a "real" therapist may be vital to enhancing and maintaining motivation and compliance. The evidence to date suggests that compliance with ICBT interventions is of importance in predicting outcome for youth, although more so with adolescents rather than children (e.g., Anderson et al. 2012). Second, there is less capacity to support the child or parent when they experience difficulties in knowledge/skill acquisition or in the application of strategies to real-life situations. Third, there are reduced opportunities to encourage generalization beyond the specific target of the intervention and assist the client to apply the learned skills to comorbid or other more complex difficulties (or common child–parent relationship problems). Although there is reduced capacity to tailor interventions to the client's needs or preferences, this is less likely to be a problem in ICBT interventions for children (as opposed to adults), due to the tendency for youth-based programs to focus on common transdiagnostic elements of CBT that relate to multiple disorders.

Of course, some of these challenges can potentially be offset in interactive programs that include therapist support components. Interestingly, despite the loss of face-to-face contact, studies have shown that a therapeutic alliance can be established in computer interventions where there is some therapist contact, even when only via e-mail (Anderson et al. 2012; Khanna and Kendall 2010), and that stronger alliance is associated with better outcomes for ICBT, at least for adolescents (Anderson et al. 2012). Therefore, clinical challenges due to the loss of real-time therapist involvement are likely to be more evident in programs that do not include therapist contact.

While it seems feasible to transfer CBT content into online packages, clinicians and researchers should be aware of the clinical challenges that accompany such

ICBT interventions. There are likely to be some children and families for whom ICBT is less suited, and future research needs to identify the specific challenges and circumstances under which ICBT is most effective for the various disorders, in order to inform clinical practice.

Dissemination and Cost-Effectiveness

Despite the growing evidence base for ICBT interventions for children and adolescents, there have been very few systematic attempts to examine models of dissemination or evaluate cost-effectiveness in this group. Although individual researchers have estimated the potential time or cost savings of their interventions (March et al. 2009; Spence et al. 2011), with respect to ICBT treatment programs, we are yet to conduct comprehensive cost-effectiveness evaluations. There is much room for further research into these issues in ICBT programs for children. Emerging findings in the adult literature demonstrate the cost-effectiveness of ICBT for depression and anxiety (Hedman et al. 2011; McCrone et al. 2004), with one study showing greater cost savings for ICBT compared to group CBT (Hedman et al. 2011).

Encouragingly, ICBT programs for childhood emotional and behavioral disorders have been generally well accepted by users, although sometimes with slightly lower satisfaction ratings given by parents (March et al. 2009; Spence et al. 2011). Unfortunately, less is known about the acceptability of Internet-based treatments by the general population and whether families would be likely to participate in interventions delivered through population-wide dissemination attempts.

While there is potential to widely disseminate ICBT programs to increase access to evidence-based treatment and provide cost-effective alternatives to face-to-face therapy, this is not achievable until we understand clearly for whom child ICBT interventions are best suited. ICBT interventions will be most cost-effective and dissemination models most effective if directed at appropriate targets. It is particularly important to prevent programs from being disseminated to the "wrong" populations: those likely to experience treatment failure and who subsequently may be unwilling to attempt CBT, ICBT, or any therapy in the future.

The purpose or objective of dissemination must also first be determined. For example, if the goal of dissemination is to enhance access to quality, gold-standard treatments for childhood emotional and behavioral disorders, then dissemination is likely to require therapist involvement and potentially lower cost savings. However, if the goal of dissemination is to provide access to lower-intensity interventions that act as a first step in a stepped-care approach, then dissemination may have a broader scope and potentially lower costs (although perhaps may not greatly reduce the impact of existing disorders). "Open access" programs are easier to disseminate (free and no participation restrictions), but also typically do not include validated diagnostic procedures and support and are not as suitable for "clinical"-level difficulties. However, they have the potential benefit of providing prevention or early intervention effects and may possibly improve acceptability of ICBT or therapy in general.

If ICBT programs are to be disseminated with the support of a therapist, it also raises the question of who is required to deliver the intervention. Fortunately, there is emerging research from the adult and child literature that demonstrates that support provided by nonprofessionals (e.g., technicians) or professionals not trained in CBT can be as beneficial as support provided by specialist CBT professionals or psychologists (Khanna and Kendall 2010; Robinson et al. 2010; Titov et al. 2010). This makes sense given that for the majority of Internet-based CBT packages, the core CBT components are built into the program and supported through multimedia mechanisms and interactive activities. Thus, specialized skills are not required from the support person and this means that dissemination models may be able to utilize nonspecialized support persons in treatment delivery (thus reducing costs further). This holds particular potential for child-based interventions as children are frequently in contact with various professionals (e.g., teachers, nurses, school counselors), all who could potentially play a role in the dissemination of ICBT programs. However, the effects of ICBT when delivered by specialist and nonspecialist support persons are yet to be determined for various child emotional and behavioral problems.

Thus, acceptability of ICBT by the general population, information about who is most suited to these interventions, and desired outcomes of dissemination models must first be determined to ensure successful and cost-effective methods for dissemination. Even if ICBT interventions are efficacious, there are still critical elements of clinical practice that are not suitable to Internet-based delivery with children (e.g., diagnosis for some childhood disorders, suicide risk assessment, family conflict) and these factors must be considered in dissemination attempts.

Conclusion

Although research and development relating to ICBT programs has mainly involved adults to date, there is rapidly increasing interest in its use with children and adolescents to treat and prevent a broad range of emotional and behavioral problems. Given that young people are experts when it comes to Internet communication, it is hardly surprising to find that they find ICBT programs to be an acceptable method of intervention and report high levels of satisfaction with the mode of therapy. What is less certain, however, is the degree to which ICBT is effective in producing long-term improvements in emotional well-being and in reducing mental health problems. Similarly, it is clear that much more research is needed to identify those contexts in which ICBT is most effective with young people and the role of therapist support or guidance.

Despite these reservations, the literature to date is extremely encouraging and suggests that ICBT offers strong promise as a therapy tool in the treatment and prevention of a wide range of emotional and behavioral problems in young people.

References

Aardoom JJ, Dingemans AE, Spinhoven P, Van Furth EF (2013) Treating eating disorders over the internet: a systematic review and future research directions. Int J Eat Disord 46:539–552

Anderson RE, Spence S, Donovan CL, March S, Prosser S, Kenardy J (2012) Working alliance in online cognitive behavior therapy for anxiety disorders in youth: comparison with clinic delivery and its role in predicting outcome. J Med Internet Res 14:e88. doi:10.2196/jmir.1848

Benford P, Standen P (2009) The internet: a comfortable communication medium for people with Asperger syndrome (AS) and high functioning autism (HFA)? J Assist Technol 3:44–53. doi:10.1108/17549450200900015

Boyd C, Francis K, Aisbett D, Newnham K, Sewell J, Dawes G, Nurse S (2007) Australian rural adolescents' experiences of accessing psychological help for a mental health problem. Aust J Rural Health 15:196–200. doi:10.1111/j.1440-1584.2007.00884.x

Bonnert M, Ljótsson B, Hedman E, Andersson J, Arnell H, Benninga M, et al. (2014) Internet-delivered cognitive behavior therapy for adolescents with functional gastrointestinal disorders. An open trial. 2014 Jul 19;1–7. Available from: http://dx.doi.org/10.1016/j.invent.2014.07.002

Calear AL, Christensen H, Mackinnon A, Griffiths KM (2009) The YouthMood Project: a cluster randomized controlled trial of an online cognitive behavioral program with adolescents. J Consult Clin Psychol 77:1021–1032. doi:10.1037/a0017391

Costello E, He J-P, Sampson NA, Kessler RC, Merikangas KR (2014) Services for adolescents with psychiatric disorders: 12-month data from the National Comorbidity Survey-Adolescent. Psychiatr Serv 65:359–366

Donovan CL, March S (2014) Online CBT for preschool anxiety disorders: a randomised control trial. Behav Res Ther 58:24–35

Enebrink P, Hogstrom J, Forster M, Ghaderi A (2012) Internet-based parent management training: a randomized controlled study. Behav Res Ther 50:240–249

Fang L, Schinke SP, Cole KCA (2010) Preventing substance use among early Asian-American adolescent girls: initial evaluation of a web-based, mother-daughter program. J Adolesc Health 47:529–532. doi:10.1016/j.jadohealth.2010.03.011

Gowers SG (2006) Evidence based research in CBT with adolescent eating disorders. Child Adolesc Mental Health 11:9–12

Hedman E, Andersson E, Ljótsson B, Andersson G, Rück C, Lindefors N (2011) Cost-effectiveness of Internet-based cognitive behavior therapy vs. cognitive behavioral group therapy for social anxiety disorder: results from a randomized controlled trial. Behav Res Ther 49:729–736. doi:10.1016/j.brat.2011.07.009

Heinicke B, Paxton S, McLean S, Wertheim E (2007) Internet-delivered targeted group intervention for body dissatisfaction and disordered eating in adolescent girls: a randomized controlled trial. J Abnorm Child Psychol 35:379–391. doi:10.1007/s10802-006-9097-9

Hoek W, Schuurmans J, Koot HM, Cuijpers P (2012) Effects of internet-based guided self-help problem-solving therapy for adolescents with depression and anxiety: a randomized controlled trial. PLoS One 7(8):e43485

James AC, James G, Cowdrey FA, Soler A, Choke A (2013) Cognitive behavioural therapy for anxiety disorders in children and adolescents (review). Cochrane Database Syst Rev 6:CD004690

Jones M, Luce KH, Osborne MI, Taylor K, Cunning D, Doyle AC, Wilfley DE, Taylor C (2008) Randomized, controlled trial of an internet-facilitated intervention for reducing binge eating and overweight in adolescents. Pediatrics 121:453–462

Kessler RC, Avenevoli S, Costello E, Georgiades K, Green JG, Gruber MJ, He J-P, Koretz D, McLaughlin KA, Petukhova M, Sampson NA, Zaslavsky AM, Merikangas KR (2012) Prevalence, persistence, and sociodemographic correlates of DSM-IV disorders in the National Comorbidity Survey Replication Adolescent Supplement. Arch Gen Psychiatry 69:372–380

Khanna MS, Kendall PC (2010) Computer-assisted cognitive behavioral therapy for child anxiety: results of a randomized clinical trial. J Consult Clin Psychol 78:737–745. doi:10.1037/a0019739

Lenhard F, Vigerland S, Andersson E, Rück C, Mataix-Cols M, Thulin U, Ljótsson B, Serlachius E (2014) Internet-delivered cognitive behavior therapy for adolescents with obsessive-compulsive disorder: an open trial. PLoS One 9(6):e100773.

Livingstone S, Bober M (2004) Taking up opportunities? Children's uses of the internet for education, communication and participation. E-learning 1(3):395–419

March S, Spence SH, Donovan CL (2009) The efficacy of an internet-based cognitive-behavioral therapy intervention for child anxiety disorders. J Pediatr Psychol 34:474–487. doi:10.1093/jpepsy/jsn099

McCrone P, Knapp M, Proudfoot J, Ryden C, Cavanagh K, Shapiro DA, Illson S, Gray JA, Goldberg D, Mann A, Marks I, Everitt B, Tylee A (2004) Cost-effectiveness of computerised therapy for anxiety and depression in primary care: randomised controlled trial. Br J Psychiatry 185:55–62. doi:10.1192/bjp.185.1.55

McDermott B, Baigent M, Chanen A, Fraser L, Graetz B, Hayman N, Newman L, Parikh N, Peirce B, Proimos J, Smalley T, Spence S (2010) Clinical practice guidelines: Depression in adolescents and young adults. Melbourne: beyondblue: the national depression initiative.

Merikangas KR, He J-P, Burstein M, Swanson SA, Avenevoli S, Cui L, Benjet C, Georgiades K, Swendsen J (2010) Lifetime prevalence of mental disorders in U.S. adolescents: results from the National Comorbidity Survey Replication-Adolescent Supplement (NCS-A). J Am Acad Child Adolesc Psychiatry 49:980–989

O'Kearney R, Gibson M, Christensen H, Griffiths KM (2006) Effects of a cognitive-behavioural internet program on depression, vulnerability to depression and stigma in adolescent males: a school-based controlled trial. Cogn Behav Ther 35:43–54. doi:10.1080/16506070500303456

O'Kearney R, Kang K, Christensen H, Griffiths K (2009) A controlled trial of a school-based Internet program for reducing depressive symptoms in adolescent girls. Depress Anxiety 26:65–72. doi:10.1002/da.20507

Patten CA, Croghan IT, Meis TM, Decker PA, Pingree S, Colligan RC, Dornelas EA, Offord KP, Boberg EW, Baumberger RK, Hurt RD, Gustafson DH (2006) Randomized clinical trial of an internet-based versus brief office intervention for adolescent smoking cessation. Patient Educ Couns 64:249–258

Pretorius N, Arcelus J, Beecham J, Dawson H, Doherty F, Eisler I, Gallagher C, Gowers S, Isaacs G, Johnson-Sabine E, Jones A, Newell C, Morris J, Richards L, Ringwood S, Rowlands L, Simic M, Treasure J, Waller G, Williams C, Yi I, Yoshioka M, Schmidt U (2009) Cognitive-behavioural therapy for adolescents with bulimic symptomatology: the acceptability and effectiveness of internet-based delivery. Behav Res Ther 47:729–736. doi:10.1016/j.brat.2009.05.006

Ritterband LM, Thorndike FP, Lord HR, Borowitz SM, Walker LS, Ingersoll KS, Sutphen JL, Cox DJ (2013) An RCT of an internet intervention for pediatric encopresis with one-year follow-up. Clin Pract Pediatr Psychol 1:68–80

Robinson E, Titov N, Andrews G, McIntyre K, Schwenke G, Solley K (2010) Internet treatment for generalised anxiety disorder: a randomized controlled trial comparing clinician vs. technician assistance. PLoS One 5:e10942. doi:10.1371/journal.pone.0010942

Sanders MR, Baker S, Turner KM (2012) A randomized controlled trial evaluating the efficacy of Triple P Online with parents of children with early-onset conduct problems. Behav Res Ther 50:675–684

Sanders MR, Dittman CK, Farruggia SP, Keown LJ (2014) A comparison of online versus workbook delivery of a self-help positive parenting program. J Prim Prev 35(3):125–133 doi: 10.1007/s10935-014-0339-2

Schinke SP, Cole KC, Fang L (2009a) Gender-specific intervention to reduce underage drinking among early adolescent girls: a test of a computer-mediated, mother-daughter program. (Report). J Stud Alcohol Drugs 70(1):70–77

Schinke SP, Fang L, Cole KC (2009b) Computer-delivered, parent-involvement intervention to prevent substance use among adolescent girls. Prev Med 49:429–435. doi:10.1016/j.ypmed.2009.08.001

Schinke SP, Fang L, Cole KC, Cohen-Cutler S (2011) Preventing substance use among Black and Hispanic adolescent girls: results from a computer-delivered, mother–daughter intervention approach. Subst Use Misuse 46:35–45. doi:10.3109/10826084.2011.521074
Schwinn TM, Schinke SP (2010) Preventing alcohol use among late adolescent urban youth: 6-year results from a computer-based intervention. (Report). J Stud Alcohol Drugs 71(4):535–538
Scott S (2008) An update on interventions for conduct disorder. Adv Psychiatr Treat 14:61–70
Spence SH, March S, Holmes JM (2005) BRAVE for children – ONLINE: an internet based program for children with anxiety. School of Psychology, University of Queensland, Brisbane
Spence SH, Holmes J, Donovan CL (2006a) BRAVE for teenagers – ONLINE: an internet based program for adolescents with anxiety. School of Psychology, University of Queensland, Brisbane
Spence SH, Holmes JM, March S, Lipp OV (2006b) The feasibility and outcome of clinic plus internet delivery of cognitive-behavior therapy for childhood anxiety. J Consult Clin Psychol 74:614–621. doi:10.1037/0022-006X.74.3.614
Spence SH, Donovan CL, March S, Gamble A, Anderson RE, Prosser S, Kenardy J (2011) A randomized controlled trial of online versus clinic-based CBT for adolescent anxiety. J Consult Clin Psychol 79(5):629–642
Stallard P, Velleman S, Richardson T (2010) Computer use and attitudes towards computerized therapy amongst young people and parents attending child and adolescent mental health services. Child Adolesc Mental Health 15:80–84
Tillfors M, Andersson G, Ekselius L, Furmark T, Lewenhaupt S, Karlsson A, Carlbring P (2011) A randomized trial of internet-delivered treatment for social anxiety disorder in high school students. Cogn Behav Ther 40:147–157. doi:10.1080/16506073.2011.555486
Titov N, Andrews G, Davies M, McIntyre K, Robinson E, Solley K (2010) Internet treatment for depression: a randomized controlled trial comparing clinician vs. technician assistance. PLoS One 5:e10939. doi:10.1371/journal.pone.0010939
Valkenburg PM, Peter J (2007) Preadolescents' and adolescents' online communication and their closeness to friends. Dev Psychol 43:267–277. doi:10.1037/0012-1649.43.2.267
van der Zanden R, Kramer J, Gerrits R, Cuijpers P (2012) Effectiveness of an online group course for depression in adolescents and young adults: a randomized trial. J Med Internet Res 14:296–309
Van Voorhees BW, Ellis J, Stuart S, Fogel J, Ford DE (2005) Pilot study of a primary care internet-based depression prevention intervention for late adolescents. Can Child Adolesc Psychiatr Rev 14:40–43
Van Voorhees BW, Vanderplough-Booth K, Fogel J, Gladstone T, Bell C, Stuart S, Gollan J, Bradford N, Domanico R, Fagan B, Ross R, Larson J, Watson N, Paunesku D, Melkonian S, Kuwabara S, Holper T, Shank N, Saner D, Butler A, Chandler A, Louie T, Weinstein C, Collins S, Baldwin M, Wassel A, Reinecke MA (2008) Integrative internet-based depression prevention for adolescents: a randomized clinical trial in primary care for vulnerability and protective factors. J Can Acad Child Adolesc Psychiatr 17:184–196
Van Voorhees BW, Vanderplough-Booth K, Fogel J, Pomper BE, Marko M, Reid N, Watson N, Larson J, Bradford N, Fagan B, Zuckerman S, Wiedman P, Domanico R (2009) Adolescent dose and ratings of an internet-based depression prevention program: a randomized trial of primary care physician brief advice versus a motivational interview. J Cogn Behav Psychother 9:1–19
Vigerland S, Thulin U, Ljótsson B, Svirsky L, Öst L, Lindefors N, Andersson G, Serlachius E (2013) Internet-delivered CBT for children with specific phobia: a pilot study. Cogn Behav Ther 42:303–314

Internet-Delivered Cognitive Behaviour Therapy (ICBT) for Older Adults with Anxiety and Depression

12

Blake F. Dear, Kristin Silfvernagel, and Vincent J. Fogliati

Abstract

Anxiety and depression are prevalent among older adults and are associated increased disability, reduced quality of life and poorer physical health. Effective psychological treatments such as cognitive behaviour therapy (CBT) are known to be effective and acceptable for older adults. However, as with younger adults, research indicates relatively few older adults access these treatments in their traditional face-to-face format. However, highlighting the potential of newer internet-delivered CBT (ICBT) approaches for increasing access to treatment, a large proportion of older adults are online and the overall proportion online is only likely to grow over time. Several clinical trials have now been conducted examining ICBT for older adults and the nature and finding of these emerging studies are reviewed in this chapter. Future directions for research focused in this area are also discussed.

Introduction

Prevalence and Burden of Anxiety and Depression

Anxiety and depression are major health issues among older adults. Epidemiological surveys indicate that 1 in 6 community-dwelling adults over the age of 65 reports symptoms consistent with a mental disorder each year and approximately 3 and 4 %

B.F. Dear (✉) • V.J. Fogliati
Department of Psychology, eCentreClinic, Macquarie University,
Sydney, NSW 2109, Australia
e-mail: blake.dear@mq.edu.au

K. Silfvernagel
Department of Behavioural Sciences and Learning, Linköping University,
Linköping SE 581 83, Sweden
e-mail: kristin.silfvernagel@liu.se

© Springer International Publishing Switzerland 2016

N. Lindefors, G. Andersson (eds.), *Guided Internet-Based Treatments in Psychiatry*, DOI 10.1007/978-3-319-06083-5_12

meet formal diagnostic criteria for affective and anxiety disorders, respectively (Trollor et al. 2007). However, it is argued that the actual prevalence rates may be underestimated in older adults and that many more likely experience clinical level symptoms of anxiety and depression (O'Connor 2006; Luppa et al. 2012). This is significant because the proportion of older adults is growing considerably in many countries and is likely to continue with increases in average life expectancies (Oeppen and Vaupel 2002). For example, in Australia, the number of adults aged 65 years and older has increased 15-fold in the last century and the percentage of adults over 65 years of age is expected to increase from 13 to 23 % by 2051 (Australian Bureau of Statistics 2009; Sachdev 2007). Similarly, the National Board of Health and Welfare in Sweden reported that 3–5 % of adults over 65 years met diagnostic criteria for generalised anxiety disorder and that 10–15 % experience late life depression (Socialstyrelsen 2009). Thus, anxiety and depression are common in older adults and the number of older adults with these conditions will almost certainly increase.

Anxiety and depression are particularly significant issues among older adults because of their association with poor physical health. Research indicates that anxiety and depression in older adults are associated with poorer physical health and the exacerbation of physical illness (Braam et al. 2005; Brenes et al. 2008) as well as reduced quality of life and increased risk of suicide (Grek 2007). There is now considerable evidence of a complex and reciprocal relationship between anxiety and depression, on the one hand, and physical illness, on the other; whereby each complicates the other (Katon and Ciechanowski 2002; Roy-Byrne et al. 2008). For example, research indicates that the risk of myocardial infarction increases fourfold among adults with symptoms of depression (Hippisley-Cox et al. 1998). Moreover, depressed patients are three times less likely to adhere to recommended medical treatment regimens for their chronic health conditions than are nondepressed patients (DiMatteo et al. 2000). Furthermore, reflecting the bidirectional relationships between psychological and physical illnesses, the prevalence of chronic health conditions increases with age and having a chronic health condition appears to be one of the strongest risk factors for anxiety and depression (Britt et al. 2008). Hence, while anxiety and depression are major health issues themselves, untreated anxiety and depression are significant issues among older adults because of their association with poor physical health.

Cognitive Behaviour Therapy (CBT) for Older Adults

Most of the evidence for the efficacy of psychological treatments, such as cognitive behaviour therapy (CBT) (e.g. Butler et al. 2006), is derived from clinical trials involving general adult cohorts which often have lower numbers of younger (e.g. 18- to 25-year-olds) or older adult populations (e.g. 60+-year-olds). CBT for older adults is very similar to CBT for adults at other ages, except that it is often modified to include gerontological knowledge and take account of cohort beliefs, physical health status and stage-of-life transitions

(Laidlaw et al. 2004). There is encouraging evidence for the efficacy of traditional CBT, which is typically delivered face-to-face in individual or group sessions, for older adults with anxiety and depression (Ayers et al. 2007; Scogin et al. 2005). For example, two recent meta-analyses found CBT to result in moderate (n = 12 RCTS; Hedge's g = .66) and large (n = 23 RCTs; Hedge's g = 1.35) effect sizes at post-treatment over waitlist control conditions for depression and anxiety, respectively (Gould et al. 2012a, b). However, many important questions do remain about the use of CBT with older adults and many of the existing studies are characterised by methodological limitations, including high dropout rates and small sample sizes (Wilkinson 2009). Despite the limited number of studies and these methodological limitations, the findings of existing studies concerning CBT for older adults with anxiety and depression are encouraging.

Internet-Delivered Cognitive Behaviour Therapy (ICBT) for Older Adults

One notable challenge facing traditional CBT is the low levels of treatment seeking among older adults. For example, in Australia, fewer than 30 % of older adults with anxiety or depression in Australia report seeking treatment for these difficulties, even when they have multiple comorbid mental health difficulties (Trollor et al. 2007). Unfortunately, the barriers against treatment seeking in this group are multiple and include stigma and shame, mobility limitations, costs of treatment, low mental health literacy and shortages of clinicians experienced in working with older adults (Cole et al. 2008). These barriers and low rates of treatment seeking among older adults have led some clinical researchers to start to explore the potential of Internet-delivered CBT (ICBT) with older adults with anxiety and depression. This interest also reflects a broader trend within the psychological literature exploring ICBT as a means of overcoming traditional barriers to treatment and increasing access to evidence-based psychological treatment (Andersson and Titov 2014). ICBT draws on the same principles as traditional face-to-face CBT but provides therapeutic information about symptoms and teaches self-management skills via the Internet and a computer. ICBT is also provided with differing levels and types of clinical support, ranging from weekly regular contact with a clinician, via telephone or email, to entirely self-guided programmes with no clinical contact.

There is now considerable meta-analytic data supporting the efficacy of ICBT for general adult populations with anxiety and depression (Andersson and Cuijpers 2009; Andrews et al. 2010; Cuijpers et al. 2009) with effect sizes comparable to traditional face-to-face interventions (Cuijpers et al. 2010) and emerging evidence cost-effectiveness (Hedman et al. 2012). However, one critical question is whether Internet delivery has the same potential to overcome barriers and increase access to effective psychological treatment among older adults as it does with younger adults. The potential does seem to exist with Internet and computer use rapidly increasing among older cohorts of adults in many countries (Ewing and Thomas 2012; Fox and Jones 2009).

For example, in Australia, estimates indicate relatively high use of the Internet among adults over 65, with more than 50 % reporting regular use of the Internet, and this proportion is growing rapidly over time (Ewing and Thomas 2012). However, while older adults appear to use the technology required for ICBT and this use is likely to increase into the future, well-designed empirical research is required to demonstrate the acceptability, efficacy and cost-effectiveness of ICBT and highlight its potential as a suitable approach to treatment for older adults with anxiety and depression.

In the next few sections, this chapter will describe the existing ICBT programmes for older adults as well as summarise existing data on clinical and cost-effectiveness. The chapter will also discuss issues of implementation and dissemination as well as future challenges facing the area. It is important to note that the present chapter focusses specifically on ICBT interventions rather than computer- or technology-delivered interventions more broadly, although a recent review of computer-delivered interventions for older adults found there was a dearth of data regarding older adults (Crabb et al. 2012).

Current ICBT Interventions

To date, very few clinical trials have examined the efficacy of ICBT programmes for older adults and there have been even fewer ICBT programmes specifically designed for older adults (Table 12.1). It is important to note that many clinical trials of ICBT do include older adults; however, a recent review of computer-delivered CBT programmes would suggest that the proportion of older adults (e.g., 60 years and older) in clinical trials of ICBT trials may be relatively low (Crabb et al. 2012). Thus, caution is needed regarding the acceptability and efficacy of general ICBT programmes for older adults and targeted research regarding older adults is required.

At the time of writing this chapter, the authors are aware of five ICBT programmes specifically designed for older adults and that have been examined via clinical trials. One further programme, while not tailored specifically for older adults, has been examined in a clinical trial consisting exclusively of adults aged between 50 and 75 years (Spek et al. 2007, 2008). These ICBT programmes are summarised below:

The Managing Stress and Anxiety and Managing Your Mood Programmes (Version 1)

The Managing Stress and Anxiety programme and the Managing Your Mood programme are two separate ICBT programmes developed for older adults with symptoms of anxiety and depression, respectively (Zou et al. 2012; Dear et al. 2013). Both programmes comprise 5 core lessons and are delivered over 8 weeks. Participants are encouraged to complete 1 core lesson every 7–10 days and the programmes are designed to prevent participants from accessing later materials before completing earlier materials. The programmes also include lesson summaries and homework tasks as well as additional resources, including assertiveness skills, problem-solving, managing beliefs and improving sleep. Participants in these

Table 12.1 Summary of current studies examining ICBT for older adults with anxiety or depression

	Sample			Results						
Authors and country	Design conditions	Primary outcome measure	Secondary outcome measure	*n*	Avg. age and range	Diagnostic tool	Response rate	Average therapist contact per participant	ES (post-tx)	ES (follow-up)
Zou et al. (2012) Australia	Open trial	GAD-7	PHQ-9	22	*M*=66 (not reported)	MINI	Post: 100 % 3 months: 95 %	78 min	*WG* GAD-7: 1.65 PHQ-9: 1.22	*WG* GAD-7: 1.03 PHQ-9: 0.53
Dear et al. (2013) Australia	Open trial	PHQ-9	GAD-7	20	*M*=63.4 (60–80)	MINI	Post: 85 % 3 months: 85 %	73.8 min	*WG* PHQ-9: 1.59 GAD-7: 1.41	*WG* PHQ-9: 1.41 GAD-7: 2.04
Dear et al. (submitted b) Australia	Two independent open trials (anxiety and depression)	*Anxiety* GAD-7 *Depression* PHQ-9	*Anxiety* PHQ-9 *Depression* GAD-7	*Anxiety* 27 *Depression* 20	*Anxiety* *M*=65.3 (60–81) *Depression* *M*=66.6 (62–76)	MINI	*Anx* Post : 85 % 3 months: 77 % *Dep* Post: 80 % 3 months: 70 %		*Anxiety WG* GAD-7: 1.17 PHQ-9: 1.26 *Depression WG* PHQ-9: 1.06 GAD-7: 0.60	*Anxiety WG* GAD-7: 0.99 PHQ-9: 1.00 *Depression WG* PHQ-9: 1.04 GAD-7: 0.59
Titov et al. (submitted) Australia	Treatment, waitlist control	PHQ-9	GAD-7	54	*M*=65.3 (61–76)	MINI	*Treatment* Post: 85 % 3 months: 74 % 12 months: 70 % *Control* Post: 88 %	45.1 min	*BW* PHQ-9: 2.08 GAD-7: 1.22	*WG (treatment)* *3 months* PHQ-9: 1.25 GAD-7: 1.00 *12 months* PHQ-9: 1.25 GAD-7: 1.12

(continued)

Table 12.1 (continued)

	Sample			Results						
Authors and country	Design conditions	Primary outcome measure	Secondary outcome measure	*n*	Avg. age and range	Diagnostic tool	Response rate	Average therapist contact per participant	ES (post-tx)	ES (follow-up)
Dear et al. (submitted a) Australia	Treatment, waitlist control	GAD-7	PHQ-9	72	*M*=65.5 (60–81)	MINI	*Treatment* Post: 90 % 3 months: 90 % 12 months: 87 % *Control* Post: 86 %	57.58 min	*BW* GAD-7: 1.43 PHQ-9: 1.79	*WG* *(treatment)* *3 months* GAD-7: 1.53 PHQ-9: 1.31 *12 months* GAD-7: 1.73 PHQ-9: 1.43
Spek et al. (2007, 2008) Netherlands	Online course, group treatment, waitlist control	BDI-II	N/A	102	*M*=55 (not reported)	WHO CIDI	*Online* Post: 66 % 12 months: 57 % *Group* Post: 57 % 12 months: 67 % *Control* Post: 58 % 12 months: 66 %	Not reported	*BW* *Online v control* BDI–II: 0.55 *BW* *Group v control* BDI–II: 0.20	*WG* *(treatment)* *Online* BDI–II: 1.22 *Group* BDI–II: 0.62
Silfvernagel et al. Unpublished Sweden	Treatment, waitlist control	BAI	GAD-7	66	*M*=66.1 (60–77)	SCID-I	Post: 82 %	100 min	*BW* BAI: 0.50 GAD-7: 0.67	

WG within-group effect sizes, *BW* between-group effect sizes programmes are provided with brief weekly contact with a clinician, via a secure messaging system or email, and also a large range of comments, feedback and suggestions from previous participants. These programmes also include a number of automatic emails, which alert participants to new content, congratulate participants for completing materials and remind participants about content that has yet to be completed.

The material in these programmes is presented in a combination of didactic and narrative formats and participants follow cartoon-based illustrated characters and stories throughout the programmes. The material in these programmes was drawn from previous programmes (Titov et al. 2011; Dear et al. 2011) but was modified to include age-appropriate characters, stories and examples and to account for issues relevant to older adults, including health status and role transitions. Importantly, the Managing Stress and Anxiety and Managing Your Mood programmes are very similar and differ only in their focus on symptoms of anxiety or depression, as well as the illustrated stories, which provide examples of older adults with either symptoms of anxiety or depression. The only other difference was the sequencing of the lessons. In particular, the presentation of information and skills for managing the physical symptoms was presented before thought challenging in the Managing Your Mood programme and vice versa in the Managing Stress and Anxiety programme. Each lesson in both programmes begins with a summary of the key information and skills described in prior lessons, provides an agenda for the current lesson and provides detailed illustrated examples of characters with similar symptoms using the skills and summary of the key points and skills covered in the lesson.

The Managing Stress and Anxiety and Managing Your Mood Courses (Version 2)

The Managing Stress and Anxiety Course and the Managing Your Mood Course are two entirely new ICBT interventions (Dear et al. (2015a) and Titov et al. (2015)), which were developed based on the structure of the earlier programmes for older adults.[1] These courses also comprise 5 core lessons and are also delivered over 8 weeks with all of the same therapeutic material and self-management skills covered. However, the materials and content were completely recreated for these newer programmes for older adults. As with the previous programmes, the materials of these newer courses were written in both a didactic format and narrative format, except that, instead of illustrated cartoons, these newer courses used detailed case studies (called Case Stories) to explain the information presented and to demonstrate the application of the skills. The Case Stories were used to facilitate learning, adherence and engagement, while reducing defensiveness and normalising the difficulties of learning the materials and applying the skills covered in the course.

[1] These courses were created because the original Managing Stress and Anxiety and Managing Your Mood programmes were not available when the researchers moved institutions.

These newer ICBT courses cover all of the same materials and skills as the previous programmes but were created in a way that they could be administered with or without clinician guidance, that is, in a clinician-guided or self-guided format. For example, *Do It Yourself Guides* were created for every lesson and these included recommendations for skills practice and detailed examples, covering a broad range of problems and symptoms, which participants could use to guide their own practice of the skills. A very comprehensive set of automatic emails was also created to more closely guide participants through the course and to support participants to consistently practice the skills taught. Specifically, as described elsewhere (Titov et al. 2013), emails were triggered (1) when participants completed a lesson during the course, (2) if a lesson was not completed within 7 days of becoming available, (3) each week when new lessons became available or to suggest some tasks for the week and (4) when participants were known to experience increases in symptoms or to have increased difficulties practicing skills. The emails were written and designed to (1) make sure participants always knew about new content available on the site, (2) remind participants about unread materials, (3) reinforce progress and skills practice, (4) 'normalise' the challenges of learning new skills and (5) emphasise and explain that symptom reduction required gentle, but consistent, practice of the skills over time.

The Individually Tailored ICBT Treatment for Older Adults with Anxiety and Depression

There is a large ongoing project focussed on developing an individually tailored Internet-based treatment for anxiety and depression by the Internet, Health and Clinical Psychology Research Group at Linköping University, Sweden (Carlbring et al. 2011; Andersson et al. 2011; Johansson et al. 2012; Bergman et al. 2013). This individually tailored treatment is designed to identify participant's unique symptom profile and to provide information and skills that were likely to be helpful based on a participant's symptom profile. Importantly, in recent years, this project has been extended to also tailor on the basis of age, specifically for adolescents (Silfvernagel et al. 2015), young adults (Silfvernagel et al. 2012) and older adults (Silfvernagel et al. unpublished).

Individually tailored ICBT aims to tailor the treatment according to the participant's needs and symptoms with transdiagnostic components (Silfvernagel et al. 2012). The goal is to identify and target participant's specific psychosocial difficulties and psychological comorbidities with the aim of increasing the relevance, comprehensiveness and clinical outcomes of ICBT treatments. Importantly, the treatment package for older adults consists of modules derived from previous ICBT treatments, which have been adapted to make them suitable for an older population (Silfvernagel et al. unpublished). The first module (i.e. the introduction module) and the last module (i.e. a relapse prevention module) are fixed and the following are optional for the therapists to prescribe within an 8-week timeframe: cognitive restructuring (2 modules), panic disorder (2 modules), agoraphobia (1 module), generalised anxiety (3 modules), social anxiety (2 modules), behavioural activation (2 modules), applied relaxation (1 module), stress (1 module), mindfulness

(1 module), problem-solving (1 module) and insomnia (1 module). There are also long and short versions for the diagnosis-specific modules for the therapist to choose from. The modules are all based on established and evidence-based CBT treatments and modules contain relevant components like psychoeducation, exposure exercises and behavioural experiments. All modules contain homework assignments for the participants, which consist of questions on the psychoeducational sections and tasks for the participant to complete, such as exposure exercises. Therapist guidance is included in the treatment and there are no automatic emails; all contact is initiated by either the therapist or the participant.

The Online Coping with Depression Course (Dutch Version)

An online version of the Dutch CWD course (Cuijpers 2000) was developed by the Trimbos Institute within the Netherlands Institute of Mental Health and Addiction (Spek et al. 2007, 2008). The original Coping with Depression (CWD) course (Lewinsohn et al. 1992) is a structured course based on CBT and social learning theory (Bandura 1977). It consists of 12 2-h group sessions over 8 weeks with sessions held twice weekly for the first 4 weeks. The course provides psychoeducation about depression as well as strategies for reducing depression, such as cognitive restructuring, pleasant activity scheduling and relapse prevention. However, the online CWD course consists of 8 online modules, delivered over 8 weeks. The online CWD comprises a mixture of didactic text, practice exercises, videos and figures. The online version of the CWD course is designed to be administered in a self-guided format with no clinician contact throughout the course. Importantly, while the original and online CWD courses were not designed for older adults, one study has examined its efficacy in reducing subclinical symptoms of depression among adults over the age of 50 and up to 75 years of age (Spek et al. 2007, 2008). Hence, the Course and the results of these trials are included in this review.

Empirical Evidence for Current ICBT Interventions

Patient Acceptability, Clinical Efficacy and Cost-Effectiveness of ICBT in Clinical Trials

The empirical evidence for the efficacy and cost-effectiveness of ICBT for older adults comes from only a small number of clinical trials conducted by a limited number of research group to date, specifically 4 open trials and 3 small randomised controlled trials (Dear et al. 2013; Dear et al. 2015 a, b; Titov et al. 2015; Zou et al. 2012; Silfvernagel et al. unpublished). A further trial has been conducted to examine the efficacy of an ICBT programme not specifically designed for older adults but evaluated in a cohort of adults aged between 50 and 65 (Spek et al. 2007, 2008). The results of these initial trials have been encouraging and highlight the potential of ICBT as an approach of increasing access to evidence-based psychological treatment among older adults.

The first two trials conducted examined the acceptability, feasibility and preliminary efficacy of ICBT for adults aged 60 years and older when provided with brief weekly contact with a clinical psychologist (Zou et al. 2012; Dear et al. 2013). These open trials examined the Managing Stress and Anxiety Programme ($n=20$) and the Managing Your Mood Programme ($n=22$) for older adults with symptoms of anxiety and low mood, respectively. Seventeen of 20 (85 %) and 21/22 (95 %) participants in the Managing Your Mood and Managing Stress and Anxiety Programmes met DSM-IV criteria for a major depressive episode and an anxiety disorder, respectively, prior to participating in the programmes. Participants were in the lower end of the upper age ranges with mean ages of 63 and 66 (SD range = 4.6–5.08; age range = 60–80). Across the two trials, approximately 60 % of participants were female, 45 % had a tertiary level education and 35 % were in full-time or part-time employment. Participants' completion rates and response rates were high for both courses, with more than 75 % of participants completing the programmes in the 8 weeks and more than 80 % of participants providing data at post-treatment and 3-month follow-up. Large effect sizes (Cohen's $d>.80$) were found on standard measures of anxiety and depression in both trials at post-treatment, and these effects were largely maintained at 3-month follow-up. High levels of satisfaction were also reported by participants, with more than 75 % of participants indicating the programmes were worth their time and that they would recommend the programmes to others. Moreover, consistent with other trials aimed at younger cohorts, these effects were obtained with an average of 73 min (SD = 36.10) and 78 min (SD = 28.48) of clinician time per participant in the Managing Your Mood Programme trial and Managing Stress and Anxiety Programmes trial, respectively.

The same research team recently conducted two randomised controlled trials (RCTs) to extend the results of the abovementioned open trials by examining the long-term clinical efficacy and cost-effectiveness of the newer Managing Your Mood ($n=54$) and Managing Stress and Anxiety Courses ($n=72$) for older adults (Dear et al. 2015 a, b; Titov et al. 2015). These RCTs employed identical designs comparing a treatment group, which received immediate access to the course, with a waitlist control group, which received access to a self-guided version of the courses after the treatment group had finished treatment. Participants in both the treatment and control groups completed questionnaires prior to treatment and at post-treatment and participants in the treatment groups completed symptom questionnaires again at 3-month and 12-month follow-up. Importantly, consistent with the earlier open trials, completion rates and response rates were high with more than 70 % of participants completing the courses within the 8 weeks and more than 80 % of participants providing data at post-treatment (Dear et al. submitted a; Titov et al. submitted). Moreover, similar clinical outcomes were obtained with large effect sizes (Cohen's $d>.80$) being obtained on standard measures of anxiety and depression at post-treatment, which were maintained at 3-month and 12-month follow-up. Relatively little clinician time was also required with the clinicians spending an average of 45 min (SD = 32.51) and 57 min (SD = 31) of time in contact with each participant during the Managing Your Mood and Managing Stress and Anxiety Courses, respectively. Reflecting this, the cost-effectiveness analyses revealed that the treatment groups in both courses incurred slightly higher costs than that of control groups as a result of providing treatment, but the costs of the treatment were relatively low (estimate: MYM = $52.91 and MSAA = $92.2 per participant) and both treatment groups had significantly higher quality-adjusted life years (QALYs) (estimate: MYM = 0.012 and MSAA = 0.010) at post-treatment. Moreover, highlighting the potential cost-effectiveness of ICBT for older adults, both courses were found to have a >95 % probability of being cost-effective at the common willingness-to-pay threshold of $50,000 per QALY.

Using the control groups from the above RCTs, the research team also sought to conduct two feasibility open trials to examine the acceptability, feasibility and preliminary efficacy of the Managing Your Mood Course ($n = 20$) and Managing Stress and Anxiety Course ($n = 27$) when delivered in a self-guided format, that is, without any contact with clinician during treatment (Dear et al. submitted b). The public health potential of self-guided ICBT treatments is considerable and, while clinician-guided treatments have traditionally resulted in greater clinical effects (Andersson and Cuijpers 2009; Andrews et al. 2010; Cuijpers et al. 2009), several recent trials have found very promising findings for certain ICBT programmes when administered in self-guided formats (Berger et al. 2011; Furmark et al. 2009; Titov et al. 2013, 2014). The results of these open trials are very encouraging. For example, 70 % and 50 % of participants completed the MYM and MSAA Courses in the 8 weeks, respectively, and more than 70 % provided data at post-treatment and 3-month follow-up. Moreover, large effect sizes (Cohen's $d > .80$) were found on standard measures of anxiety for participants in the MSAA Course and standard measures of depression for participants in the MYM Course. These reductions in symptoms were maintained at 3-month follow-up and participants in both courses reported improvements in health-related QALYs, while the costs of treatment were relatively low, highlighting the potential clinical and cost-effectiveness of self-guided ICBT for older adults with anxiety and depression.

The third two-group RCT was conducted in Sweden with older adults (mean age = 66.1; SD = 4.15) who were randomised to either a treatment group or control group (Silfvernagel et al. unpublished). The treatment group ($n = 33$) received individually tailored Internet-based ICBT for symptoms of anxiety and depression while the control group ($n = 33$) received general support from a psychologist. The control group was offered the same treatment after the initial trial period, that is, after the treatment group had finished the 8-week treatment. Participants completed questionnaires prior to treatment and at post-treatment. Out of the 33 participants, 67 % completed 50 % of the treatment in the 8 weeks and 82 % of participants provided post-treatment data. Moderate to large effect sizes (Cohen's $d > .50$) being obtained on standard measures of anxiety and depression at post-treatment and the treatment were rated as highly acceptable. These results were obtained with an estimated average of 100 min of clinician contact per participant.

Finally, although the online CWD course was not specifically designed for older adults, its efficacy has been measured in a population of Dutch adults between the ages of 50 and 75 years (Spek et al. 2007, 2008). Specifically, one RCT ($n=301$) to date has been conducted to measure the efficacy of the online CWD ($n=102$) compared to a waitlist control group ($n=100$) and a traditional face-to-face CWD group treatment ($n=99$) in reducing subclinical symptoms of depression. Participants had a mean age of 55 (SD=4.6) in the online CWD course. Approximately 67.6 % of participants in the online CWD course were female, 62 % were in full-time or part-time employment and 87 % were described as having medium to high levels of education. Completion rates were lower in the online CWD course (i.e. 48.3 %) than in the face-to-face group-based CWD treatment (i.e. 94.5 %) (Spek et al. 2007). However, large within-group effect sizes were found for the online CWD treatment at post-treatment (Cohen's $d=1.00$) and there was a moderate between-group effect size for the comparison between the online CWD treatment and the waitlist control (Cohen's $d=0.55$). No significant difference was found between the group-based and online CWD treatments and this pattern of results was maintained at 12-month follow-up (Spek et al. 2008). Importantly, a numbers-needed-to-treat analysis found that 3.85 people would need to be treated to avert one case of subclinical depression compared to 14.29 needed to treat in the traditional group-based CWD treatment.

Discussion and Future Directions

The prevalence of untreated anxiety and depression represents a critical public health issue in older adults and the proportion of older adults is set to grow over the coming decades. Unfortunately, despite their clinical efficacy, there are numerous barriers to traditional face-to-face psychological treatments and few older adults currently seek treatment. Internet-delivered cognitive behaviour therapy (ICBT) represents one potential approach for increasing access to treatment and several clinical trials have now been conducted with encouraging results. The findings of these trials indicate that ICBT is acceptable to older adults and can result in clinically significant reductions in levels of anxiety and depression, which are maintained up to 12 months following treatment. These trials also indicate that ICBT requires relatively little clinician time per person (i.e. less than 1 h on average) and is a cost-effective approach to treatment with some emerging evidence that ICBT treatment may be acceptable and effective without clinician contact. The available evidence is, therefore, supportive of the acceptability, clinical efficacy and cost-effectiveness of ICBT for older adults with symptoms of anxiety and depression. There is also evidence to suggest that ICBT programmes that are not specifically designed for older adults can be effective for reducing subclinical symptoms of depression (Spek et al. 2007) and that these improvements are maintained for up to a year after treatment (Spek et al. 2008).

Despite the positive findings of existing studies, there is a need for much more work examining the acceptability, efficacy and cost-effectiveness of ICBT for older adults with anxiety and depression. To date, while consistent results have been obtained across trials, all of the research on ICBT programmes specifically designed for older adults has been conducted by a limited number of research groups and the clinical trials have involved relatively small numbers of participants. There is, therefore, a strong need for independent replication by other research groups, especially outside of Australia and Sweden, and the implementation and evaluation of larger trials involving much larger numbers of participants to establish the robustness of observed clinical effects. Alongside this, there is also a need for studies examining the implementation of ICBT for older adults into routine practice, particularly where participants are referred to ICBT treatment rather than seeking ICBT as is often the case in clinical trials. While a growing number of researchers are starting to report the results of ICBT when used in routine clinical practice and many of these reports likely include older adults (Andersson and Hedman 2013), there have been no specific reports about the acceptability, efficacy or cost-effectiveness of ICBT for older adults in routine practice.

Several key questions also remain unexplored in the current literature and would benefit from further consideration and attention in future studies. For example, while many of the existing studies include older adults with broad age ranges, the mean age of participants has fallen within a younger cohort of older adults, that is, adults in their mid to late 60s. Moreover, given the smaller number of participants in existing trials, there has not been the ability to examine whether the various age cohorts of older adults differ in terms of how acceptable they find ICBT or how they respond to ICBT.

Related to this issue, there are limited empirical data to clearly indicate whether, and if so when, older adults might require or might benefit from ICBT programmes designed specifically for them (e.g. providing age-appropriate examples, dealing with cohort beliefs, life transitions), that is, compared with programmes designed generally for adults with anxiety and depression. This issue is highlighted by the findings of the trial examining the online CWD course, which was not specifically designed for older adults (Spek et al. 2007, 2008). However, it is important to note that this research did not examine the effect of the course on clinical levels of depression and the average age of participants in the trial was very low at 55 years. The degree to which online treatments need to be modified for older adults holds important implications for the implementation of ICBT into routine care for older adults with anxiety and depression. Another interesting future research direction is exploring the benefit of ICBT for older adults with chronic physical health conditions, such as diabetes mellitus, cardiovascular diseases, respiratory diseases, neurological disorders, cancer and chronic pain. Chronic health conditions can have a very significant impact on all aspects of life and they become more common with age. It is widely acknowledged that there is a complex interrelationship between anxiety and depression and chronic physical health conditions. Reflecting this, chronic physical health conditions are strong risk factors for anxiety and depression (Wells et al. 1988) and, conversely, anxiety and depression are strong risk factors for poor physical health (Roy-Byrne et al. 2008; Katon and Ciechanowski 2002). There is emerging evidence for the use of ICBT for people with some chronic health conditions (Beatty and Lambert 2013), but very little research has examined ICBT for older adults with chronic health conditions. Moreover, the research regarding ICBT for older adults has focussed purely on adults with anxiety and depression without exploring the issue of physical health. Consequently, there is a significant opportunity and considerable benefit in future research exploring ICBT for improving emotional health but also assisting in the adjustment and management of chronic physical health conditions.

In summary, there are strong reasons for exploring ICBT as an approach to increasing access to evidence-based treatment for older adults with anxiety and depression. To date, only a limited number of clinical trials have examined ICBT for older adults. However, the results of existing trials are promising and support ICBT as an acceptable, clinically efficacious and cost-effective approach to providing treatment to older adults.

References

Andersson G, Cuijpers P (2009) Internet-based and other computerized psychological treatments for adult depression: a meta-analysis. Cogn Behav Ther 38:196–205

Andersson G, Hedman E (2013) Effectiveness of guided internet-based cognitive behaviour therapy in regular clinical settings. Verhaltenstherapie 23:140–148

Andersson G, Titov N (2014) Advantages and limitations of Internet-based interventions for common mental disorders. World Psychiatry 13:4–11

Andersson G, Estling F, Jakobsson E, Cuijpers P, Carlbring P (2011) Can the patient decide which modules to endorse? An open trial of tailored internet treatments of anxiety disorders. Cogn Behav Ther 40:57–64

Andrews G, Cuijpers P, Craske MG, McEvoy P, Titov N (2010) Computer therapy for the anxiety and depressive disorders is effective, acceptable and practical health care: a meta- analysis. PLoS One 5(10):e13196

Australian Bureau of Statistics (2009) Australian Social Trends, cat no 4102.0. Australian Bureau of Statistics, Canberra

Ayers CR, Sorrell JT, Thorp SR, Wetherell JL (2007) Evidence-based psychological treatments for late-life anxiety. Psychol Aging 22:8–17

Bandura A (1977) Social learning theory. Prentice Hall, Englewood Cliffs

Beatty L, Lambert S (2013) A systematic review of internet-based self-help therapeutic interventions to improve distress and disease control among adults with chronic health conditions. Clin Psych Rev 33:609–622

Berger T, Hammerli K, Gubser N, Andersson G, Caspar F (2011) Internet-based treatment of depression: a randomized controlled trial comparing guided with unguided self-help. Cogn Behav Ther 40:251–266

Bergman NL, Carlbring P, Linna E, Andersson G (2013) Role of the working alliance on treatment outcome in tailored internet-based cognitive behavioural therapy for anxiety disorders: randomized controlled pilot trial. JMIR Res Protoc 2(1):e4

Braam AW, Prince MJ, Beekman ATF et al (2005) Physical health and depressive symptoms in older Europeans. Br J Psychiatry 187:35–42

Brenes GA, Penninx BW, Judd PH, Rockwell E, Sewell DD, Wetherell JL (2008) Anxiety, depression and disability across the lifespan. Aging Ment Health 12:158–163

Britt HC, Harrison CM, Miller GC, Knox SA (2008) Prevalence and patterns of multimorbidity in Australia. Med J Aust 189:72–77

Butler AC, Chapman JE, Forman EM, Beck AT (2006) The empirical status of cognitive behavioral therapy: a review of meta-analyses. Clin Psychol Rev 26:17–31

Carlbring P, Maurin L, Törngren C, Linna E, Eriksson T, Sparthan E et al (2011) Individually-tailored, internet-based treatment for anxiety disorders: a randomized controlled trial. Behav Res Ther 49:18–24

Cole MG, McCusker J, Sewitch M, Ciampi A, Dyachenko A (2008) Health services use for mental health problems by community-living seniors with depression. Int Psychogeriatr 20:554–570

Crabb RM, Cavanagh K, Proudfoot J, Learmonth D, Rafie S, Weingradt KR (2012) Is computerized cognitive-behavioural therapy a treatment option for depression in late-life?: a systematic review. Br J Clin Psychol 51:459–464

Cuijpers P (2000) In de put, uit de put: zelf depressiviteit overwinnen 55+. Trimbos-instituut, Utrecht

Cuijpers P, Marks IM, van Straten A, Cavanagh K, Gega L, Andersson G (2009) Computer-aided psychotherapy for anxiety disorders: a meta-analytic review. Cogn Behav Ther 38:66–82

Cuijpers P, Donker T, van Straten A, Li J, Andersson G (2010) Is guided self-help as effective as face-to-face psychotherapy for depression and anxiety disorders? A systematic review and meta-analysis of comparative outcome studies. Psychol Med 40:1943–1957

Dear BF, Zou J, Ali S, Lorian C, Johnston L, Sheehan J, Staples LG, Gandy M, Fogliati V, Klein B, Titov N (2015a) Clinical and cost-effectiveness of clinician-guided internet-delivered cognitive behaviour therapy program for older adults with symptoms of anxiety: a randomised controlled trial. Behavior Therapy 46:206–217

Dear BF, Zou J, Ali S, Lorian C, Johnston L, Terides MD, Staples LG, Gandy M, Fogliati V, Klein B, Titov N (2015b) Examining self-guided internet-delivered cognitive behaviour therapy for older adults with symptoms of anxiety and depression: Two feasibility open trials. Internet Interventions 2:17–23

Dear BF, Titov N, Schwencke G, Andrews G, Johnston L, Craske MG, McEvoy P (2011) An open trial of a brief transdiagnostic treatment for anxiety and depression. Behav Res Ther 49:830–837

Dear BF, Zou JB, Titov N, Lorian C, Johnston L, Spence J, Anderson T, Sachdev P, Brodaty H, Knight RG (2013) Brief internet-delivered cognitive behavioural therapy for depression: a feasibility open trial for older adults. Aust N Z J Psychiatry 47:169–176

DiMatteo RM, Lepper HS, Croghan TW (2000) Depression is a risk factor for noncompliance with medical treatment: meta-analysis of the effects of anxiety and depression on patient adherence. Arch Intern Med 160:2101–2107

Ewing S, Thomas J (2012) CCi Digital Futures 2012: the Internet in Australia. ARC Centre of Excellence for Creative Industries and Innovation, Kelvin Grove

Fox S, Jones S (2009) The social life of health information. http://www.pewinternet.org/Reports/2009/8-The-Social-Life-of-Health-Information.aspx

Furmark T, Carlbring P, Hedman E, Sonnenstein A, Clevberer P et al (2009) Guided and unguided self-help for social anxiety disorder: randomised controlled trial. Br J Psychiatry 195:440–447

Gould RL, Coulson MC, Howard RJ (2012a) Efficacy of cognitive behavioral therapy for anxiety disorders in older people: a meta-analysis and meta-regression of randomized controlled trials. J Am Geriatr Soc 60:218–229

Gould RL, Coulson MC, Howard RJ (2012b) Cognitive behavioral therapy for depression in older people: a meta-analysis and meta-regression of randomized controlled trials. J Am Geriatr Soc 60:1817–1830

Grek A (2007) Clinical management of suicidality in the elderly: an opportunity for involvement in the lives of older patients. Can J Psychiatry 52(6 Suppl 1):47S–57S

Hedman E, Ljotsson B, Lindfors N (2012) Cognitive behaviour therapy via the internet: a systematic review of applications, clinical efficacy and cost-effectiveness. Expert Rev Pharmacoecon Outcomes Res 12:745–764

Hippisley-Cox J, Fielding K, Pringle M (1998) Depression as a risk factor for ischaemic heart disease in men: population based case-control study. Br Med J 316:1714–1719

Johansson R, Sjöberg E, Sjögren M, Johnsson E, Carlbring P, Andersson T, Rousseau A, Andersson G (2012) Tailored vs. standardized internet-based cognitive behavior therapy for depression and comorbid symptoms: a randomized controlled trial. PLoS One 7(5):e36905

Katon W, Ciechanowski P (2002) Impact of major depression on chronic medical illness. J Psychosom Res 53:859–863

Laidlaw K, Thompson LW, Gallagher-Thompson D (2004) Comprehensive conceptualization of cognitive behavior therapy for late life depression. Behav Cogn Psychother 32:389–399

Lewinsohn PM, Munoz RF, Youngren MA, Zeiss AM (1992) Control your depression. Fireside, New York

Luppa M, Sikorski C, Luck T et al (2012) Age- and gender-specific prevalence of depression in latest-life: systematic review and meta-analysis. J Affect Disord 136:212–221

O'Connor DW (2006) Do older Australians truly have low rates of anxiety and depression?: a critique of the 1997 National Survey of Mental Health and Wellbeing. Aus N Z J Psychiatry 40:623–631

Oeppen J, Vaupel JW (2002) Broken limits to life expectancy. Science 296:1029–2031

Roy-Byrne PP, Davidson KW, Kessler RC, Asmundson GJG, Goodwin RD, Kubzansky L, Lydiard RB, Massie MJ, Katon W, Laden SK, Stein MB (2008) Anxiety disorders and comorbid medical illness. Gen Hosp Psychiatry 30:208–225

Sachdev PS (2007) Geriatric psychiatry research in Australia. Am J Geriatr Psychiatry 15:451–454

Scogin F, Welsh D, Hanson A et al (2005) Evidence-based psychotherapies for depression in older adults. Clin Psychol Sci Pract 12:222–237

Silfvernagel K, Carlbring P, Kabo J, Edström S, Eriksson J, Månson L, Andersson G (2012) Individually tailored internet-based treatment for young adults and adults with panic attacks: randomized controlled trial. J Med Internet Res 14(3):e65

Silfvernagel K, Gren-Landell M, Emanuelsson M, Carlbring P, Andersson G (2015) Individually tailored internet-based cognitive behavior therapy for adolescents with anxiety disorders: A pilot effectiveness study. Internet Interventions 2(3):297–302

Socialstyrelsen (2009) Folkhälsorapport 2009. Edita Västra Aros, Västerås

Spek V, Nylkíček I, Smits N, Cuijpers P, Riper H, Keyzer J, Pop V (2007) Internet-based cognitive behavioral therapy for subthreshold depression in people over 50 years old: a randomized controlled trial. Psychol Med 37:1797–1806

Spek V, Cuijpers P, Nylkíček I, Smits N, Riper H, Keyzer J, Pop V (2008) One-year follow-up results of a randomized controlled trial on internet-based cognitive behavioural therapy for subthreshold depression in people over 50 years. Psychol Med 38:635–639

Titov N, Dear BF, Ali S, Zou J, Lorian C, Johnston L, Terides MD, Kayrouz R, Klein B, Gandy M, Fogliati V (2015) Clinical and cost-effectiveness of clinician-guided internet-delivered cognitive behaviour therapy program for older adults with symptoms of depression: a randomised controlled trial. Behavior Therapy 46:193–205

Titov N, Dear BF, Schwencke G, Andews G, Johnston L, Craske MG, McEvoy P (2011) Transdiagnostic treatment for anxiety and depression: a randomised controlled trial. Behav Res Ther 49:331–452

Titov N, Dear BF, Johnston L, Lorian C, Zou J, Wootton B, McEvoy PM, Rapee RM (2013) Improving adherence and clinical outcomes in self-guided internet treatment for anxiety and depression: randomised controlled trial. PLoS One 8:262873

Titov N, Dear BF, Johnston L, McEvoy PM, Wootton B, Terides MD, Gandy M, Fogliati V, Kayrouz R, Rapee RM (2014) Improving adherence and clinical outcomes in self-guided internet treatment for anxiety and depression: a 12 month follow-up of a randomised controlled trial. PLoS One 9(2):e89591

Trollor JN, Anderson TM, Sachdev PS, Brodaty H, Andrews G (2007) Prevalence of mental disorders in the elderly: the Australian National Mental Health and Well-Being Survey. Am J Geriat Psychiatry 15:455–466

Wells KB, Golding JM, Burnham MA (1988) Psychiatric disorder in a sample of the general population with and without medical disorder. Am J Psychiatry 145:876–981

Wilkinson P (2009) Cognitive behavioural therapy with older adults: enthusiasm without the evidence? Cogn Behav Ther 2:75–82

Zou JB, Dear BF, Titov N, Lorian CN, Johnston L, Spence J, Knight RG, Anderson T, Sachdev P (2012) Brief internet-delivered cognitive behavioural therapy for anxiety in older adults: a feasibility trial. J Affect Disord 26:650–655

Index

© Springer International Publishing Switzerland 2016

N. Lindefors, G. Andersson (eds.), *Guided Internet-Based Treatments in Psychiatry*, DOI 10.1007/978-3-319-06083-5